Lecture Notes in Computer Science 6204

Commenced Publication in 1973
Founding and Former Series Editors:
Gerhard Goos, Juris Hartmanis, and Jan van Leeuwen

W0016605

Bernd Fischer   Benoît M. Dawant
Cristian Lorenz (Eds.)

Biomedical Image Registration

4th International Workshop, WBIR 2010
Lübeck, Germany, July 11-13, 2010
Proceedings

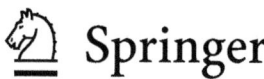 Springer

Volume Editors

Bernd Fischer
University of Lübeck
Institute of Mathematics and Image Computing
23560 Lübeck, Germany
E-mail: bernd.fischer@mic.uni-luebeck.de

Benoît M. Dawant
Vanderbilt University
Department of Electrical Engineering and Computer Science
Nashville, TN 37240-1662, USA
E-mail: benoit.dawant@vanderbilt.edu

Cristian Lorenz
Philips Research Europe - Hamburg
Sector Medical Imaging Systems
22335 Hamburg, Germany
E-mail: cristian.lorenz@Philips.com

Library of Congress Control Number: 2010930227

CR Subject Classification (1998): I.4, I.5, H.3, I.3.5, J.3

LNCS Sublibrary: SL 6 – Image Processing, Computer Vision, Pattern Recognition, and Graphics

ISSN   0302-9743
ISBN-10   3-642-14365-2 Springer Berlin Heidelberg New York
ISBN-13   978-3-642-14365-6 Springer Berlin Heidelberg New York

springer.com

© Springer-Verlag Berlin Heidelberg 2010
Printed in Germany

Typesetting: Camera-ready by author, data conversion by Scientific Publishing Services, Chennai, India
Printed on acid-free paper   06/3180

Preface

Welcome to the proceedings of the 4th Workshop on Biomedical Image Registration (WBIR). Previous WBIRs took place in Bled, Slovenia (1999), at the University of Pennsylvania, USA (2003) and in Utrecht, The Netherlands (2006). This year, WBIR was hosted by the Institute Mathematics and Image Processing and the Fraunhofer Project Group on Image Registration and it was held in Lübeck, Germany. It provided the opportunity to bring together researchers from all over the world to discuss some of the most recent advances in image registration and its applications.

We had an excellent collection of papers that were reviewed by at least three reviewers each from a 35-member Program Committee assembled from a worldwide community of registration experts. This year 17 papers were accepted for oral presentation, while another 7 papers were accepted as poster papers. We believe all of the conference papers were of excellent quality.

Registration is a fundamental task in image processing used to match two or more pictures taken, for example, at different times, from different sensors, or from different viewpoints. Establishing the correspondence of structures within medical images is fundamental to diagnosis, treatment planning, and surgical guidance. The conference papers address state-of-the-art techniques for providing reliable and efficient registration techniques, thereby imposing relationships between specific application areas and appropriate registration schemes.

We are grateful to all those who contributed to the success of WBIR 2010. In particular, we would like to thank the organization staff and members of the Program Committee for their work. We also thank Philips Medical Systems for kind and generous financial support. For those who did not attend, we hope this publication provides a good view into the research presented at the conference, and we look forward to meeting you at the next WBIR workshop.

July 2010

Bernd Fischer
Benoit Dawant
Cristian Lorenz

Organization

The 4th Workshop on Biomedical Image Registration was organized by the Institute of Mathematics and Image Computation (MIC), University of Lübeck and Fraunhofer MEVIS Project Group Image Registration, Lübeck.

Executive Committee

Bernd Fischer	University of Lübeck, Germany
Benoit Dawant	Vanderbilt University, USA
Cristian Lorenz	Philips Research Europe - Hamburg, Germany

Program Committee

Christian Barillot	INRIA, France
Faisal Beg	Simon Fraser University, Canada
Nathan Cahill	Rochester Institute of Technology, USA
Gary Christensen	University of Iowa, USA
Mike Fitzpatrick	Vanderbilt University, USA
Jim Gee	University of Pennsylvania, USA
Martin Groher	Technical University of Munich, Germany
Eldad Haber	Emory University, USA
David Haynor	University of Washington, USA
Stefan Heldmann	Fraunhofer MEVIS, Germany
Joachim Hornegger	University of Erlangen-Nuremberg, Germany
Ali Kamen	Siemens Corporate Research, USA
Rasmus Larsen	Technical University of Denmark, Denmark
Bostjan Likar	University of Ljubljana, Slovenia
Dirk Loeckx	K.U. Leuven, Belgium
Frederik Maes	K.U. Leuven, Belgium
Calvin Maurer Jr.	Accuray, Inc., USA
Jan Modersitzki	University of Lübeck, Germany
Nassir Navab	Technical University of Munich, Germany
Wiro Niessen	University Medical Center Rotterdam, The Netherlands
Sebastien Ourselin	University College London, UK
Nils Papenberg	Fraunhofer MEVIS, Germany
Xavier Pennec	INRIA, France
Graeme Penney	Kings College London, UK
Josien Pluim	University Medical Center Utrecht, The Netherlands
Torsten Rohlfing	SRI International, USA

Karl Rohr   University of Heidelberg and DKFZ Heidelberg,
                                     Germany
Daniel Rueckert   Imperial College London, UK
Oskar Skrinjar   Georgia Institute of Technology, USA
Colin Studholme   University of California, San Francisco, USA
Philippe Thévenaz   École polytechnique fédérale de Lausanne
                                     (EPFL), Switzerland
Max Viergever   University Medical Center Utrecht,
                                     The Netherlands
Simon Warfield   Harvard Medical School, USA
Wolfgang Wein   Siemens Corporate Research, USA
Sandy Wells   Harvard Medical School and Brigham and
                                     Women's Hospital, USA

Sponsoring Institutions

Philips Research Europe - Hamburg, Germany

Table of Contents

Applications

Poster Session

Evaluation

Methods Part I

Model Based Registration

Methods II

Unifying Vascular Information in Intensity-Based Nonrigid Lung CT Registration

Kunlin Cao[1], Kai Ding[2], Gary E. Christensen[1], Madhavan L. Raghavan[2], Ryan E. Amelon[2], and Joseph M. Reinhardt[2,*]

[1] Department of Electrical and Computer Engineering
[2] Department of Biomedical Engineering
The University of Iowa, Iowa City, 52242

Abstract. Image registration plays an important role within pulmonary image analysis. Accurate registration is critical to post-analysis of lung mechanical properties. To improve registration accuracy, we utilize the rich information of vessel locations and shapes, and introduce a new similarity criterion, sum of squared vesselness measure difference (SSVMD). This metric is added to three existing intensity-based similarity criteria for nonrigid lung CT image registration to show its ability in improving matching accuracy. The registration accuracy is assessed by landmark error calculation and distance map visualization on vascular tree. The average landmark errors are reduced by over 20% and are within 0.7 mm after adding SSVMD constraint to three existing intensity-based similarity metrics. Visual inspection shows matching accuracy improvements in the lung regions near the thoracic cage and near the diaphragm. Experiments also show this vesselness constraint makes the Jacobian map of transformations physiologically more plausible and reliable.

1 Introduction

The respiratory system provides gas exchange during breathing cycles. Many pulmonary diseases can alter the material properties and mechanics of lung tissue. Therefore, understanding the ventilation patterns of lung parenchyma is important for disease detecting, tracking and radiotherapy planning.

Imaging allows non-invasive study of lung behaviors and image registration can be used to match images acquired at different inflation levels to examine the mechanical properties of lung parenchyma and pulmonary functions [1,2,3]. Coselmon et al. [4] used mutual information based registration to model deformation of lung CT images between exhale and inhale breathing states. Christensen et al. [5] used the sum of squared intensity difference (SSD) consistent linear elastic image registration to match images across cine-CT sequences, and estimate rates of local tissue expansion and contraction. Gorbunova et al. [6] developed a weight preserving image registration method for monitoring disease progression. Yin et al. [7] proposed a new similarity cost preserving the lung

---

* Joseph M. Reinhardt is a shareholder in VIDA Diagnostics, Inc.

B. Fischer, B. Dawant, and C. Lorenz (Eds.): WBIR 2010, LNCS 6204, pp. 1–12, 2010.
© Springer-Verlag Berlin Heidelberg 2010

tissue volume, and compared the new cost function driven registration method with SSD driven registration in the estimation of regional lung function.

All these methods utilize their own assumption about the underlying process of lungs during gas exchange. However, as an important part of the respiratory system, the pulmonary blood vessels have not attracted enough attention in lung image registration problem. During the respiration cycles, blood vessels keep their tree structures and tube-like shapes. The location and shape information of vessels can be used to help guide the registration process.

In this paper, we describe a similarity criterion utilizing the information of vessel locations and shapes in the registration process. This metric is added to three existing intensity-based similarity metrics and comparison experiments show that this criterion helps improve the registration accuracy. Higher matching accuracy makes the post-analysis of regional tissue mechanical properties more plausible and reliable.

2   Methods

2.1   Data Acquisition

Pairs of volumetric CT data sets from three normal human subjects scanned at supine orientation on a Siemens Sensation 64 multi-detector CT scanner are used in the study. For subject 1, data sets were acquired at functional residual capacity (FRC) with 26.3% of the vital capacity (VC) and total lung capacity (TLC) with 95.7% of the VC. For subject 2, data sets were acquired at FRC with 21.8% of the VC and TLC with 95.6% of the VC. For subject 3, data sets were acquired at FRC with 11.0% of the VC and TLC with 68.9% of the VC. Volumetric data were acquired at a section spacing of 0.5 mm and a reconstruction matrix of 512 × 512. In-plane pixel spatial resolution is 0.6 mm × 0.6 mm.

The parenchyma regions in the FRC and TLC data sets were segmented using the method described in [8]. An expert selected more than 100 landmark pairs for each subject. The landmarks in FRC image were selected as the bifurcations of the airway and vascular trees. A semi-automatic system [9] was used to guide the observer to find the corresponding landmarks in the TLC image.

2.2   Image Registration and Transformation Parameterization

Image registration is used to find an optimal spatial transform that maps points from the template image I_1 to the corresponding points in the target image I_2. Let $\mathbf{x} = (x_1, x_2, x_3)^T$ define a voxel coordinate in the image domain. The transformation $\mathbf{h}$ is a (3×1) vector-valued function defined on the voxel lattice of target image and $\mathbf{h}(\mathbf{x})$ gives its corresponding location in template image.

The B-spline based parameterization is chosen to represent the transformation. Let $\phi_i = [\phi_x(\mathbf{x}_i), \phi_y(\mathbf{x}_i), \phi_z(\mathbf{x}_i)]^T$ be the coefficients of the i-th control point $\mathbf{x}_i$ on the spline lattice G along each direction. The transformation is represented as $\mathbf{h}(\mathbf{x}) = \mathbf{x} + \sum_{i \in G} \phi_i \beta^{(3)}(\mathbf{x} - \mathbf{x}_i)$, where $\beta^{(3)}(\mathbf{x}) = \beta^{(3)}(x)\beta^{(3)}(y)\beta^{(3)}(z)$

is a separable convolution kernel. $\beta^{(3)}(x)$ is the uniform cubic B-spline basis function.

2.3 Matching Similarity Criteria

Many criteria have been suggested as the metrics for aligning two images. In this paper, three intensity-based metrics and a vesselness similarity metric are used to register a pair of lung CT images at different inflation levels.

Sum of Squared Difference (SSD). A simple and common metric is the sum of squared difference (SSD), which measures the intensity difference at corresponding points between two images. Mathematically, it is defined by

$$C_{\text{SSD}} = \int_{\Omega} [I_2(\mathbf{x}) - I_1(\mathbf{h}(\mathbf{x}))]^2 \, d\mathbf{x}, \tag{1}$$

where I_1 and I_2 are the template and target image intensity functions, respectively. Ω denotes the lung region of target image. However, the underlying assumption of SSD is that the image intensity at corresponding points between two images should be similar. Considering the change in CT intensity as air inspired and expired during the respiratory cycle, a histogram matching procedure is used before SSD registration to modify the histogram of template image so that it is similar to that of target image.

Mutual Information (MI). As mentioned above, CT intensity is a measure of tissue density and therefore changes as the tissue density changes during inflation and deflation. The registration problem under this circumstance is similar to the multi-modality image registration, where mutual information (MI) is well suited and widely used as the similarity metric. In the image registration field, mutual information expresses the amount of information that one image contains about the other one. Analogous to the Kullback-Leibler measure, the negative mutual information cost of two images is defined as [10,11]

$$C_{\text{MI}} = -\sum_i \sum_j p(i,j) \log \frac{p(i,j)}{p_{I_1 \circ h}(i) p_{I_2}(j)}. \tag{2}$$

where $p(i,j)$ is the joint intensity distribution of transformed template image $I_1 \circ h$ and target image I_2; $p_{I_1 \circ h}(i)$ and $p_{I_2}(j)$ are their marginal distributions, respectively. The histogram bins of $I_1 \circ h$ and I_2 are indexed by i and j. The experiments in this paper use 50×50 histogram bins to estimate joint distribution. Misregistration results in a decrease in the mutual information, and thus, increases the similarity cost C_{MI}.

Sum of Squared Tissue Volume Difference (SSTVD). A recently developed similarity metric, the sum of squared tissue volume difference (SSTVD) [7], accounts for the variation of intensity in the lung CT images during respiration.

This similarity criterion minimizes the local difference of tissue volume inside the lungs scanned at different pressure levels. Assume the Hounsfield units (HU) of CT lung images are primarily contributed by tissue and air. Then, the tissue volume in a voxel at position $\mathbf{x}$ can be estimated as $V(\mathbf{x}) = v(\mathbf{x}) \frac{HU(\mathbf{x}) - HU_{air}}{HU_{tissue} - HU_{air}}$ where $v(\mathbf{x})$ is the volume of voxel $\mathbf{x}$. It is assumed that $HU_{air} = -1000$ and $HU_{tissue} = 55$. The intensity similarity metric SSTVD is defined as [7]

$$C_{\text{SSTVD}} = \int_{\Omega} [V_2(\mathbf{x}) - V_1(\mathbf{h}(\mathbf{x}))]^2 \, d\mathbf{x}$$

$$= \int_{\Omega} \left[v_2(\mathbf{x}) \frac{I_2(\mathbf{x}) + 1000}{1055} - v_1(\mathbf{h}(\mathbf{x})) \frac{I_1(\mathbf{h}(\mathbf{x})) + 1000}{1055} \right]^2 d\mathbf{x} \quad (3)$$

The Jacobian of a transformation $J(\mathbf{h})$ estimates the local volume changes resulted from mapping an image through the deformation. Thus, the tissue volumes in image I_1 and I_2 are related by $v_1(\mathbf{h}(\mathbf{x})) = v_2(\mathbf{x}) \cdot J(\mathbf{h}(\mathbf{x}))$.

Sum of Squared Vesselness Measure Difference (SSVMD). Feature information extracted from the intensity image is important to help guide the image registration process. During the respiration cycle, blood vessels keep their tubular shapes and tree structures. Therefore, the spatial and shape information of blood vessels can be utilized to help improve the registration accuracy. Blood vessels have larger HU values than that of parenchymal tissues. This intensity contrast is low at small vessels and thus gives almost no contribution to intensity-based similarity metrics. A better way to use the information of vessel locations is computing the vesselness measure (VM) from intensity images, and then registering similar vesselness patterns in two images.

The vesselness measure is based on the analysis of eigenvalues of the Hessian matrix of image intensity. The eigenvalues, ordered by magnitude $|\lambda_1| \leq |\lambda_2| \leq |\lambda_3|$, can be used to indicate the shape of underlying object. In 3D lung CT images, isotropic structures such as parenchymal tissues are associated with three similar non-zero positive eigenvalues while tubular structures such as blood vessels are associated with one negligible eigenvalue and two similar non-zero negative eigenvalues [12]. The vesselness measure is computed from the Frangi's vesselness function [12]

$$F(\lambda) = \begin{cases} (1 - e^{-\frac{R_A^2}{2\alpha^2}}) \cdot e^{\frac{-R_B^2}{2\beta^2}} \cdot (1 - e^{-\frac{S^2}{2\gamma^2}}) & \text{if } \lambda_2 < 0 \text{ and } \lambda_3 < 0 \\ 0 & \text{otherwise} \end{cases} \quad (4)$$

with $R_A = \frac{|\lambda_2|}{|\lambda_3|}$, $R_B = \frac{|\lambda_1|}{\sqrt{|\lambda_2 \lambda_3|}}$, $S = \sqrt{\lambda_1^2 + \lambda_2^2 + \lambda_3^2}$, and α, β, γ control the sensitivity of the vesselness measure. The experiments in this paper use $\alpha = 0.5$, $\beta = 0.5$, and $\gamma = 5$.

The vesselness image is rescaled to $[0, 1]$ and can be considered as a probability-like estimate of vesselness features. Larger vesselness value indicates the underlying object is more likely to be a vessel structure, as shown in Figure 1. The sum of squared vesselness measure difference (SSVMD) is designed to match similar

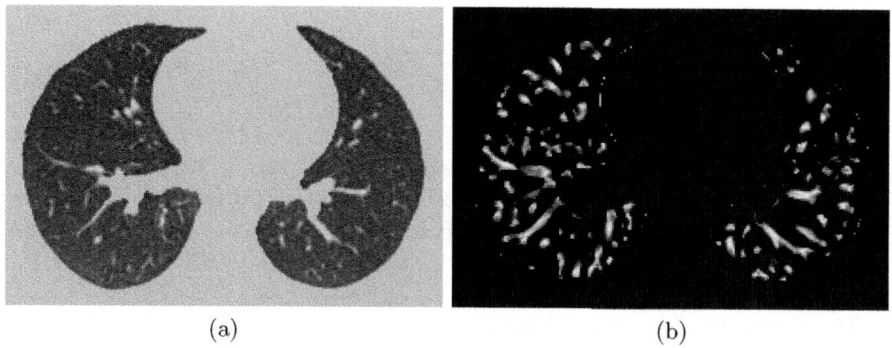

(a) (b)

Fig. 1. The vesselness images calculated from lung CT grayscale images. (a) A transverse slice of FRC data. (b) The vesselness measure of slice in (a). Vesselness measure is computed in multiscale analysis and rescaled to [0, 1].

vesselness patterns in two images. Given F_1 and F_2 as the vesselness measures of images I_1 and I_2, respectively, this cost function is formed as

$$C_{\mathrm{SSVMD}} = \int_\Omega \left[F_2(\mathbf{x}) - F_1(\mathbf{h}(\mathbf{x})) \right]^2 . \tag{5}$$

For each pair of data sets, registrations using six similarity cost functions are performed for comparison. They are three basic registration methods driven by: (i) C_{SSD}, (ii) C_{MI}, (iii) C_{SSTVD}; and three registration methods with SSVMD build in and thus driven by: (iv) $C_{\mathrm{SSD}} + C_{\mathrm{SSVMD}}$, (v) $C_{\mathrm{MI}} + C_{\mathrm{SSVMD}}$, (vi) $C_{\mathrm{SSTVD}} + C_{\mathrm{SSVMD}}$. In this paper, the weights of C_{SSVMD} to costs (iv)-(vi) are selected by trial to give the best improvement on landmark matching accuracy for one subject, and are applied on experiments for all three subjects.

2.4 Multi-resolution Scheme and Estimation

A spatial multiresolution procedure from coarse to fine is used in the registration in order to improve speed, accuracy and robustness. The basic idea is that registration is first performed at a coarse scale and the transformation estimated at the coarse scale is used to initialize registration at the next finer scale. This process is repeated until it reaches the finest scale. The multiresolution strategy used in the experiments proceeds from low to high image resolution starting at one-eighth the spatial resolution and increases by a factor of two until the full resolution is reached. Meanwhile, a hierarchy of B-spline grid spaces from large to small is used. The finest B-spline grid space used in the experiments is 8 mm. The images and grid space are refined alternatively.

The similarity cost is optimized using a limited-memory, quasi-Newton minimization method with bounds (L-BFGS-B) [13] algorithm and a sufficient condition is used in the optimization to constrain the B-splines coefficients so that the transformation maintains the topology of two images [14].

3 Experiments and Results

3.1 Landmark Matching Accuracy

For each subject, the six registration methods described in Section 2 were used to register the parenchyma region imaged at TLC to FRC. Landmarks such as branch points of the airway and vascular tree were utilized to evaluate registration accuracy. 100-150 landmark pairs were chosen for each subject. Figure 2(a) shows an example of landmark distribution on a FRC data from one subject.

The landmark error for a landmark on one image measures the Euclidean distance from its estimated position to real position on the second image. Table 1 shows the mean and standard deviation of landmark errors through all three subjects after using different registration methods. Figure 2(b) shows the box-plot of landmark errors.

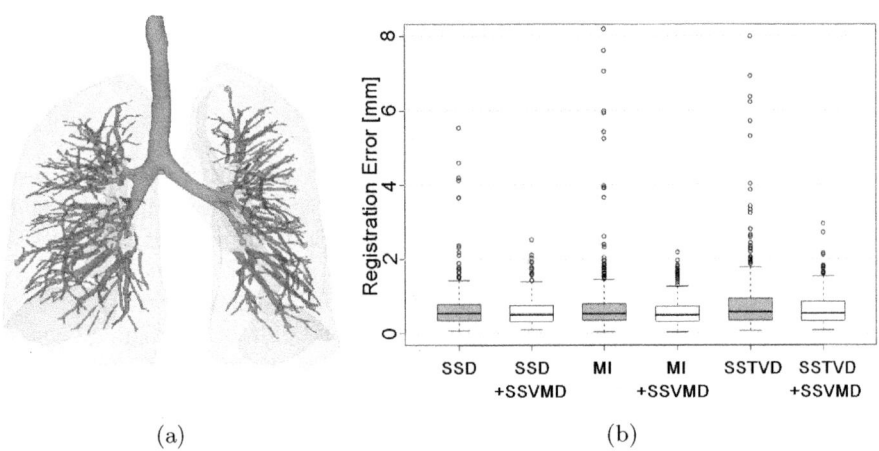

(a)   (b)

Fig. 2. (a) Distribution of landmark (green points) on one FRC data. (b) Box-plot of landmark errors through three subjects after using six registration methods. Results from SSD method and MI method contain outliers beyond the error range in (b).

Table 1. Landmark errors (mm) through three subjects after using different registration methods. The original average landmark error (after rigid registration) was $25.25 \pm 12.67\ mm$ with a maximum landmark error of 61.87 mm.

	SSD		MI		SSTVD	
	Avg.	Max	Avg.	Max	Avg.	Max
Without SSVMD	0.74 ± 1.09	15.66	1.05 ± 2.49	25.49	0.83 ± 0.93	7.99
With SSVMD	0.59 ± 0.37	2.52	0.58 ± 0.36	2.19	0.65 ± 0.42	2.95

3.2   Vessel Matching Accuracy

The registration accuracy on the vessel tree was evaluated by vessel matching distance, which is calculated as the distance between a point on FRC vessel tree and its closet point on warped TLC vessel tree. Figure 3 shows the distance map on FRC vessel tree from one subject after using six different registration methods. Large errors between the deformed source and target vessel trees were reduced after adding the SSVMD constraint.

3.3   Jacobian Comparison

Both landmark error and vessel matching distance evaluate the registration accuracy at vessel locations. Good matching accuracy on vessels does not guarantee that the parenchymal tissues are correctly aligned. In order to reveal the lung tissue deformation pattern, the Jacobian of the transformation field derived by image registration was used to estimate the local tissue deformation [2]. Using a Lagrangian reference frame, local tissue expansion corresponds to a Jacobian greater than one and local tissue contraction corresponds to a Jacobian less than one. Figure 4 shows the Jacobian maps resulted from six registration methods.

3.4   Correlation between Lung Expansion and Xe-CT Estimates of Specific Ventilation

Previous studies have shown that the degree of regional lung expansion is directly related to specific ventilation (sV) [2]. In order to evaluate how SSVMD affects the resulting deformation field and estimates of regional lung tissue deformation, we compared lung expansion measured by the Jacobian with Xe-CT estimates of sV on lung CT data sets from one sheep.

The adult sheep was anesthetized using intravenous pentobarbital and mechanically ventilated during the experiment. CT scans were acquired with the sheep in the supine orientation and with a static protocol at 10 cm (P10) and 25 cm (P25) H_2O airway pressure. For Xe-CT studies, twelve contiguous axial locations and approximately 40 breaths were selected from the whole lung volumetric scan performed near end-expiration. Both types of images were acquired at a reconstruction matrix of 512×512. The sV was computed using the Pulmonary Analysis Software Suite 11.0 (PASS) [15]. To compare the Jacobian values with the sV, the static scan P10 was registered to the Xe-CT scan using rigid affine registration. The Xe-CT data was subdivided into 30 slabs along the y (ventral–dorsal) direction. The average Jacobian within each slab was compared to the corresponding average sV measurement in the Xe-CT images. The Jacobian and sV measurements are shown on a transverse slice in Figure 5. Table 2 shows the correlation coefficient r value between sV and Jacobian derived from six registration methods.

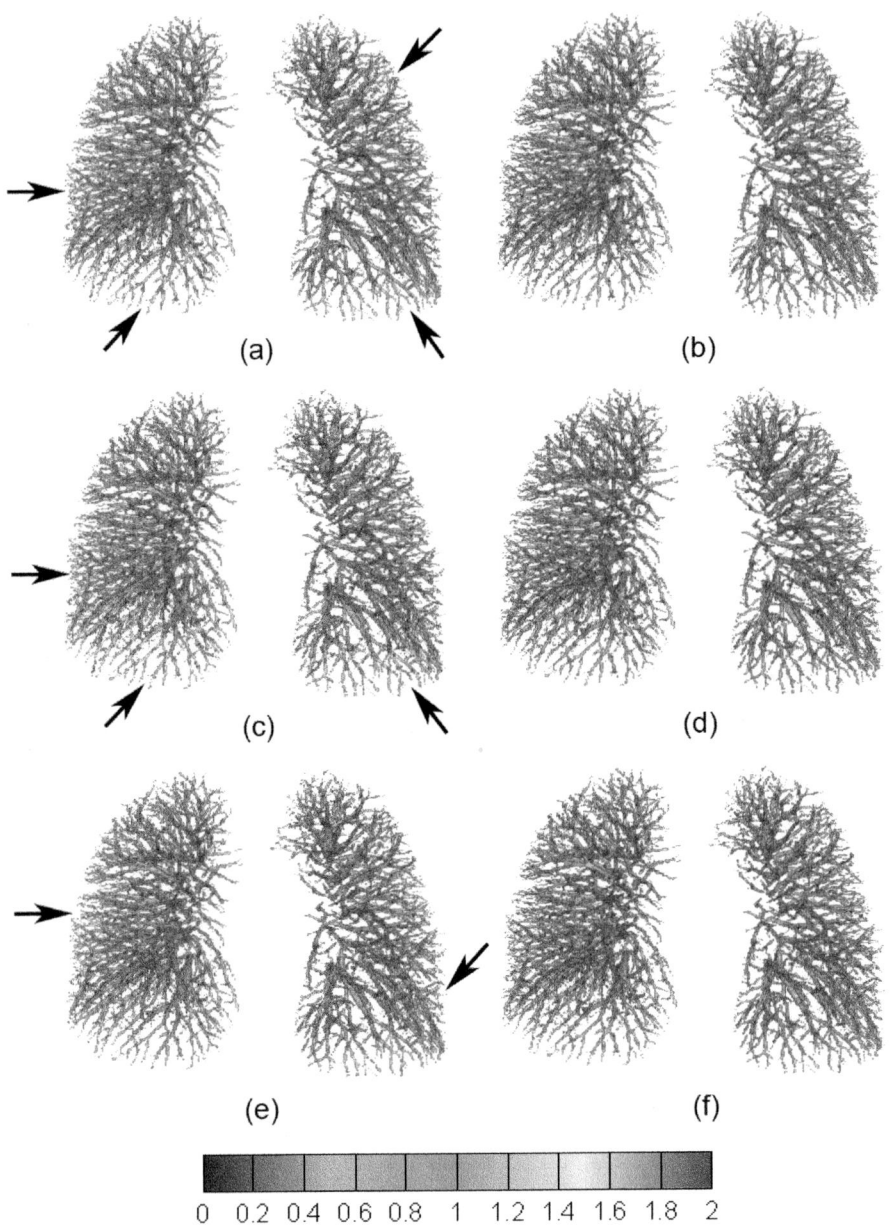

Fig. 3. Vessel matching distance (mm) on target vessel tree resulted from six registration methods: (a) SSD, (b) SSD + SSVMD, (c) MI, (d) MI + SSVMD, (e) SSTVD, and (f) SSTVD + SSVMD. Arrows denote regions of large discrepancies between the deformed source and target vessel trees. Note that the errors in these regions were reduced after adding the SSVMD constraint to the registration algorithms.

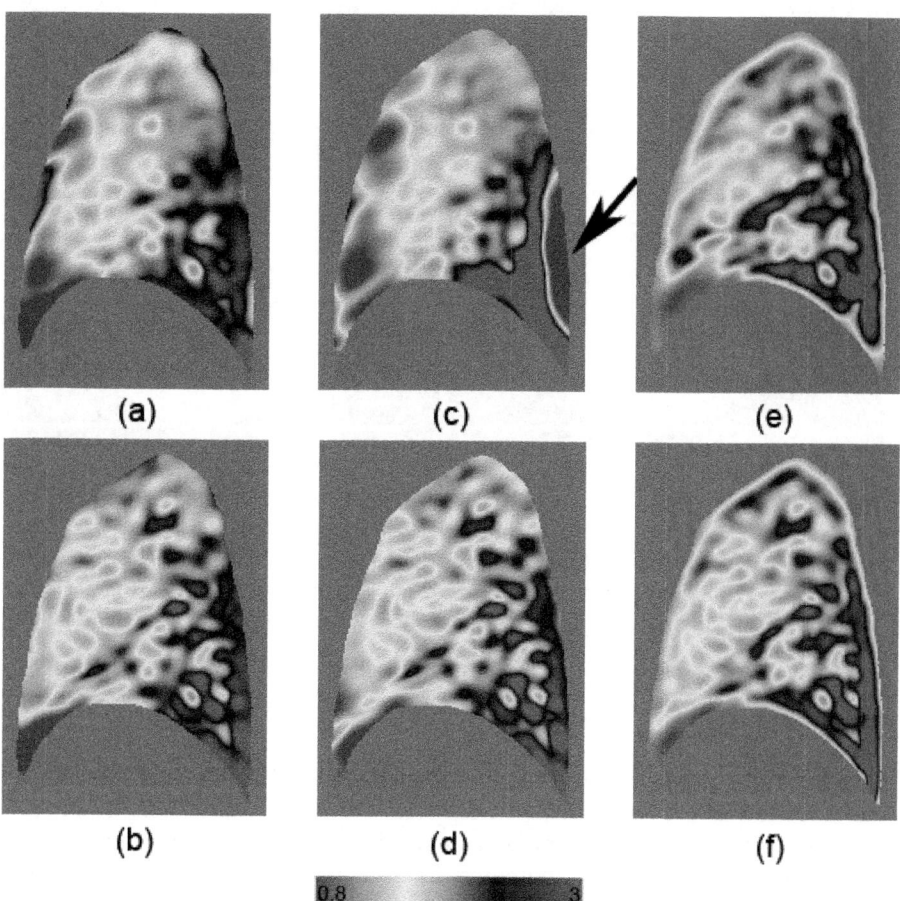

Fig. 4. The color-coded Jacobian maps of a sagittal slice resulted from six registration methods: (a) SSD, (b) SSD + SSVMD, (c) MI, (d) MI + SSVMD, (e) SSTVD, and (f) SSTVD + SSVMD. Blue and purple regions have larger lung deformation, while red and orange regions are deforming less. The arrow points to a region where Jacobian pattern is suspected to be incorrect.

Table 2. Correlation coefficient r between sV and Jacobian derived from six registration methods

	SSD	MI	SSTVD
Without SSVMD	0.72	0.60	0.92
With SSVMD	0.88	0.87	0.91

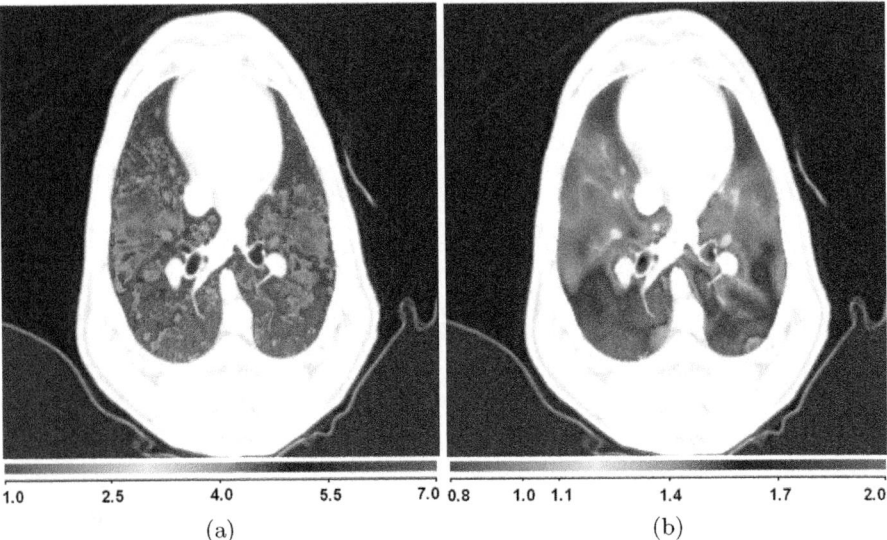

1.0   2.5   4.0   5.5   7.0 0.8   1.0 1.1   1.4   1.7   2.0

(a)   (b)

Fig. 5. Color-coded maps overlaid on a transverse slice from the sheep lung data showing (a) specific ventilation (1/min) and (b) the Jacobian of transformation between P10 and P25. Blue and purple regions show higher ventilation in (a) and larger deformation in (b), while red and orange regions show lower ventilation in (a) and smaller deformation in (b).

4   Discussion

Table 1 and Figure 2(b) show that adding the SSVMD cost function reduced the mean landmark errors of the three basic registration methods. Landmarks with large errors, shown as outliers in the box-plot, are aligned much better when SSVMD is used. Vessel matching distance maps in Figure 3 reflect the fact that SSVMD constraint helps improve matching accuracy over all three basic methods on small vessels, around lung boundaries and in the region near diaphragm. The reason for this is that blood vessels in those regions are usually small and have low intensity contrast, and thus they contribute little to conventional intensity similarity criteria. The vesselness measurement enhances blood vessel information and strengthens contribution of small vessels to registration process when using the SSVMD similarity metric.

Although SSD method (after histogram matching) has smaller mean landmark error than SSTVD method, its accuracy in the inferior region of the lung is not as good as that of SSTVD method. The reason may be that SSTVD cost function contains a local Jacobian factor which can constrain incorrect displacement and capture large deformation in the region near diaphragm with higher accuracy. However, after adding SSVMD on the three basic methods, the vessels are generally aligned better and the resulting vessel matching distance maps (Figure 3 right column) look similar.

The top row in Figure 4 shows that the Jacobian maps generated by the three registration methods without SSVMD have a similar ventral to dorsal gradient as expected since the subjects were imaged in the supine orientation. However, the local tissue deformation patterns derived from these methods are different even in the methods pair SSD and SSTVD which have similar landmark errors as shown in Table 1. This is consistent with the findings that while the inter-method variability on the landmark error is small there may be discriminating difference in the Jacobian maps [16]. The Jacobian from MI method is strikingly different in the region pointed by an arrow, which may be due to the differences in convergence speed among registration methods. The Jacobian maps from SSD and SSTVD methods show more local structure in the dorsal region, but they are of different patterns, especially in the region around lung boundaries. The bottom row in Figure 4 shows that adding the SSVMD constraint produces Jacobian images that are very similar across the three registration methods and reveal more detailed deformation patterns especially near vessel locations. Generally, vessels have smaller volume changes comparing with parenchymal tissues during breathing cycles. The three Jacobian maps produced using registration methods with SSVMD are very similar which may imply that the derived local deformation patterns are more reliable.

Regional lung expansion should correlate with regional ventilation measured by Xe-CT estimates of sV. As shown in Figure 5, both sV and Jacobian maps show a similar ventral to dorsal gradient. High specific ventilation should correspond with large tissue expansion. Table 2 shows that SSVMD improves the correlation results for both SSD and MI methods. For SSTVD, there is little change in the correlation. This may result from the accurate regional model of the intensity change in SSTVD method, and it is difficult to achieve additional improvement. These results suggest that SSVMD helps generate more physiologically meaningful transformations.

5 Conclusion

We have described a vesselness preserving constraint that can be used to improve the registration of similar vesselness patterns in two lung CT images. Results were presented to show that adding the SSVMD constraint to existing similarity metrics such as SSD, MI, and SSTVD reduces landmark error and improves vascular tree overlap. The purpose of adding this metric in registration process is that it can help correct the mismatches of small vessels and their surrounding lung tissues. The SSVMD constraint was shown to produce a more detailed expansion pattern for local tissue, especially near vessel locations. In addition, adding the SSVMD constraint was shown to improve the correlation between Jacobian and specific ventilation after registration. This demonstrates that using the SSVMD constraint not only helps match vessel structures, but it also helps align corresponding parenchymal tissues providing a more reliable pattern of local lung tissue deformation.

Acknowledgments

This work was supported by the NIH grants HL079406, HL64368, EB004126, HL080285, and CA129022.

References

1. Guerrero, T., Sanders, K., Castillo, E., Zhang, Y., Bidaut, L., Pan, T., Komaki, R.: Dynamic ventilation imaging from four-dimensional computed tomography. Phys. Med. Biol. 51(4), 777–791 (2006)
2. Reinhardt, J.M., Ding, K., Cao, K., Christensen, G.E., Hoffman, E.A., Bodas, S.V.: Registration-based estimates of local lung tissue expansion compared to xenon-CT measures of specific ventilation. Medical Image Analysis 12(6), 752–763 (2008)
3. Ding, K., Bayouth, J.E., Buatti, J.M., Christensen, G.E., Reinhardt, J.M.: 4DCT-based measurement of changes in pulmonary function following a course of radiation therapy. Medical Physics 37(3), 1261–1272 (2010)
4. Coselmon, M.M., Balter, J.M., McShan, D.L., Kessler, M.L.: Mutual information based CT registration of the lung at exhale and inhale breathing states using thin-plate splines. Medical Physics 31(11), 2942–2948 (2004)
5. Christensen, G.E., Song, J.H., Lu, W., Naqa, I.E., Low, D.A.: Tracking lung tissue motion and expansion/compression with inverse consistent image registration and spirometry. Medical Physics 34(6), 2155–2165 (2007)
6. Gorbunova, V., Lo, P., Ashraf, H., Dirksen, A., Nielsen, M., de Bruijne, M.: Weight preserving image registration for monitoring disease progression in lung CT. In: Metaxas, D., Axel, L., Fichtinger, G., Székely, G. (eds.) MICCAI 2008, Part II. LNCS, vol. 5242, pp. 863–870. Springer, Heidelberg (2008)
7. Yin, Y., Hoffman, E.A., Lin, C.L.: Mass preserving non-rigid registration of CT lung images using cubic B-spline. Medical Physics 36(9), 4213–4222 (2009)
8. Hu, S., Hoffman, E.A., Reinhardt, J.M.: Automatic lung segmentation for accurate quantitation of volumetric X-ray CT images. IEEE Trans. on Medical Imaging 20, 490–498 (2001)
9. Murphy, K., van Ginneken, B., Pluim, J., Klein, S., Staring, M.: Semi-automatic reference standard construction for quantitative evaluation of lung CT registration. In: Metaxas, D., Axel, L., Fichtinger, G., Székely, G. (eds.) MICCAI 2008, Part II. LNCS, vol. 5242, pp. 1006–1013. Springer, Heidelberg (2008)
10. Thevenaz, P., Unser, M.: Spline pyramids for inter-modal image registration using mutual information. In: Proc. SPIE, vol. 3169, pp. 236–247 (1997)
11. Mattes, D., Haynor, D., Vesselle, H., Lewellen, T., Eubank, W.: PET-CT image registration in the chest using free-form deformations. IEEE Transactions on Medical Imaging 22(1), 120–128 (2003)
12. Frangi, A.F., Niessen, W.J., Vincken, K.L., Viergever, M.A.: Multiscale vessel enhancement filtering. In: Wells, W.M., Colchester, A.C.F., Delp, S.L. (eds.) MICCAI 1998. LNCS, vol. 1496, pp. 130–137. Springer, Heidelberg (1998)
13. Byrd, R.H., Lu, P., Nocedal, J., Zhu, C.: A limited memory algorithm for bound constrained optimization. SIAM J. Sci. Comput. 16(5), 1190–1208 (1995)
14. Choi, Y., Lee, S.: Injectivity conditions of 2d and 3d uniform cubic b-spline functions. Graphical Models 62(6), 411–427 (2000)
15. Guo, J., Fuld, M.K., Alford, S.K., Reinhardt, J.M., Hoffman, E.A.: Pulmonary analysis software suite 9.0: Integrating quantitative measures of function with structural analyses. In: First International Workshop on Pulmonary Image Analysis, New York, pp. 283–292 (2008)
16. Kabus, S., Klinder, T., Murphy, K., van Ginneken, B., Lorenz, C., Pluim, J.P.W.: Evaluation of 4D-CT lung registration. In: Yang, G.-Z., Hawkes, D., Rueckert, D., Noble, A., Taylor, C. (eds.) MICCAI 2009. LNCS, vol. 5761, pp. 747–754. Springer, Heidelberg (2009)

Deformable Image Registration of Follow-Up Breast Magnetic Resonance Images

Tobias Boehler[1], Kathy Schilling[2], Ulrich Bick[3], and Horst K. Hahn[1]

[1] Fraunhofer MEVIS, Bremen 28359, Germany
[2] Boca Raton Community Hospital, FL 33486, USA
[3] Charité Universitätsmedizin, Berlin 10117, Germany
tobias.boehler@mevis.fraunhofer.de

Abstract. A novel method for the deformable image registration of follow-up breast magnetic resonance (MR) images is proposed, aimed at an automatic synchronization of temporal images. To compensate potentially large breast deformations and differences among device coordinates, an initial linear alignment of each individual breast, a combination of both transformations using thin-plate splines, as well as a subsequent linear-elastic registration are performed in sequence. Complementary to algorithmic details, an overview of modality-specific factors influencing follow-up registration accuracy is given. The proposed method was evaluated on 20 clinical datasets annotated with landmarks by an expert radiologist. Despite large variations among the MR images, accuracy of the method was sufficient to allow spatial synchronization, with remaining target registration errors of $< 32\%$. Concluding, potential enhancements to further increase robustness and accuracy are discussed.

1 Introduction

For breast magnetic resonance imaging, comparative examination of currently and previously acquired images provides valuable diagnostic information. Subsequent follow-up imaging and reading take place several months after the preceding acquisition. The temporal interval is chosen patient-specifically. Corresponding consecutive image pairs are also referred to as current-prior images.

Contrary to conventional x-ray mammography (MG), the role of diagnostic software supporting follow-up imaging for breast MRI is less established. Follow-up MR images have complemented MG for long-term classifications of lesions over several years time or to detect potential recurrent diseases [1]. Rather than long-term, short-term follow-up imaging is more frequently applied to assess interventional or medicamentous treatment of lesions by chemotherapy [2,3]. Furthermore, it was shown that additional retrospective follow-up examinations allow the detection of contralateral breast cancers and might even lead to changes in treatment planning and management for early-cancer patients [4]. Moreover, a review of different follow-up schedules has been published recently [5].

The value of follow-up investigations for diagnostics stems from its temporal range: observation of regions of the breast over a longer period of time allows the

B. Fischer, B. Dawant, and C. Lorenz (Eds.): WBIR 2010, LNCS 6204, pp. 13–24, 2010.
© Springer-Verlag Berlin Heidelberg 2010

radiologist to track pathological and morphological changes in the breast tissue. In particular, such an analysis facilitates the detection of malignant cancers originally graded as "probably benign". Visual appearance of these cancers often varies significantly over time, so that growth patterns and lesion-typical signs are perceived. These visual cues might then lead to a different rating of the lesion.

In addition, follow-up investigations support the radiologist when some uncertainty with respect to grading remains. Frequently, lesions which are difficult to grade are classified as belonging to BI-RADS category 3, rated as "unclear" or as "probably benign" [6]. For a final assessment of the lesion, a biopsy must be performed. Consequently, the number and expense of evitable biopsies could be reduced by the examination of current-prior images. Routinely and repeatedly conducted follow-up diagnostics are therefore required [7,6].

Registration of follow-up images is complicated by numerous unpredictable factors determined both by breast physiology as well as image acquisition. These issues must be considered in addition to geometric changes of the breast tissue. Table 1 shows the main issues to be regarded. Accordingly, the visual appearance of current and prior images is subject to substantial change.

In particular, tissue deformation, different patient placement and changes of the field-of-view make the reading tedious for the radiologist. Even coarse alignment of such images will therefore offer important support. Spatially-synchronized, simultaneous viewing of current and prior images allows the clinician to quickly establish correspondence between time points and to correlate lesions.

Registration of follow-up MRI is a novel field of research. To our knowledge, only two other contributions have been published before, focused on the quantification of neoadjuvant chemotherapy. Chittineni et al. performed an automatic delineation of the air-breast boundary and chestwall, followed by non-rigid registration [8]. Recently, Li et al. proposed a registration algorithm for short-term follow-up therapy monitoring based on the adaptive bases algorithm [9].

In the following sections, we propose a method that performs an automatic preprocessing and registration of long-term follow-up breast MR images in order to synchronize them. Contrary to [8], no additional segmentation is required. The method extends a previously published registration technique by adding an intermediate thin-plate spline interpolation to ensure consistency of the deformation [10]. We evaluated the method on 20 clinical breast datasets and quantitatively assessed its accuracy using expert-annotated landmark locations. Finally, current limitations and future enhancements of the method are discussed.

2   Methods

Application of current-prior registration is a sequential procedure that addresses issues listed in Table 1. In particular, dislocation of the current breast image with respect to the MR device coordinates of the prior image must be compensated. This is achieved by two independent linear image registration tasks, after the breasts have been preprocessed. Remaining local tissue variations are then corrected using non-linear registration to establish further spatial correspondence.

Table 1. Overview of patient-specific and general issues for the reading of breast MRI follow-up (current-prior) images, including exemplary images for each described issue. Images courtesy of U. Bick, Charité Berlin.

Issue	Description	Source	Prior image	Current image
Devices	Image characteristics (noise, resolution, inhomogeneities etc.), different breast shapes or larger deformations.	Different coils, different pressure to stabilize the breasts, different MRI scanners, different vendors or technology, change of device co-ordinate systems.		
Fields-of-view	Either whole thorax, both breasts or single breast (e.g., biopsy imaging), orthogonally reformatted views.	Adjustment of the field-of-view depending on the diagnostic or interventional task, as well as the applied imaging protocol.		
Resolution	Different in-plane and out-of-plane resolutions, as well as voxel size and slice thickness.	Protocol- and device-dependent settings.		
Pathology	Visible lesions or biopsy scars, different appearances in both images.	Interventions, new or recurrent lesions visible in the breast tissue.		
Artifacts	Different MRI artifacts visible in the images.	MR-specific reconstruction artifacts.		
Intensities	Different voxel intensities, local variation and misaligned regions.	Various reasons, such as field inhomogeneities, contrast enhancement, image noise or tissue changes (due to elasticity, relation of fibrotic to adipose or glandular tissue).		
Geometry	Different breast geometry.	Post-interventional (lumpectomy, mastectomy or biopsy) examination of the breast.		

2.1 Preprocessing

Initially, each image is divided into two images containing disjunct halves of the breast using an automatic cropping method. The motivation behind this is to perform two separate linear registrations constrained to each breast in order to compensate deformations more effectively. Particularly, different compression applied to each individual breast cannot be modeled by a single affine-linear transformation, since the breast-individual change in pose is frequently dissimilar. The computation of two unconnected transformations is therefore better suited to provide a good initialization for the subsequent linear-elastic image registration. The latter in turn is able to compensate only small non-linear deformations, and therefore requires a preceding alignment.

Consequently, each breast is registered separately after a division of the images. The breasts are separated using a dedicated breast MRI cropping method, which is more accurate in dividing the images than simply splitting along the image centerline [11]. As the reference image **R** for the registration, the follow-up image was selected, whereas the original prior image was taken as the template image **T** to be registered onto the follow-up image. For dynamic contrast-enhanced (DCE) sequences, the first, unenhanced images were selected.

2.2 Linear Image Registration

The affine-linear transformation is restricted to a similarity transform with seven degrees of freedom, modeling rotation and translation, as well as isotropic scaling. Therefore, applied transformations retain most of the original breast geometry while allowing deviations from the original size. On the other hand, relative orientation and pose must be modified liberally in order to model different device coordinate systems and independent deformations of each breast.

Assuming that the distribution of glandular, adipose and fibrotic breast tissue remains approximately consistent, intensities of the current and prior images will be closely related. Predominantly, images will be subject to low-frequency intensity changes induced by the breast coil setup. Therefore, it is assumed that the expected intensity change roughly approximates a linear function, and the normalized cross-correlation coefficient

$$e_{ncc}(\mathbf{R}, \mathbf{T}) = 1 - \frac{(cov(\mathbf{R}, \mathbf{T}))^2}{\sigma^2(\mathbf{R})\sigma^2(\mathbf{T})} \in [0, 1] \tag{1}$$

can be used to measure image dissimilarity [12]. The coefficient is subtracted from unity to assume highest similarity for $e_{ncc} \to 0$. Minimization of equation (1) is achieved by numerical optimization using an iterative Levenberg-Marquardt optimization scheme until convergence is reached [13]. Appropriate iteration step widths are estimated using Armijo's line search strategy [14]. Convergence is declared when suitable stopping criteria are met [15].

Subsequently, deformation fields are computed for each affine-linear registration. To avoid undefined regions of the deformation, the individual fields are

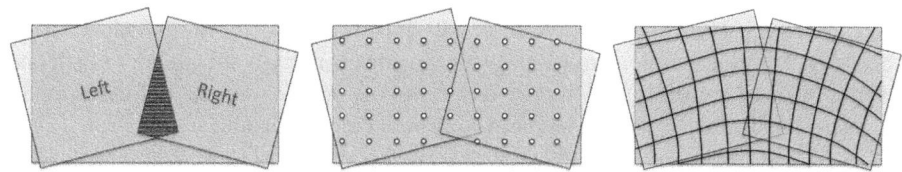

Fig. 1. Concatenation of the linear deformation fields. Overlap regions (striped) are neglected (left), and regular grid points are sampled in valid regions (middle). After back-transformation, the two point sets are interpolated using a thin-plate spline transformation, the resulting deformation completely covers the template image (right).

combined to one joint field. However, this combination requires dedicated handling, since the deformation fields are derived from disjunct transformations. Consequently, concatenation by averaging or addition of the two fields will result in a joint field that does not necessarily cover the entire image (see Fig. 1, left). Transformation of the template image with such a deformation will distort the image, because some image regions are not transformed.

Therefore, a thin-plate spline (TPS) interpolation is used to combine both deformation fields and retain a maximum of the original deformations [16]. Although specific poly-affine methods exist [17], the TPS method is employed due to its simplicity and inherent treatment of affine-linear transformations. First, corresponding points before and after linear registration are computed. For this purpose, both breasts and their linear transformations are considered independently to identify point pairs for each transformation. A sparse set of n and m regular grid points $\{\mathbf{p}_i^{left}, \mathbf{p}_j^{right}\} \in \mathbb{R}^3, i = \{1 \ldots n\}, j = \{1 \ldots m\}$ are defined in regions for which the corresponding deformation field is known, for the left and right breast, respectively. Given the computed homogenous 4×4 matrices $\mathbf{M}^{left}$ and $\mathbf{M}^{right}$ for each linear transformation, the points (in homogenous notation) are back-projected by left-multiplying the inverse transformations so that

$$\forall i : \mathbf{q}_i^{left} = (\mathbf{M}^{left})^{-1}\mathbf{p}_i^{left} \quad \text{and} \quad \forall j : \mathbf{q}_j^{right} = (\mathbf{M}^{right})^{-1}\mathbf{p}_j^{right} \quad (2)$$

yield the transformed points. Concatenation of the transformed and untransformed point lists creates the two point lists $\mathbf{P} = \{\mathbf{p}^{left}\} \cup \{\mathbf{p}^{right}\}$ and $\mathbf{Q} = \{\mathbf{q}^{left}\} \cup \{\mathbf{q}^{right}\}$ with identical sizes $s = n + m$. The deformation field is then interpolated using the thin-plate functional

$$u(\mathbf{x}) = \sum_{\nu=1}^{4} a_\nu \phi_\nu(\mathbf{x}) + \sum_{\mu=1}^{s} w_\mu U(|\mathbf{x} - \mathbf{p}_\mu|_2) \quad (3)$$

with the 3-D radial basis functions $U(r) = -\frac{1}{8\pi}r, r \in \mathbb{R}$, monomials $\phi_\nu \in \mathbb{R}$ and $\mathbf{p} \in \mathbf{P}$ [18]. Solving for the linear coefficients a_ν and non-linear coefficients w_μ in equation (3) using the point set $\mathbf{Q}$ is achieved by solving an appropriate equation system, using the conjugate gradient method [18]. Subsequently, the dense deformation field can be computed by directly evaluating the functional (3) at each image coordinate. After interpolation, the resulting joint field contains both the affine-linear deformations as well as intermediate non-linear transitions. The joint field is applied to the original template image and the deformed image is passed as input to the subsequent non-linear deformation.

2.3   Linear-Elastic Image Registration

After application of the joint linear transformations, both breasts are roughly aligned. Remaining dissimilarities of image regions are primarily caused by local tissue deformations. For this reason, a linear-elastic transformation model is employed for the non-linear registration [12]. The transformation model enforces the regularization of computed deformations in each iteration similar to the demon's algorithm [19,20].

For the non-linear registration, a reference image $\mathbf{R}$ and a template image $\mathbf{T}$ with n voxels each are given. For each voxel position $\mathbf{x}_i \in \mathbb{R}^3, i = 0, \ldots, n - 1$, a local non-linear deformation $\mathbf{u}(\mathbf{x}_i) = (u_x, u_y, u_z)^T$, $\mathbf{u} : \mathbb{R}^3 \longrightarrow \mathbb{R}^3$ is computed. The local deformation $\mathbf{u}(\mathbf{x}_i)$ compensates tissue deformation and is defined by a corresponding displacement field $\mathbf{u}$. The local error measure

$$e = \frac{1}{2n} \sum_{i=0}^{n-1} e_{\text{local}}(\mathbf{x}_i, \mathbf{x}_i + \mathbf{u}(\mathbf{x}_i)) \tag{4}$$

depends on the spatial image coordinates $\mathbf{x}_i$, the transformed coordinates $\mathbf{x}_i + \mathbf{u}(\mathbf{x}_i)$, as well as the reference and template images. Instead of defining a measure of similarity, we thus consider the equivalent minimization of a local error e_{local}.

For the linear-elastic registration, an intensity-based similarity measure was selected. The sum of squared differences (SSD) measure is defined as

$$e_{\text{ssd}}(\mathbf{x}_i, \mathbf{x}_i + \mathbf{u}(\mathbf{x}_i)) = [\mathbf{R}(\mathbf{x}_i) - \mathbf{T}(\mathbf{x}_i + \mathbf{u}(\mathbf{x}_i))]^2. \tag{5}$$

Although the measure assumes a constant intensity relation, it was successfully employed in the current-prior registration: Assuming that motion correction has been previously performed, it is sufficient to register only the unenhanced base images. Remaining images are already in the identical coordinate space of the base image. As no local high-frequency temporal enhancement is apparent for these current-prior base image pairs, intensity-based registration is applicable. This does not hold for the global affine-linear registration which considers the entire image. In addition, unlike contrast-enhanced MRI, rapid brightness changes of lesions do not occur. Registration is achieved by minimization of equation (4) using a gradient descent method and explicit Euler integration [20].

To ensure consistency of the computed deformation field, explicit *a posteriori* regularization is employed in each iteration [19,20]. For the registration of breast tissue, regularization with the linear elastic potential defines an appropriate elastic model. An iterative solution was derived by Gramkow [21], employing convolution of the deformation with a linear filter in analogy to the demon's algorithm [19]. For this purpose, a complex-valued $7 \times 7 \times 7$ filter-response kernel

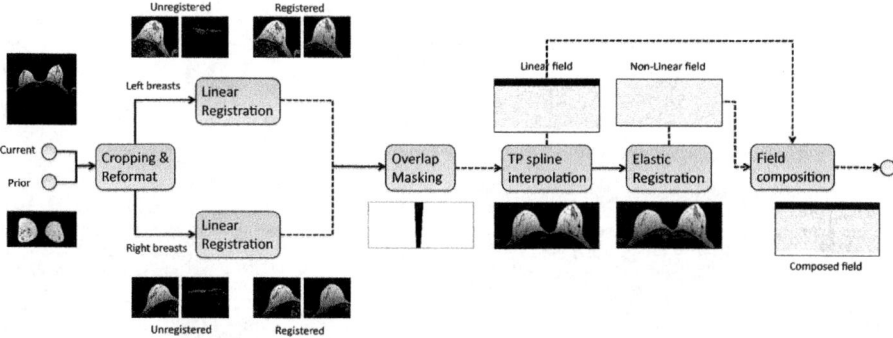

Fig. 2. The computational processing pipeline for the proposed method (dashed lines illustrate processing of deformation fields, solid lines image processing)

is generated from the linear-elastic potential [21]. Lamé parameters were set to $\mu = 500, \lambda = 0.1$. Convolution of the updated deformation field with the kernel enforces explicit linear-elastic regularization. The deformation is updated by composing it with the update force field, identical to the compositive demon's algorithm [22]. After the linear-elastic registration has been performed, computed deformations for both linear and non-linear registration need to be composed in order to jointly apply them to the input image. The composed deformation is generated by addition of both deformation fields. Finally, the resulting transformed template image and the composed deformation are stored. The complete image processing scheme is illustrated in Fig. 2.

Synchronization of cursor positions requires that for a selected voxel position $\mathbf{v} \in \mathbb{R}^3$ in one image a corresponding position $\hat{\mathbf{v}} \in \mathbb{R}^3$ is computed in the other image. This mapping is defined by the deformation field computed in the previous steps. Given the joint displacement $\mathbf{u}(\mathbf{v})$ at voxel $\mathbf{v}$, we simply compute $\hat{\mathbf{v}} = \mathbf{v} + \mathbf{u}(\mathbf{v})$ as the corresponding position and reposition the cursor accordingly.

2.4   Evaluation

Accuracy of the method was evaluated on clinical datasets, using visual inspection as well as landmark-based measurement of the target registration error [23]. An expert breast radiologist annotated corresponding landmarks in both current and prior images. For this annotation task, a dedicated application had been developed. While the assessment of landmarks alone provides only limited insight into the accuracy of a non-linear image registration, the combination with visual inspection of the registered images allows an overall evaluation. For the visual inspection, reference and template images were inspected as checkerboard-like views. A standalone, synchronized viewing application was evaluated by radiologist experts. Additionally, the deformation fields were displayed as discrete grid overlays, in order to reveal implausible deformations and misregistrations.

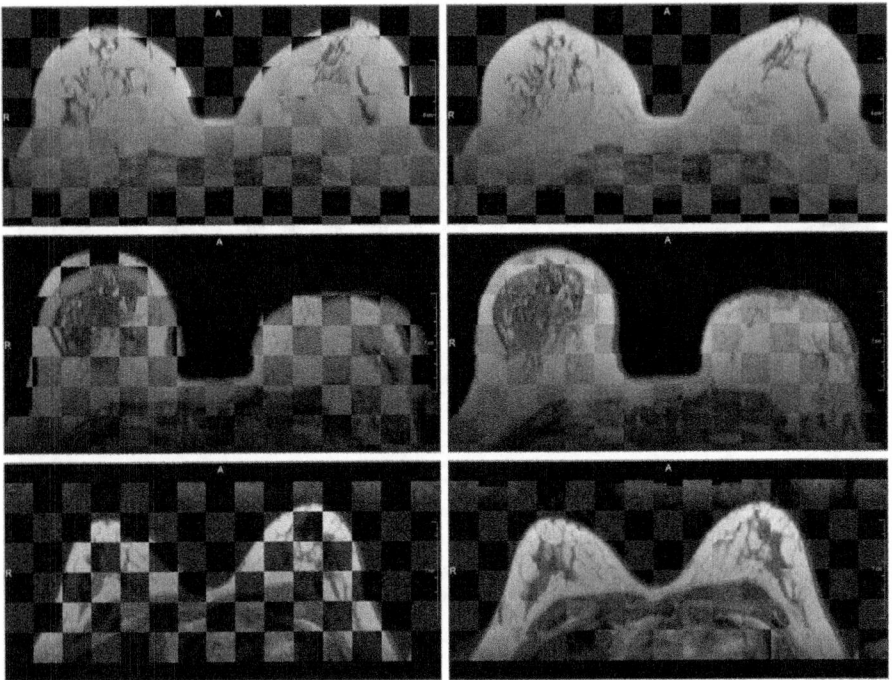

Fig. 3. Checkerboard-like overlays of exemplary current-prior images before (left) and after (right) registration with the proposed method. Images courtesy of U. Bick, Charité Berlin.

3   Results

The proposed method was evaluated on 20 pairs of clinical T1-weighted MR images acquired from 17 patients using standard DCE protocols and double breast coils. The images were acquired on four different MR scanning systems (Siemens Magnetom and Symphony Vision, Avanto, Sonata) with varying resolutions ($256 \times 128 \times 64$ to $560^2 \times 120$ voxels) and voxel sizes ($1.25^2 \times 2.844mm$ to $0.625^2 \times 2mm$). Biopsy images were removed from the test set prior to processing.

Initially, visual inspection of the current-prior images before and after registration was conducted. The images were displayed to breast radiologists as checkerboard-like overlays. Figure 3 shows three exemplary registration results. After registration, the alignment of internal breast structures and tissue boundaries has improved significantly. Complementarily, the annotated landmarks were transformed with respect to the deformation fields computed by the image registration. In particular, for a given set of reference landmarks, the corresponding transformed reference landmarks were determined. This mapping effectively positions the reference landmarks in the template space. Since a non-symmetric image registration method was applied, the mapping is generally not bijective.

Table 2. Resulting distances (in mm) between landmarks after registration, including minimum (underlined) and maximum (bold) values

Datasets (1-10)	B1	B2	B3	B4	B5	B6	B7	B8	B9	B10
Mean	7.28	5.88	8.98	12.56	5.41	13.74	6.06	14.02	10.31	16.07
Std.dev.	2.14	0.68	4.23	4.87	1.47	7.53	2.62	6.07	11.09	4.91
Minimum	4.72	4.86	3.6	7.39	3.38	7.02	3.44	7.37	<u>1.35</u>	9.16
Maximum	9.96	6.86	13.94	19.01	6.86	24.25	9.64	22.04	25.94	20.13

Datasets (11-20)	B11	B12	B13	B14	B15	B16	B17	B18	B19	B20
Mean	19.2	12.08	10.36	15.32	16.1	15.35	5.53	**24.61**	11.37	<u>3.17</u>
Std.dev.	3.21	2.24	4.09	<u>0.32</u>	7.26	7.36	0.72	**16.5**	7.21	1.55
Minimum	**15.4**	9.02	5.4	14.91	7.84	9.1	4.52	1.43	5.72	1.44
Maximum	23.25	14.33	15.42	15.69	25.51	25.69	6.14	**38.27**	21.54	<u>5.2</u>

Euclidean distance measurements were then taken between the mapped reference landmarks and the template landmarks in the template coordinate system. Results of these measurements for the SSD-driven linear-elastic regularizer are shown in Table 2.

For each dataset pair, the average, minimum and maximum distance as well as the standard deviation were computed. Subsequently, average values for all datasets were derived. Overall, the mean distance between landmarks was $11.67\pm 5.36mm$, including all datasets. The minimum average distance was $3.17mm$, while the maximum average distance was $24.64mm$. The minimum overall distance was $1.35mm$, the maximum overall distance $38.27mm$. Standard deviations for these values were at $3.91mm$ and $8.63mm$, respectively. Table 3 summarizes the overall distance statistics.

In addition, the relative improvement of landmark distances was estimated by comparison of the original distances with the distances after registration. The resulting values in mm and percentages are shown in Table 4. After registration, the mean overall distance was reduced to 31.73% of the original average distance. Standard deviation for the mean values was reduced to 13.36% of its original value. The average minimum and maximum distances were reduced to 27.53% and 35.47% of those for the unregistered images.

Table 3. Average distances (in mm) over all measurements after registration with the proposed method

Distance (mm)	Post-registration measurements			
	Mean	Std.dev.	Minimum	Maximum
Mean overall	11.67	4.81	6.53	17.49
Std.dev. overall	5.36	3.97	3.91	8.63
Minimum overall	3.17	0.32	1.35	5.2
Maximum overall	24.64	16.5	15.39	38.27

Table 4. Original average distances (in mm) over all measurements prior to registration, and relative percentages of the remaining distances after registration

Distance (mm)	Pre-registration measurements			
	Mean	Std.dev.	Minimum	Maximum
Mean overall	36.77	11.27	23.08	49.3
Std.dev. overall	40.13	18.91	17.43	58.56
Minimum overall	9.56	0.93	4.95	11.73
Maximum overall	159.63	69.72	70.49	240.69
Percentage (%)	Relative remaining distances			
Mean overall	31.74	42.69	27.53	35.47
Std.dev. overall	13.36	21.0	22.43	14.73
Minimum overall	33.15	34.28	27.21	44.33
Maximum overall	15.43	23.66	21.84	15.9

4   Discussion

Considering the quantitative and qualitative evaluation, the proposed method effectively reduced the average distance between landmarks to under a third of the original distance. Given the obviously large dislocations and deformations, this reduction greatly improves the spatial correlation. Variation in distance among the set of landmarks was reduced to 13.36% of the original standard deviation, on average. In addition to the reduced minimum and maximum distances, the narrowed range of standard deviations indicates that the registration performed well for the given datasets.

The average distance after registration was $11.67mm$, compared to $36.77mm$ before processing. Considering the voxel size of $1.25^2 \times 2mm$ for most of the datasets, the achieved improvement already allows to establish synchronization of current and prior datasets. Moreover, the visual inspection of results confirmed that the method aligned images in some cases very accurately.

The method performed worse on datasets containing large changes in breast tissue and geometry, such as post-interventional images. For these datasets, the linear-elastic small-deformation assumption is violated, resulting in imprecise registration results of both the linear and non-linear registrations. Notably, the linear registration often already failed to determine a plausible pre-registration. While the linear-elastic regularization is adequate for small deformations of the breast, its usage for follow-up registration must be supplemented by methods providing custom transformation models to reduce larger variations. Alternatively, diffeomorphic hyper-elastic registration methods must be implemented.

Currently, the non-symmetric mapping of the non-linear registration limits the applicability of the method in that two independent registration tasks need to be performed to allow bidirectional synchronization. A symmetric registration with ensured invertible mapping is currently being developed for this task.

Accuracy of the target registration error measurements depends on the placement of landmark points at feature positions in the images. This annotation is highly subjective and therefore landmark positions might not be exact, causing larger distance values. Following future evaluations will therefore also consider the fiducial registration error by comparing annotations of multiple experts [23].

5   Conclusion

A novel image registration method for the synchronization of breast MRI follow-up images has been proposed, along with an overview of registration-relevant issues. The method was qualitatively and quantitatively evaluated on 20 clinical datasets showing significant variation in breast geometry and image appearance. Accuracy of the registration method in terms of landmark-distances was in the range of $11.67 \pm 4.81mm$, corresponding to a decrease of the initial distances to only 31.74%. Variation was furthermore reduced to 13.36% of the original value. Consequently, the accuracy is sufficient to synchronize follow-up images and support the radiologist during reading. The computationally intensive registration tasks can be precomputed efficiently. At present, the main limitation of the method is the usage of an unspecific linear-elastic image registration method, whose capture range is insufficient for very large deformations of the breast. Therefore, current work aims at improving the method with the integration of prior initialization of the deformation to improve robustness and precision. In addition, the method will be extended to be fully symmetric to ensure an inverse-consistent mapping of the non-linear transformation.

Acknowledgements

Parts of this work have been funded as part of the HAMAM project by the European Union's 7th Framework Programme, ICT-2007.5.3, grant no. 224538.

References

1. Kuhl, C., Mielcareck, P., Klaschik, S., Leutner, C., Wardelmann, E., Gieseke, J., Schild, H.: Dynamic Breast MR Imaging: Are Signal Intensity Time Course Data Useful for Differential Diagnosis of Enhancing Lesions? Radiology 211(1), 101–110 (1999)
2. Kuhl, C., Schrading, S., Leutner, C., Morakkabati-Spitz, N., Wardelmann, E., Fimmers, R., Kuhn, W., Schild, H.: Mammography, breast ultrasound, and magnetic resonance imaging for surveillance of women at high familial risk for breast cancer. Journal of Clinical Oncology 23(33), 8469–8476 (2005)
3. Viehweg, P., Rotter, K., Laniado, M., Lampe, D., Buchmann, J., Kölbl, H., Heywang-Köbrunner, S.: MR imaging of the contralateral breast in patients after breast-conserving therapy. European Radiology 14(3), 402–408 (2004)
4. Lehman, C., Gatsonis, C., Kuhl, C., Hendrick, R., Pisano, E., Hanna, L., Peacock, S., Smazal, S., Maki, D., Julian, T., et al.: MRI evaluation of the contralateral breast in women with recently diagnosed breast cancer. The New England Journal of Medicine 356(13), 1295–1303 (2007)

5. Montgomery, D., Krupa, K., Cooke, T.: Alternative methods of follow up in breast cancer: a systematic review of the literature. British Journal of Cancer 96(11), 1625 (2007)
6. Varas, X., Leborgne, J., Leborgne, F., Mezzera, J., Jaumandreu, S., Leborgne, F.: Revisiting the mammographic follow-up of BI-RADS category 3 lesions. American Journal of Roentgenology 179(3), 691–695 (2002)
7. Sickles, E.: Periodic mammographic follow-up of probably benign lesions: results in 3,184 consecutive cases. Radiology 179(2), 463–468 (1991)
8. Chittineni, R., Su, M., Nalcioglu, O.: Breast Delineation using Active Contours to Facilitate Coregistration of Serial MRI Studies for Therapy Response Evaluation. In: IEEE International Conference on Image Processing, vol. 6, pp. 261–264 (2007)
9. Li, X., Dawant, B., Welch, E., Chakravarthy, A., Freehardt, D., Mayer, I., Kelley, M., Meszoely, I., Gore, J., Yankeelov, T.: A nonrigid registration algorithm for longitudinal breast MR images and the analysis of breast tumor response. Magnetic Resonance Imaging 27(9), 1258–1270 (2009)
10. Boehler, T., Bick, U., Hahn, H.: Assessment of image registration for follow-up MR mammography. European Radiology Supplements 19(4), 961–963 (2009)
11. Koenig, M., Kohle, S., Peitgen, H.O.: Automatic Cropping of Breast Regions for Registration in MR Mammography. In: Proceedings of SPIE of Medical Imaging 2005, pp. 1563–1570 (2005)
12. Modersitzki, J.: Numerical Methods for Image Registration. Oxford University Press, New York (2004)
13. Thevenaz, P., Ruttimann, U., Unser, M.: A pyramid approach to subpixel registration based on intensity. IEEE Transactions on Image Processing 7(1), 27–41 (1998)
14. Armijo, L.: Minimization of functions having Lipschitz continuous first partial derivatives. Pacific Journal of Mathematics 16(1), 1–3 (1966)
15. Gill, P., Murray, W., Wright, M.: Practical optimization. Academic Press, London (1981)
16. Bookstein, F.: Principal Warps: Thin-Plate Splines and the Decomposition of Deformations. IEEE Transactions on Pattern Analysis and Machine Intelligence 11(6), 567–585 (1989)
17. Commowick, O., Arsigny, V., Isambert, A., Costa, J., Dhermain, F., Bidault, F., Bondiau, P., Ayache, N., Malandain, G.: An efficient locally affine framework for the smooth registration of anatomical structures. Medical Image Analysis 12(4), 427–441 (2008)
18. Rohr, K.: Landmark-based image analysis: using geometric and intensity models. Kluwer Academic Pub., Dordrecht (2001)
19. Thirion, J.P.: Image Matching as a Diffusion Process: An Analogy with Maxwell's Demons. Medical Image Analysis 2(3), 243–260 (1998)
20. Pennec, X., Cachier, P., Ayache, N.: Understanding the Demon's Algorithm: 3D Non-Rigid Registration by Gradient Descent. In: Taylor, C., Colchester, A. (eds.) MICCAI 1999. LNCS, vol. 1679, pp. 597–605. Springer, Heidelberg (1999)
21. Gramkow, C., Bro-Nielsen, M.: Comparison of Three Filters in the Solution of the Navier-Stokes Equation in Registration. In: Proceedings of the Scandinavian Conference on Image Analysis, pp. 795–802 (1997)
22. Vercauteren, T., Pennec, X., Perchant, A., Ayache, N.: Non-parametric diffeomorphic image registration with the demons algorithm. In: Ayache, N., Ourselin, S., Maeder, A. (eds.) MICCAI 2007, Part II. LNCS, vol. 4792, pp. 319–326. Springer, Heidelberg (2007)
23. Hajnal, J., Hawkes, D., Hill, D.: Medical image registration. CRC Press, Boca Raton (2001)

3D-Reconstruction of Basal Cell Carcinoma
A Proof-of-Principle Study

Patrick Scheibe[1], Tino Wetzig[2], Jens-Peer Kuska[3], Markus Löffler[4],
Jan C. Simon[2], Uwe Paasch[2], and Ulf-Dietrich Braumann[3]

[1] Translational Centre for Regenerative Medicine (TRM Leipzig),
Universität Leipzig, Philipp-Rosenthal-Straße 55, 04103 Leipzig
pscheibe@trm.uni-leipzig.de
[2] Department of Dermatology, Venerology and Allergology, Universität Leipzig,
Philipp-Rosenthal-Straße 23-25, 04103 Leipzig
[3] Interdisciplinary Centre for Bioinformatics (IZBI), Universität Leipzig,
Härtelstraße 16-18, 04107 Leipzig, Germany
[4] Institute for Medical Informatics, Statistics, and Epidemiology (IMISE),
Universität Leipzig, Härtelstraße 16-18, 04107 Leipzig

Abstract. This work presents a complete processing-chain for a 3D-reconstruction of Basal Cell Carcinoma (BCC). BCC is the most common malignant skin cancer with a high risk of local recurrence after insufficient treatment. Therefore, we have focused on the development of an automated image-processing chain for 3D-reconstruction of BCC using large histological serial sections. We introduce a novel kind of image-processing chain (core component: non-linear image registration) which is optimised for the diffuse nature of BCC.

For full-automatic delineation of the tumour within the tissue we apply a fuzzy c-means segmentation method, which does not calculate a hard segmentation decision but class membership probabilities. This feature moves the binary decision tumorous vs. non-tumorous to the end of the processing chain, and it ensures smooth gradients which are needed for a consistent registration.

We used a multi-grid form of the nonlinear registration effectively suppressing registration runs into local minima (possibly caused by diffuse nature of the tumour). To register the stack of images this method is applied in a new way to reduce a global drift of the image stack while registration.

Our method was successfully applied in a proof-of-principle study for automated tissue volume reconstruction followed by a quantitative tumour growth analysis.

Keywords: Non-linear Image Registration, Image Segmentation, 3D-Reconstruction.

1 Introduction

Basal Cell Carcinoma (BCC) is the most common skin cancer worldwide in Caucasian populations [1]. It is a slow-growing epithelial malignant skin cancer,

B. Fischer, B. Dawant, and C. Lorenz (Eds.): WBIR 2010, LNCS 6204, pp. 25–36, 2010.
© Springer-Verlag Berlin Heidelberg 2010

which tends to infiltrate the surrounding tissues and it is strongly associated with exposure to UV-irradiation [2]. The most common localisation (80 %) for BCC is the head and neck [3]. Lesions located in the mid-face or ear (so called H-zone) have a high risk of local recurrence after treatment [4]. BCC exists in different subtypes and a deeper understanding of the spatial shape is important when analysing patterns of invasion.

For other types of cancer, 3D-reconstruction methods have already been established successfully in the past [5,6]. For the 3D-reconstruction of BCCs up to now only basic attempts were made to explore spatial features of tumour growth [7,8]. The scattered structure of the BCC requires a new registration strategy for the sequence of image registration steps. In this paper we introduce a novel registration strategy for image slice stacks appropriate for diffuse cancer structures and present a proof-of-principle study for a new automated image processing chain for 3D-reconstruction as well as for the certain directional and angular morphometric growth analyses of BCC.

2   Methods

2.1   Image Acquisition

Excised tissue blocks were routinely fixed and embedded in paraffin. To obtain the maximum information on the tumour, the volumes of interest (VOI) of the specimens were consecutively sliced in vertical direction with a thickness of 6 μm.

For routine, haematoxylin-eosin (H&E) staining of all slides were subjected to automated staining using a linear stainer (Microm, Germany). Histological examination following finalisation of the processing by automated covering using standard glass cover slips was performed by an independent investigator who checked whether or not the lesions were completely excised.

Whole histological specimens with verified tumour tissue were subjected for scanning with an automated system for digital pathology (MIRAX MIDI, Carl Zeiss, Germany). For the reconstruction a downscaled version of colour-images was used, each with a resolution of 1000×400 pixels and a nominal pixel size of 15 μm × 15 μm.

Not all images are appropriate for the reconstruction due to heavy folds in the slices which sometimes appear in the process of slicing and staining. The images of these slices were not used and finally filled with their neighbouring slice.

2.2   Preprocessing

The first step of the processing chain is a rigid registration. It roughly co-registers consecutive image pairs by applying a combination of translation, rotation and scaling. For a reference image $R(x)$ and a deformable template image $T(x)$ this registration step tries to find the optimal parameters of a transformation $u(x) : \Omega \to \Omega$ with $x = (x_1, x_2)^\top \in \Omega \subset \mathbb{R}^2$. In the case of a rigid registration the transformation is given by

$$u(x) = Ax + b_r \quad \text{with} \quad A = \begin{pmatrix} s_r & 0 \\ 0 & s_r \end{pmatrix} \begin{pmatrix} \cos \alpha_r & -\sin \alpha_r \\ \sin \alpha_r & \cos \alpha_r \end{pmatrix} \tag{1}$$

and the optimal parameters are found when a certain distance measure $\mathcal{D}$ between the images $R(x)$ and $T(u(x))$ is minimised, which is here the sum of squared differences between the images

$$\mathcal{D}(u) = \frac{1}{2} \int_{\Omega} [T(x - u(x)) - R(x)]^2 \, dx. \tag{2}$$

Throughout this work we tried to be consistent with the notation-style of Modersitzki [9]. This first rigid registration step is fundamental to the success of the second non-linear registration which follows after the segmentation. This is caused by the fact that it is more likely that the following non-linear registration succeeds when the images are already near the solution and the registration has to compensate for small local differences only.

The effect of the rigid registration can be observed in fig. 1(a). The top image shows an unregistered set of slides, whereas the bottom image clearly documents that after registration the slides fit quite well onto another.

All images are now filtered through a total variation (TV) filter suggested by Chan et al. [10] to reduce noise in images while preserving structure edges. This step is necessary since the segmentation preferably needs images of smooth tissue areas with clear edges to succeed. Other edge preserving denoising operators like median filters or non-linear diffusion filters preserve the edges not so well (median filter) or need more parameter (non-linear diffusion filter). The only parameter the TV filter requires is the estimated standard deviation of the noise whereas this feature is easy to be estimated from background parts of a typical image.

2.3   Tumour Segmentation

The smoothed images are the basis for the fuzzy c-means segmentation [11,12]. The reasons for choosing the fuzzy c-means algorithm are threefold: This algorithm does not make a sharp decision which area in the image belongs to which class in the segmentation result but rather provides a probability of the membership. This is crucial since the H&E-staining produces violet images with different saturations for tumorous and non-tumorous parts. These parts sometimes overlap in colour-space and at this stage of the reconstruction a sharp decision for a pixel which is given by other segmentation methods is not adequate. Therefore, segmentations like c-means or mean shift cannot be used.

The second reason is that the colour saturation of the slices changes due to instabilities in the staining procedure. Therefore, an overall (3D) segmentation of the colour space is not possible, because the same colour can correspond to different tissue types in different slices due to different slice thickness and exposure time to the staining chemicals. The fuzzy c-means segmentation does solve this problem by an adaptation of already calculated segmentation-class-distributions and therefore provides constantly good tissue segmentation results throughout the whole image stack.

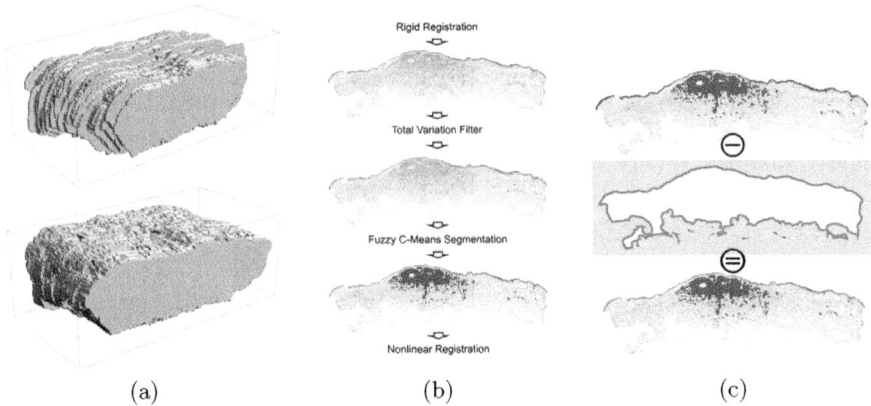

Fig. 1. (a) Shape of an unregistered (top) and the rigid registered (bottom) image-stack. (b) The flowchart shows the main steps of the tumour segmentation. To demonstrate the edge-preserving behaviour of the Total Variation Filter we took extreme filter parameters for this example. Those are not necessary in the real process chain. (c) The automatic extraction of the epidermis is possible with the grown background-mask of the segmentation. This mask is grown by the size of the epidermis and is then used to mask out the regions in the segmentation result.

The third reason for the choice of the fuzzy c-means method is that segmentation results are approximated memberships of the pixels to colour classes. Since these membership probabilities are represented as grey-levels and not as binary-values they provide smooth gradients which are important for the non-linear image registration.

As mentioned before, the used fuzzy c-means method is able adapt a given set of colour-centres as starting point for a new image and calculate a segmentation on this basis. Therefore, in the segmentation-process of the complete image stack we had to verify only one segmentation-result and for the rest of the images it was not necessary to adjust any parameters.

In fig. 1(b) the main steps of the image processing chain are depicted, in particular both the smoothing and segmentation step. The small layer of the epidermis and the adjacent tumour tissue are too close together in colour-space and are not separable by the segmentation. However, it was possible to extract this layer automatically by taking the mask of the background of each slide and enlarge it by the size of the epidermis. This step which is depicted in fig. 1(c) completes the extraction of the tumour.

2.4   Reconstruction

At this point it is necessary to re-align local differences in tumorous parts of consecutive slides. During preparation, inevitable deformations occur, which need to get compensated. For this purpose a non-linear registration step was applied which was working on intensity images resulting from a combination of the approximate class membership for the cancer class obtained from the fuzzy c-means segmentation and a low-level intensity image of the slide itself. Primarily we are interested in a mapping of the tumour regions, but to get a consistent result, the usage of the slide intensity in regions without tumour is essential.

As already mentioned in the segmentation section the registration of the approximate class membership from the segmentation procedure provides smoother gradients which means less local gradients for the non-linear registration procedure than one would obtain by hard segmented images.

The non-linear registration after the rigid registration step is necessary since this method can stretch and bend parts of the image to bring the tumour tissue of adjacent slides onto another. The method of choice at this point bases on the optical flow and was firstly mentioned by Amit [13] and Modersitzki [9] and later extensively used by others [5,14].

In the process of registration the required displacement field $\boldsymbol{u}(\boldsymbol{x}) : \Omega \rightarrow \Omega$ is found by minimising a joint registration criterion

$$\min_{\boldsymbol{u}} \left(\mathcal{D}(\boldsymbol{u}) + \alpha \mathcal{S}(\boldsymbol{u}) \right) \tag{3}$$

consisting of the already mentioned distance measure

$$\mathcal{D}(\boldsymbol{u}) = \frac{1}{2} \int_{\Omega} \left[T(\boldsymbol{x} - \boldsymbol{u}(\boldsymbol{x})) - R(\boldsymbol{x}) \right]^2 d\boldsymbol{x} \tag{4}$$

and smoothing term

$$\mathcal{S}(\boldsymbol{u}) = \frac{1}{2} \sum_{i=1}^{2} \int_{\Omega} (\Delta u_i)^2 d\boldsymbol{x}. \tag{5}$$

Using the calculus of variations, the solution for equation (3) will require to solve a system of 4th order partial differential equations. Different approaches are possible but in this work we used the multi-grid implementation which is described in more detail in [5].

Likewise, we registered the whole set of images so that every slide is co-registered onto its predecessor. Usually the image-stack is processed in a single run and one (forward) direction. This procedure excels the chosen direction over the opposite one, which is adequate for relatively solid structures and tissue types. The diffuse nature of the BCC and the fact that the skin is not completely surrounded by stabilising tissue require a more symmetrical alignment of the slices which is in this work ensured by not processing the images of the stack in one registration run. Instead, we registered at first each image pair-wise with its neighbour starting at the first image and processing in forward direction through the stack breaking up the registration before it converges. Thereafter we proceed backwards through the image stack with the same approach and repeated the whole procedure three times.

2.5   Visualisation

After this last step the reconstruction chain is finished and the result is a 3D-tumour-density field which is the basis for further morphological analysis and

3D-visualisation. In the case of this work we calculated an iso-surface of the largest connected component of the tumour. For that purpose a 3D total variation filter on the tumour density was used in order to smooth the data for visualisation.

After that, a volume labelling algorithm was utilised to mark connected parts with an ID and calculate their volume. With position and volume of all objects we could verify that the biggest component was the main tumour-object (see fig. 3).

2.6   Quantification

To characterise the tumour we want to determine the dependency of the distance distribution with respect to different angles and radii in spherical and cylindrical coordinates, respectively. For both approaches we have chosen the point of origin to be the centre of masses of the tumour projected onto the topmost horizontal plane of the bounding-box (the xy-plane in our coordinate system). This centre is depicted in figure 2(a) as point of intersection of the radii and in figure 2(c) as centre of the concentric circles. It can be obtained by

$$m = P_{xy} \left(\frac{1}{N} \sum_{i=1}^{N} x_i \right), \tag{6}$$

where x_i are all positions of tumour in the data set and P_{xy} is the projection onto the xy-plane.

In this work the primary focus is put on the invasion of BCC in the surrounding tissue whereas the lateral propagation *direction* is not in the main focus. Therefore, we are in the first rank rather interested in the dependency on the polar angle as depicted in figure 2(a). With

$$t_{\mathrm{sp}}(x) = \left(\arctan \left(\frac{\sqrt{x_1^2 + x_2^2}}{x_3} \right), \sqrt{x_1^2 + x_2^2 + x_3^2} \right)^{\mathsf{T}} \tag{7}$$

we can transform all positions x_i of tumour in the data set by calculating

$$r_i = t_{\mathrm{sp}}(m - x_i). \tag{8}$$

This list is now quantised into different angular intervals. Note that the angles in this list are all in the main interval $[0, \pi/2]$ since (i) in the hemisphere above the centre m (a region outside the skin) there is no tumour and (ii) corresponding radii left and right of m in figure 2(a) represent the same polar angles.

All collected radii of an angular interval can be treated as realisation of a Γ-distributed random variable, since the Γ-distribution is the only distribution going along with the power of the random variable. The probability density function of a gamma distribution is given by

$$f_\Gamma(r; k, \Theta) = r^{k-1} \frac{\Theta^{-k} \exp(-r/\Theta)}{\Gamma(k)} \quad \text{where} \quad \Gamma(k) = \int_0^\infty t^{k-1} \exp(-t) \mathrm{d}t \tag{9}$$

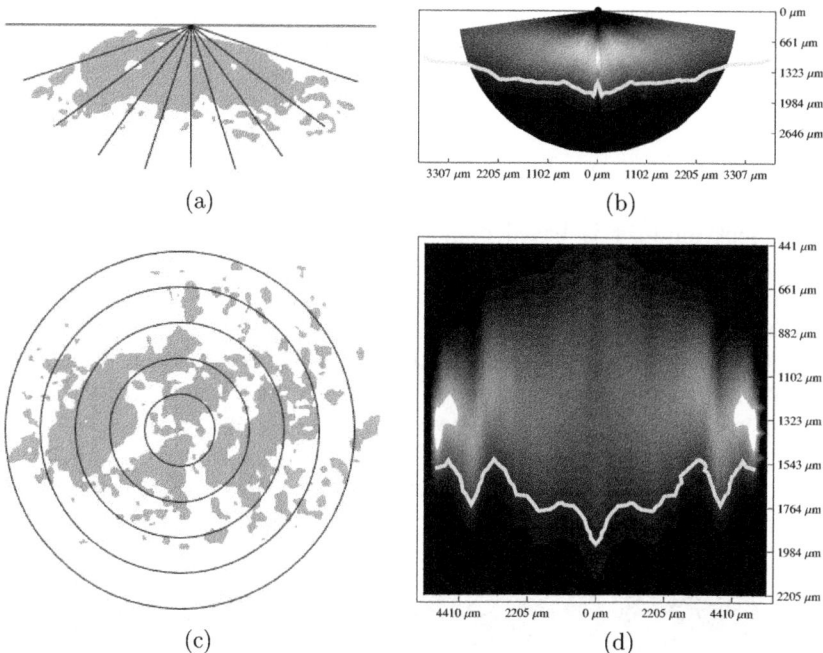

Fig. 2. While (a) is a sectional view of a virtual cutting plane orthogonal to the skin surface, where the lines indicate different polar angles, (c) shows a plane parallel to the skin with different radii. The different angles and radii are used in the density plots (b) and (d) of probability distributions obtained by the quantification methods. The origin of the coordinate system is in both cases the reference point $\boldsymbol{m}$. The yellow lines denote the $P(X \leq 0.95)$ border. (b) is a plot of the angular distribution where angles are transformed back to Cartesian coordinates and (d) is a plot of the depth distribution.

with the parameters (k, Θ). In order to estimate values for these parameters we used an iterative maximum likelihood estimation (MLE) scheme [15]. The parameters found by the MLE algorithm are the basis for distribution analysis as is detailed in the following section.

Going beyond the angular analysis, more information can be extracted using a method reflecting the depth distribution of BCC. We step in after the calculation of the reference point $\boldsymbol{m}$ (eq. 6), but now we are interested in the probability of the tumour depth at a given distance from $\boldsymbol{m}$. Therefore we use cylindrical coordinates and analyse the depth distribution of different range intervals as basically depicted in figure 2(c).

In this approach all positions $\boldsymbol{x}_i$ of tumour are transformed by

$$\boldsymbol{r}_i = \boldsymbol{t}_{\mathrm{cy}}(\boldsymbol{m} - \boldsymbol{x}_i) \quad \text{where} \quad \boldsymbol{t}_{\mathrm{cy}}(\boldsymbol{x}) = \left(\sqrt{x_1^2 + x_2^2} \, , \, x_3 \right) \tag{10}$$

which are the first and the last component of cylindrical coordinates. The rest of the approach is similar to the first method besides the fact that the estimated tumour depth distribution is normal distributed.

3   Results

The present data-set is based on a serial section of a complete BCC which consists of 193 slices. From this data-set 43 slices had to be excluded due to folds or artifacts. The specimen has a volume of 80 mm^3 and contains a segmented tumour of about 2.6 mm^3.

The 3D-iso-surface plot depicts the tumour component (fig. 2.6). To enhance illustration it was artificially enlarged and embedded behind the surface of the tissue specimen. Since we only have visualised the largest component, we had to verify that all small segments previously masked out were indeed false positives, i.e., 3D-coordinates of them were taken, thereafter the dermatologist classified all segments to be false positive.

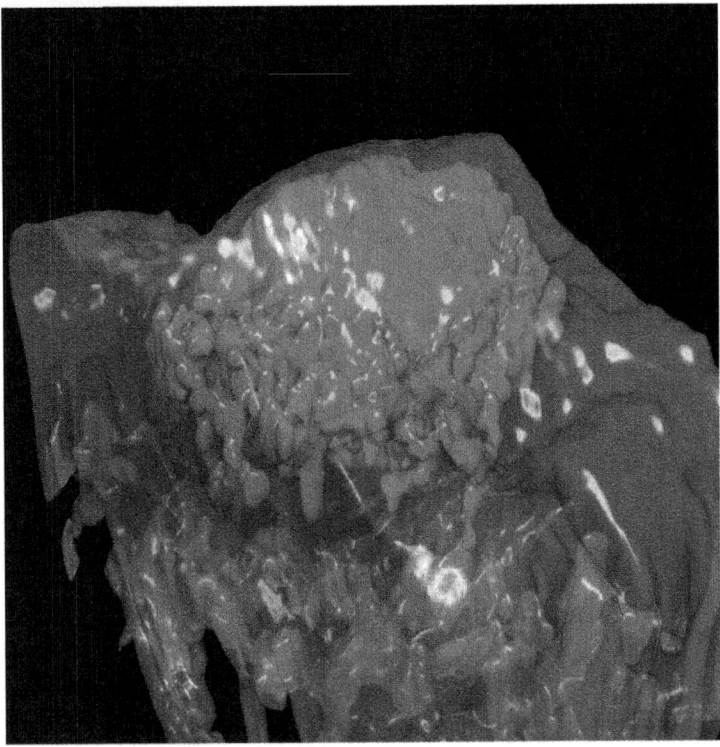

Fig. 3. An iso-surface plot of the reconstructed BCC (red) embedded behind the surface of the tissue specimen (green)

As already mentioned, epidermis and tumour are not well separable in H&E-stained slices using the applied staining-based segmentation method. Another source for false-positive segmentation are hair follicles. While the epidermis can be identified by its closeness to the tissue boundary and therefore can be masked out by the above mentioned steps, hair follicles are identifiable due to their characteristics in the final reconstruction.

A hair follicle is an epidermal sheath that surrounds the hair. Sebaceous glands are usually attached to the side of a follicle. Their oily secretion enters the follicle and follows it to the surface. The hair grows from the bulb, swollen lower end of the follicle. The bulb is invested with blood vessels and nerves. Due to these typical histological characteristics they can easily be identified and extracted from the volume.

Generally speaking, a new method for the non-linear registration of a stack of slice images applying several runs with alternating directions in the stack has been introduced. The new method has shown to work well even under the presence of diffuse cancer structures as appearing in BCC.

4   Discussion

This work has successfully given a proof-of-principle for an image processing chain for a 3D-reconstruction of BCC. The starting point was an H&E stained large serial histological section from paraffin embedded specimen.

Unlike established microscopic imaging techniques such as confocal laser scanning microscopy (CLSM), or the "bread leaf" sectioning technique as applied in histopathological routine, in Moh's micro-graphic surgery [4] used by Braun [7], our new approach relying on histological serial sections allows for (i) a complete tissue volume reconstruction, (ii) visualisation of the whole tumour including surrounding tissue and (iii) quantification of statistical properties.

CLSM, however, cannot provide a sufficient penetration depth of several millimetres. The "bread leaf" sectioning obviously takes far too less (non-adjacent!) sections for registration-based reconstructions. Moh's surgery relies on cryosections and uses horizontal sectioning, hence the method, besides the flat-bed scanning and manual tumour delineation as done by Braun [7], will not provide sufficient preparation quality as can be obtained using paraffin embedding and vertical sectioning, the latter preserving the epidermis.

Instead, our approach utilises virtual microscopy for image capture as well as state-of-the-art image processing methods for the successive image series registration in order to re-establish a 3D histological data-set. We therefore applied a sophisticated non-linear image registration algorithm (optical flow method) in order to ensure that unavoidable distortions as occur during manual sectioning and further slice preparation (staining-induced partial shrinking) can be compensated within the image data.

Even though captured virtual microscopy images typically come along with raw pixel sizes below 1 μm^2, since our intention was to segment and reconstruct *tissue* volumes, during the pre-processing we had to downscale the images in order to avoid sub-cellular resolution. Moreover, the application of the edge-preserving TV filter to compensate for staining inhomogeneities is another important pre-processing step with respect to a reliable tissue segmentation.

Further, the staining-based automatic tumour segmentation (fuzzy c-means method), even though ending up with a few false-positives as e.g. hair follicles, is essential to treat data-sets consisting of hundreds of images per series. To replace the remaining minimum of manual interaction to sort out respective false positive regions would require knowledge-based approaches to get eliminated in future, but this was not the focus of this work.

However, since segmentation quality is crucial for our method, in preliminary work we have evaluated the reliability of tumour segmentation in H&E stained single sections of 10 randomly selected BCCs of different sub-types. After careful inspection of the results by the dermatologist it turned out that the segmentation is appropriate to detect all tumorous parts. The sources of false positive segmented tissue remained restricted to parts of epidermis, sebaceous gland, and hair follicles.

Concerning the treatment of images with damaged slices (folds, fissures) which occasionally occur during the preparation process, we avoided to do some interpolation as was proposed in [16] and instead have done an image replacement from neighbouring sections to fill such gaps. To us, interpolation appears not appropriate within a reference-free consecutive image registration framework.

The present proof-of-principle study demonstrates the first feasible approach to elucidate the 3D tumour growth of a complete BCC in microscopic resolution. The volume data obtained by the presented method is considered highly appropriate for further phenotypical investigations in order to morphometrically describe tumour growth.

One such detail of interest is e.g. how an objective description of the spatial tumour distribution can be obtained. For this purpose it is possible to determine the dependence of the distance distribution with respect to different polar angles in spherical coordinates. Through such a characterisation distances from the centre of the BCC can be calculated which have a certain probability that none of the tumorous tissue infiltrates into deeper regions of the skin.

For this approach we chose the origin m of the spherical coordinate system to be the centre of masses of the tumour projected onto the topmost horizontal plane of the bounding-box. This choice is motivated by the idea that it is possible for the surgeon to identify this centre on the skin. After the transformation in spherical coordinates the data-set is quantised into different angular intervals. Note that these angles are all in the main interval $[0, \pi/2]$ since (i) on the hemisphere above m there is no tumour and (ii) corresponding radii left and right of m represent the same polar angles, since the azimuth dependence is not taken into account.

The next step is to treat all collected radii of an angular interval as realisation of a Γ-distributed random variable, since the Γ-distribution is the only distribution going along with the power of the random variable. In order to estimate values for these parameters we used an iterative maximum likelihood estimation (MLE) scheme [15]. The parameters found by the MLE algorithm are the base for distribution visualisation given in fig. 2(b). Since the dependence on the azimuth was not taken into account, the visualisation is symmetric to the centre. The colour ranges from black to white and denotes the probability interval $[0, 0.03]$. The yellow line is the P_{95} border which states 95% of the tumour is below this radius.

With methods like the presented one, another future application is the validation of new non-invasive high-resolution skin imaging techniques. Nevertheless, the next steps following this work are to process several samples of each BCC-subtype to capture important statistical properties. In general, for detailed objective insights into shape, structure and growth patterns further investigations in quantification techniques for BCC are required.

Obituary

The authors are very grateful for having had the opportunity to work with Dr. rer. nat. Jens-Peer Kuska, whose ideas and contributions have incomparably influenced our research activities for many years. On July 1st, 2009, he has passed away at the age of just 45.

References

1. Raasch, B.A., Buettner, P.G., Garbe, C.: Basal cell carcinoma: histological classification and body-site distribution. Br. J. Dermatol. 155(2), 401–407 (2006)
2. Rigel, D.S.: Cutaneous ultraviolet exposure and its relationship to the development of skin cancer. J. Am. Acad. Dermatol. 58(5 Suppl. 2), 129–132 (2008)
3. Woerle, B., Heckmann, M., Konz, B.: Micrographic surgery of basal cell carcinomas of the head. Recent Results Cancer Res. 160, 219–224 (2002)
4. Swanson, N.A.: Mohs surgery. technique, indications, applications, and the future. Arch. Dermatol. 119(9), 761–773 (1983)
5. Braumann, U.D., Kuska, J.P., Einenkel, J., Horn, L.C., Löffler, M., Höckel, M.: Three-dimensional reconstruction and quantification of cervical carcinoma invasion fronts from histological serial sections. IEEE Transactions on Medical Imaging 24(10), 1286–1307 (2005)
6. Braumann, U.D., Scherf, N., Einenkel, J., Horn, L.C., Wentzensen, N., Loeffler, M., Kuska, J.P.: Large histological serial sections for computational tissue volume reconstruction. Methods Inf. Med. 46(5), 614–622 (2007)
7. Braun, R., Klumb, F., Bondon, D., Salomon, D., Skaria, A., Adatto, M., French, L., Saurat, J., Vallee, J.: Three-Dimensional Reconstruction of Basal Cell Carcinomas. Derma Surg. 31(5), 562–569 (2005)
8. Matsumura, T., Sato-Matsumura, K.C., Yokota, T., Kobayashi, H., Nagashima, K., Ohkawara, A.: Three-dimensional reconstruction in dermatopathology–a personal computer-based system. J. Cutan. Pathol. 26(4), 197–200 (1999)
9. Modersitzki, J.: Numerical Methods for Image Registration, Numerical Mathematics and Scientific Computation. Oxford University Press, USA (2004)
10. Chan, T., Osher, S., Shen, J.: The digital TV filter and non-linear denoising (2001)
11. Bezdek, J.: Pattern Recognition with Fuzzy Objective Function algorithms. Plenum, New York (1981)

12. Dunn, J.C.: A fuzzy relative of the ISODATA process and its use in detecting compact well-separated clusters. Journal of Cybernetics 3, 32–57 (1973)
13. Amit, Y.: A nonlinear variational problem for image matching. SIAM Journal on Scientific Computing 15(1), 207–224 (1994)
14. Braumann, U.D., Kuska, J.P.: Influence of the boundary conditions on the result of non-linear image registration. In: Proceedings of the IEEE International Conference on Image Processing, pp. I-1129–I-1132. IEEE Signal Processing Society, Los Alamitos (September 2005)
15. Choi, S., Wette, R.: Maximum likelihood estimation of the parameters of the gamma distribution and their bias. Technometrics 11(4), 683–690 (1969)
16. Gaffling, S., Jäger, F., Daum, V., Tauchi, M., Lütjen-Drecoll, E.: Interpolation of Histological Slices by means of Non-rigid Registration. In: Meinzer, H.P., Deserno, T.M., Handels, H., Tolxdorff, T. (eds.) Bildverarbeitung für die Medizin 2009 – Algorithmen, Systeme, Anwendungen, Informatik aktuell, pp. 267–271. Springer, Heidelberg (March 2009)

Monocular Deformable Model-to-Image Registration of Vascular Structures

Martin Groher, Maximilian Baust, Darko Zikic, and Nassir Navab

Computer Aided Medical Procedures (CAMP),
Technische Universität München, Germany

Abstract. The registration of 3D vasculature to 2D projections is the key for providing advanced systems for image-based navigation and guidance. In areas with non-rigid patient motion, however, it is very difficult to accurately perform the registration if only one 2D view is available.

We propose a method for deformable registration of a 3D vascular model extracted from an angiographic scan to a single 2D Digitally Subtracted Angiogram (DSA). Different to existing approaches, our method does not require a segmentation of 2D vasculature. In consequence, our method can be used without manual interaction during medical treatment.

Formulated as an energy minimization problem, our approach combines a novel data term with the length regularization proposed in [1] which removes the ill-posedness of this monocular scenario. Besides attracting projected 3D centerline points to locations with high vessel probability the proposed data term ensures an injective projection of the centerline points.

Due to our novel image-based data term, we achieve a considerable gain in performance compared to feature-based approaches.

Accuracy, robustness to outliers, as well as performance issues are analyzed through tests on synthetic and real data within a controlled environment.

1 Introduction

Image-based guidance on angiographic images has become a standard technique in modern hospitals. Needles, catheters, guide wires, or other instruments are injected into the patient vessel system and their progression is usually monitored by 2D angiography and fluoroscopy. Most procedures are carried out with a mono-plane device, which produces 2D images from one view only. Efforts have been made to bring 3D angiographic scans into the 2D guidance process in order to constantly provide spatial details on vasculature [2,3].

One of the main obstacles to be overcome here is an accurate 2D-3D registration of vessel images. Only then, a correct fusion of the available information can create a benefit in terms of depth perception or augmentation. Especially in abdominal or cardiac procedures, vessels are subject to non-rigid motion, which has to be considered by the registration process.

B. Fischer, B. Dawant, and C. Lorenz (Eds.): WBIR 2010, LNCS 6204, pp. 37–47, 2010.
© Springer-Verlag Berlin Heidelberg 2010

While rigid 2D-3D vessel registration has been addressed extensively in the literature [4,5,6,7], deformable registration is mostly tackled only if multi-plane X-ray devices are available [8,9,10]. For a single view scenario, a method has been proposed recently, which aligns centerline features of 3D vasculature by minimizing the Euclidean distance of projected centerline points to their nearest 2D pendants [1]. The data term alone cannot solve for displacements in projection direction. By adding a length preservation together with a smoothing regularization term this issue is met and the registration is driven to the accurate solution.

This approach successfully recovers a non-rigid transformation from only one view, but requires an extraction of centerline features in 3D and in 2D. Due to a uniform contrast propagation, the 3D extraction can be carried out with quite simple processing methods; 2D angiograms, however, include regions with inhomogeneous contrast distribution and vessel overlays, which may lead to erroneous results when creating a vascular model. Moreover, such extraction techniques often require a certain amount of user interaction, which is undesired during medical procedures.

We address this issue by proposing a method which registers a 3D vascular model to a vessel image, e.g. a DSA, without any prior geometric extraction step in 2D. To this end, we define a circular region around each projected centerline point in which intensities of the 2D image are accumulated. The region is formalized using a level set function, which inherently penalizes solutions where multiple regions project onto the same part of the image. The accumulated intensities, together with a length preservation in 3D, define an energy, whose optimization attracts projected centerline points towards 2D vessel centers. In order to keep our computed transformations smooth we regularize the updates of a gradient descent scheme using approximating thin-plate splines [11,12].

Tests on synthetic examples and a comparison with the feature-based approach from [1] show the high accuracy as well as the improved runtime of our approach. Additional to the synthetic data, we conduct an experiment with patient data, where two 3D data sets are available, one preoperative Computed Tomography Angiogram (CTA) and an intraoperative 3D reconstruction.

2   Method

Our method optimizes an energy, which is defined on a vascular model extracted from a 3D angiographic scan, a 2D image where noise is reduced and tubular structures are enhanced, and a projection function, which relates each 3D point to a corresponding 2D point in the image plane.

In order to create the vascular model consisting of centerline points and their associated radii, a region growing algorithm is applied to the 3D data. Due to uniform contrast propagation, this basic method yields a good segmentation result, which is used to compute centerline points (via a topological thinning algorithm) and associated radii (via a Euclidean distance transformation), see Fig. 1.

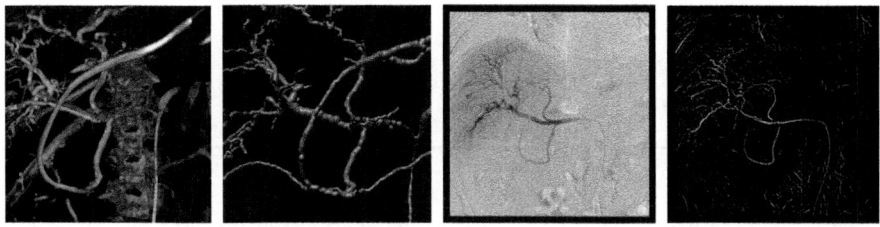

Fig. 1. From left to right: 3D input volume showing liver arteries and spine; 3D vascular model, where centerline points and radii are extracted from the input volume; 2D DSA of the same patient; 2D DSA with enhanced tubular structures

For noise reduction and vessel enhancement of the 2D DSA we use a filter which enhances tubular structures in a multi-scale approach [13]. This is accomplished by a pixel-wise comparison of the gradient vector and the eigenvector of the Hessian associated to the larger eigenvalue at a distance equal to the expected radius of the vessel. The more parallel the two vectors, the higher the response of the filter, compare Fig. 1.

The projection parameters are assumed to be given by the device. This is achieved either by machine-based geometric calibration [2], or by a rigid registration step [6], which is carried out prior to the deformable registration.

2.1 Energy Formulation

Let $\{\mathbf{X}_i\}$ be the set of n centerline points in 3D. Each centerline point $\mathbf{X}_i$ has an associated vessel radius R_i. We denote our vascular model with the tuples $\{(\mathbf{X}_i, R_i)\}$. For each $\mathbf{X}_i$ we define a displacement vector φ_i and a displaced location $\mathbf{Y}_i = \mathbf{X}_i + \varphi_i$. The vector including all entries of the displacement vectors φ_i is denoted by φ.

Now we want to find the displacement φ' minimizing the following energy:

$$\varphi' = \arg\min_{\varphi} E_E + \alpha E_I, \tag{1}$$

where E_E defines the external energy, and E_I represents the internal (regularizing) energy. The weighting parameter α controls the impact of the regularization.

External Energy. Let $p : \mathbb{R}^3 \to \mathbb{R}^2$ be a perspective projection function. We denote projected centerline points by $\mathbf{x}_i = p(\mathbf{X}_i)$ and their projected radii by $r_i = \|p(\mathbf{X}_i) - p(\mathbf{X}_i + R_i\mathbf{V})\|$, where $\mathbf{V}$ is a 3D unit vector parallel to the image plane in device coordinates[1].

We want to encourage each 3D centerline point $\mathbf{X}_i$ to project onto the center of a 2D vessel. As centerline points correspond to high values in the enhanced

---

[1] The device coordinate system has its origin in the center of projection, spans the x-y-plane parallel to the image plane and the z-axis points towards the image plane. If p is described by a projection matrix $\mathsf{P} = \mathsf{K}[\mathsf{R}|\mathbf{t}] \in \mathbb{R}^{3\times4}$, world coordinates are transformed to device coordinates by applying rotation R and translation $\mathbf{t}$.

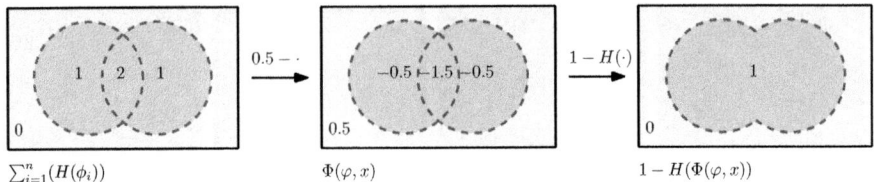

Fig. 2. illustration of the selection term of Eq. (7)

2D image $\mathcal{I}_f : \Omega \subseteq \mathbb{R}^2 \to \mathbb{R}$ (Fig. 1) the following data term seems to be a reasonable choice:

$$\widehat{E}_E(\varphi) = -\sum_{i=1}^{n} \int_{D_i} \mathcal{I}_f(\mathbf{x})\, d\mathbf{x}, \qquad (2)$$

where $D_i = D(p(\mathbf{X}_i + \varphi_i), r_i)$ denotes the disk with radius r_i centered at the ith projected centerline point. In order to obtain a formulation where the integration domain is independent of φ_i and r_i we rewrite $\widehat{E}_E$ in terms of level set functions:

$$\widehat{E}_E(\varphi) = -\sum_{i=1}^{n} \int_{\Omega} \mathcal{I}_f(\mathbf{x}) \cdot H(\phi_i(\mathbf{x}))\, d\mathbf{x}, \qquad (3)$$

where

$$\phi_i(\mathbf{x}) = r_i - \|\mathbf{x} - p(\mathbf{X}_i + \varphi_i)\| \qquad (4)$$

is a level set function whose zero level set is the boundary of the disk D_i and

$$H(x) = \begin{cases} 0, & x \le 0, \\ 1, & x > 0, \end{cases} \qquad (5)$$

denotes the Heaviside function. Unfortunately $\widehat{E}_E$ does not prevent all centerline points from being projected onto the same point in 2D, because the area of the projected disks $\sum_i \int_\Omega H(\phi_i)$ is always constant regardless of the position of the projected points $p(\mathbf{X}_i + \varphi_i)$. Consequently an overlap of the disks D_i is not penalized by $\widehat{E}_E$. In order to resolve this issue we define the level set function

$$\Phi(\mathbf{x}, \varphi) = 0.5 - \sum_{i=1}^{n} H(\phi_i(\mathbf{x})). \qquad (6)$$

Now the area $\int_\Omega 1 - H(\Phi)$ defined by Φ shrinks when the projected disks D_i overlap as depicted in Fig. 2. Thus an improved data term is given by

$$E_E(\varphi) = -\int_\Omega \mathcal{I}_f(\mathbf{x}) \cdot (1 - H(\Phi(\mathbf{x}, \varphi)))\, d\mathbf{x}. \qquad (7)$$

Internal Energy. Similar to [1] we add a length preservation term to induce transformations in projection direction. To each centerline point $\mathbf{X}_i$ we define a squared distance to left and right centerline neighbors, denoted by $d(\mathbf{X}_i, \mathbf{X}_{i\pm1})$. E_I is then given by the relative change in length after deformation

$$E_I = \frac{1}{n} \sum_{i=1}^{n} \left[\frac{d(\mathbf{X}_i, \mathbf{X}_{i\pm1}) - d(\mathbf{Y}_i, \mathbf{Y}_{i\pm1})}{d(\mathbf{X}_i, \mathbf{X}_{i\pm1})} \right]^2, \tag{8}$$

where $\mathbf{Y}_i = \mathbf{X}_i + \varphi$ as defined above. To impose transformation smoothness, there are two approaches that can be followed in general. Either a penalizing term is added to the internal energy, or a regularizing operator is directly applied to the updates that are computed in the optimization procedure [12]. We choose the second approach, and realize it by computing an *approximating* thin-plate spline (TPS) from the displacement updates in each iteration. The displacements are then smoothed by recalculating their values from the TPS. By choosing the TPS basis function $U(r) = -|r|$ we minimize the second derivatives of the 3D displacement field [14].

2.2   Optimization

We employ two different gradient-based optimization methods. One is a steepest descent approach, the second is a BFGS optimization [15], which usually yields faster convergence.

The first derivative of E_E with respect to parameters φ_k is given by

$$\frac{\partial E_E}{\partial \varphi_k} = - \int_{\Omega} \mathcal{I}_f(\mathbf{x}) \delta(\Phi(\mathbf{x}, \varphi)) \delta(r_k - ||\mathbf{x} - p(\mathbf{Y}_k)||) \frac{(\mathbf{x} - p(\mathbf{Y}_k))^{\top}}{||\mathbf{x} - p(\mathbf{Y}_k)||} J(\mathbf{Y}_k) \, d\mathbf{x}, \tag{9}$$

where $J(\mathbf{Y}_k) \in \mathbb{R}^{2\times3}$ is the Jacobian of the projection function p evaluated at $\mathbf{Y}_k$, and δ is the Dirac delta-function.

The first derivative of E_I with respect to parameters φ_k is given by

$$\frac{\partial E_I}{\partial \varphi_k} = -\frac{8}{n} [\kappa_k^-(\mathbf{Y}_k - \mathbf{Y}_{k-1}) + \kappa_k^+(\mathbf{Y}_k - \mathbf{Y}_{k+1})], \tag{10}$$

where $\kappa_k^{\pm} = (d(\mathbf{X}_k, \mathbf{X}_{k\pm1}) - d(\mathbf{Y}_i, \mathbf{Y}_{k\pm1}))/d(\mathbf{X}_i, \mathbf{X}_{k\pm1})$ [1].

The gradients of external and internal energy are normalized such that the gradient of φ_j, which has the highest magnitude is normalized to one:

$$\frac{\partial}{\partial \varphi_k} E_E / \max_{j=1\ldots n} ||\frac{\partial}{\partial \varphi_j} E_E||, \text{ and } \frac{\partial}{\partial \varphi_k} E_I / \max_{j=1\ldots n} ||\frac{\partial}{\partial \varphi_j} E_I||. \tag{11}$$

With this, we ensure normalization throughout different units (E_E is computed on image intensities in 2D space, E_I is computed in 3D space), which makes a combination of the two energy terms more tractable. Given the partial derivatives, our registration algorithm can be summarized in Algorithm 1.

Algorithm 1 Monocular Deformable 2D-3D Registration

INPUT: Given a vascular model $\{(\mathbf{X}_i, R_i)\}$, $i = 1, \ldots, n$, an enhanced image $\mathcal{I}$, and a projection function p
OUTPUT: A transformation φ
1: $\varphi_0 = \mathbf{0}$
2: **repeat**
3:     compute gradients $\nabla E = \nabla E_E + \alpha \nabla E_I$ using Eqs. (9), (10), and (11)
4:     compute update $\Delta\varphi$ using gradient direction
5:     compute TPS warp $\mathbf{W}$ given $\{\mathbf{X}_i\}, \{\mathbf{X}_i + \Delta\varphi_i\}$, $i = 1, \ldots, n$ and a smoothing parameter λ
6:     smooth displacement update using warp: $\Delta\tilde{\varphi} = \mathbf{W}(\mathbf{X}_i) - \mathbf{X}_i$
7:     $\varphi_{t+1} = \varphi_t + \Delta\tilde{\varphi}$
8: **until** convergence

2.3   Implementation

In our implementation we use smeared-out versions of Heaviside and Dirac delta-function as described in [16], i.e.

$$H(x) = \begin{cases} 0, & x < -\epsilon, \\ \frac{1}{2} + \frac{x}{2\epsilon} + \frac{1}{2\pi} \sin\left(\frac{\pi x}{\epsilon}\right), & -\epsilon \geq x \geq \epsilon, \\ 1, & \epsilon < x, \end{cases} \tag{12}$$

and

$$\delta(x) = \begin{cases} \frac{1}{2\epsilon} + \frac{1}{2\epsilon} \cos\left(\frac{\pi x}{\epsilon}\right), & |x| \leq \epsilon, \\ 0, & |x| > \epsilon. \end{cases} \tag{13}$$

In Eqs. (12) and (13) ϵ is set to 1.5 [16]. We follow the description of the BFGS optimization procedure from [15]. For increasing the capture range of our algorithm we use an image pyramid, which is traversed during optimization. For each pyramid level we update the projection matrix by multiplying $D = \mathrm{diag}(0.5, 0.5, 1) \in \mathbb{R}^{3\times 3}$ from the left. Instead of evaluating the gradient at every pixel in the image domain, we use a narrow band technique, whose boundaries are given by the radii around each projected centerline point.

3   Evaluation

We evaluate our algorithm through tests on synthetic and real data. Artificial data is created such that contains a deformation component in projection direction. We analyze two error measures. The first is the mean Euclidean distance to a ground truth vascular model in 3D. The second error is the deviation from angles defined between vectors to neighboring points in the vascular model. Again, the deviation from the ground truth values is computed. Finally, we compare our method to the feature-based approach [1] in terms of accuracy and runtime. Runtime is evaluated on an Intel Core2Duo 2.6GHz machine. We were kindly provided with data and code by the authors of [1].

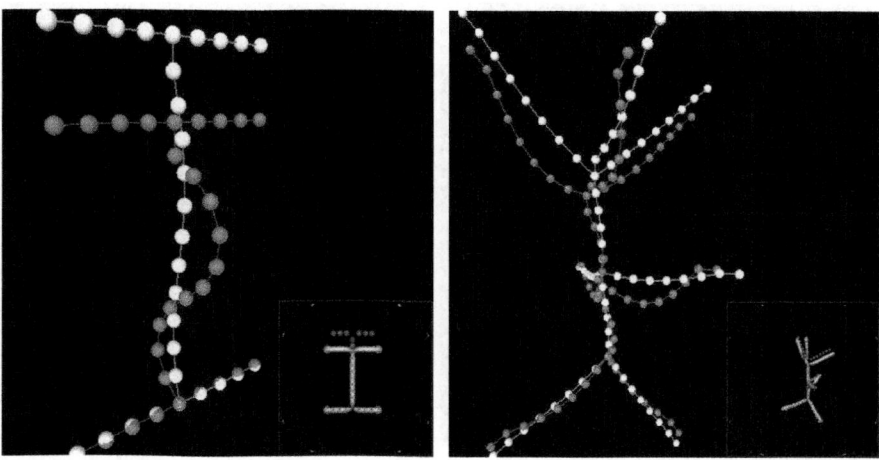

Fig. 3. Two synthetic data sets, denoted S2 and S3 in table 1. The white spheres represent the input vascular model, the gray spheres show the deformed input model (the ground truth) from which the projection image has been generated. The lower right sub-images visualize the enhanced projection images, where dark gray disks are drawn at all projected centerline points at the beginning of the registration.

In all our experiments the input 2D image is enhanced as described in Sec. 2. This fully automatic filter takes approximately 3 *sec* on an image of size 1024×1024 pixels. The parameter α, which controls the length preservation term, is set between 0.5 and 2.0, the smoothing parameter λ (see Algorithm 1) is set to 10.0. We use 5 pyramid levels in all our experiments with a downsampling factor of 2.

3.1   Tests on Synthetic Data

Synthetic test data is created from an artificial vascular model, which is deformed in a length-preserving manner. Moreover, the deformation is chosen such that its major part occurs orthogonal to the image plane, see Fig. 3.

From this deformed model we compute a 2D projection using projection parameters from a calibrated C-arm device. The projected vascular model $\{(\mathbf{x}_i, r_i)\}$ is used to compute an artificial DSA image in the following way. We first use a background image, which contains noise and collimator masks similar to a real DSA. Then, we draw disks at each $\mathbf{x}_i$ with radius r_i. Intensities of disk pixels $\mathbf{x}_d$ are assigned proportional to the radius r_i:

$$\mathcal{I}(\mathbf{x}_d) = c - \frac{1}{2r_i}, \tag{14}$$

where c is an intensity constant, which represents the maximal value a contrasted vessel should have. This way we assure higher intensities at thin vessels and lower intensities at thicker vessels, which stems from the observation that X-rays get

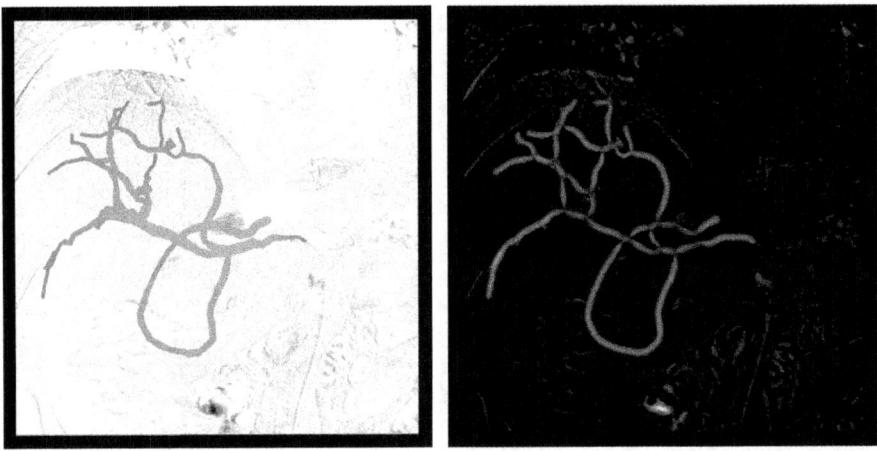

Fig. 4. A synthetic DSA created from the vasculature of an intraoperative CBR. The background image has been generated from two X-ray projections of the same patient. The right image shows the DSA after tubular structure enhancement. Note that, due to the background image, artifacts remain, which are similar to the ones in real DSA images.

more attenuated the more contrast agent they traverse, i.e. the thicker the vessel structure. Thereafter the intensities are smoothed using an averaging filter and Gaussian noise (with a standard deviation of 5% of the intensity range) is added.

We test three synthetic vascular models with increasing complexity and deformation, see Fig. 3. We compute Euclidean errors, angle errors, and runtime for our technique and for the feature-based approach. Input for the feature-based approach are the 2 vascular models $\{(\mathbf{X}_i, R_i)\}$, $\{(\mathbf{x}_i, r_i)\}$, and the projection function p. Table 1 illustrates errors with relative improvement compared to the initial situation as well as algorithm runtime in seconds.

3.2   Tests on Real Data

For the experiment similar to a clinical scenario we use two 3D data sets, a CTA, which has been acquired before an abdominal intervention, and a 3D CBR, which has been acquired with a C-arm during the intervention while a catheter was inserted. Both data sets visualize liver arteries of the same patient, which are extracted as described above to create two vascular models, $\{(\mathbf{X}_i^{CTA}, R_i^{CTA})\}$ and $\{(\mathbf{X}_i^{CBR}, R_i^{CBR})\}$. In a first step the two models are rigidly registered using a closed-form least-squares method [17] on manually assigned bifurcation correspondences. Then, more correspondences are manually assigned to compute a reference deformation via an interpolating TPS. The vascular model, which is extracted from the CBR, is projected using a calibrated projection matrix from the intraoperative C-arm. The projection matrix is chosen in anteroposterior position, which is a typical pose for the acquisition of DSA images during

Table 1. The first 6 rows show results on synthetic, the 2 lower rows on real data sets. Data with 'M2I' suffix show values for the proposed method, data with 'M2M' suffix show comparison values of the feature-based approach [1]. The second column shows the number of centerline points included in the 3D vascular model. The remaining rows show values for Euclidean and Angle error together with a relative improvement compared to the initial error as well as runtime (Intel Core2Duo 2.6GHz) results.

Data	$|\{\mathbf{X}_i\}|$	Euclidean error $[mm]$	Angle error $[rad]$	Runtime $[sec]$
S1-M2I	22	0.24 (77.7%)	0.04 (75.6%)	0.39
S1-M2M	22	0.31 (72.1%)	0.02 (85.5%)	2.67
S2-M2I	23	0.43 (68.0%)	0.07 (78.4%)	0.43
S2-M2M	23	0.40 (70.8%)	0.04 (88.7%)	3.27
S3-M2I	59	1.04 (26.7%)	0.34 (2.5%)	4.01
S3-M2M	59	0.86 (39.3%)	0.32 (6.7%)	17.90
R1-M2I	318	9.13 (16.3%)	0.22 (-0.2%)	184.1
R1-M2M	318	11.67 (-6.9%)	0.23 (-4.1%)	679.3

abdominal procedures. A synthetic DSA image is created from the projected vascular model as described above. Here, we obtain the background image by subtracting two high-dose X-ray images of the same patient, see Fig. 4. Again, tests were conducted using the proposed method and using the feature-based approach whose results are summarized in table 1.

Our experiments show that the new algorithm can cope with different deformations and has an accuracy similar to the feature-based approach. Moreover, when applied to the real data set, we improve the error by 16.3%, whereas the feature-based approach yields results worse than the initial situation. Please note that our algorithm decreases the runtime by a factor between 3 and 6 compared to the feature-based algorithm.

4   Conclusion

In this paper we propose a new method for deformable 2D-3D registration of vascular structures in a one-view scenario. Due to the combination of our novel image-based external energy term and a length preservation in 3D we create a well-posed problem, which can be solved via gradient descent optimization. Different to existing methods for 2D-3D non-rigid vascular registration, we define our energy on the image intensities, which both decreases runtime and increases ease of use. At the same time, we preserve accuracy as well as capture range due to a pyramidal implementation.

It should be noted that some approximative assumptions are made in our method. First, 3D centerlines are not projectively invariant, i.e. if registered, 3D centerlines do not necessarily project onto centerlines extracted in 2D. Only if the center of the 3D vessel intersects with the principal ray[2], projected and 2D centerline would overlap. The same applies to the projection of radii as mentioned in Sec. 2.1: in general, the perspective projection of a ball is a conic, only in the aforementioned special case it becomes a disk. These two issues, however, are marginal since angiographic devices have a focal length, which is much larger than the extents of a volumetric data set. In such scenarios, the error which is introduced can be neglected. Finally, we leave the projected radius r_i constant throughout the optimization. When a centerline point is displaced the projection of its associated radius will also change, which consequently changes the size of the disks D_i, see Eq. (2). We also neglect this issue using the same argument as above.

Encouraged by the promising results we intend to run more extensive tests on real data, not only on abdominal but also on heart anatomy, where deformation is increased due to immanent heart beat.

References

1. Groher, M., Zikic, D., Navab, N.: Deformable 2d-3d registration of vascular structures in a one view scenario. IEEE Trans. Med. Imag. 28(6), 847–860 (2009)
2. Gorges, S., Kerrien, E., Berger, M.O., Trousset, Y., Pescatore, J., Anxionnat, R., Picard, L.: Model of a vascular C-Arm for 3D augmented fluoroscopy in interventional radiology. In: Duncan, J.S., Gerig, G. (eds.) MICCAI 2005. LNCS, vol. 3750, pp. 214–222. Springer, Heidelberg (2005)
3. Bender, F., Groher, M., Khamene, A., Wein, W., Heibel, T., Navab, N.: 3D dynamic roadmapping for abdominal catheterizations. In: Metaxas, D., Axel, L., Fichtinger, G., Székely, G. (eds.) MICCAI 2008, Part II. LNCS, vol. 5242, pp. 668–675. Springer, Heidelberg (2008)
4. Hipwell, J., Penney, G., McLaughlin, R., Rhode, K., Summers, P., Cox, T., Byrne, J., Noble, J., Hawkes, D.: Intensity based 2D-3D registration of cerebral angiograms. IEEE Trans. Med. Imag. 22, 1417–1426 (2003)
5. Turgeon, G.A., Lehmann, G., Guiraudon, G., Drangova, M., Holdsworth, D., Peters, T.: 2D-3D registration of coronary angiograms for cardiac procedure planning and guidance. Medical Physics 32, 3737–3749 (2005)
6. Jomier, J., Bullitt, E., van Horn, M., Pathak, C., Aylward, S.: 3D/2D model-to-image registration applied to TIPS surgery. In: Larsen, R., Nielsen, M., Sporring, J. (eds.) MICCAI 2006. LNCS, vol. 4191, pp. 662–669. Springer, Heidelberg (2006)
7. Metz, C.T., Schaap, M., Klein, S., Neefjes, L.A., Capuano, E., Schultz, C., van Geuns, R.J., Serruys, P.W., van Walsum, T., Niessen, W.J.: Patient specific 4D coronary models from ECG-gated CTA data for intra-operative dynamic alignment of CTA with X-ray images. In: Yang, G.-Z., Hawkes, D., Rueckert, D., Noble, A., Taylor, C. (eds.) MICCAI 2009. LNCS, vol. 5761, pp. 369–376. Springer, Heidelberg (2009)
8. Benameur, S., Mignotte, M., Parent, S., Labelle, H., Skalli, W., de Guise, J.: 3D/2D registration and segmentation of scoliotic vertebra using statistical models. Computerized Medical Imaging and Graphics 27, 321–337 (2003)

---

[2] The principal ray is the line, which connects the center of projection with the center of the image.

9. Tang, T.S.Y., Ellis, R.E.: 2D/3D deformable registration using a hybrid atlas. In: Duncan, J.S., Gerig, G. (eds.) MICCAI 2005. LNCS, vol. 3750, pp. 223–230. Springer, Heidelberg (2005)

10. Yao, J., Taylor, R.: Assessing accuracy factors in deformable 2D/3D medical image registration using a statistical pelvis model. In: International Conference on Computer Vision (ICCV), Washington, DC, USA, p. 1329. IEEE Computer Society, Los Alamitos (2003)

11. Rohr, K., Stiehl, H.S., Sprengel, R., Buzug, T.M., Weese, J., Kuhn, M.H.: Landmark-based elastic registration using approximating thin-plate splines. IEEE Trans. Med. Imag. 20(6), 526–534 (2001)

12. Chefd'hotel, C., Hermosillo, G., Faugeras, O.: Flows of diffeomorphisms for multimodal image registration. In: Proceedings of IEEE International Symposium on Biomedical Imaging, pp. 753–756 (2002)

13. Koller, T.M., Gerig, G., Szekely, G., Dettwiler, D.: Multiscale detection of curvilinear structures in 2-D and 3-D image data. In: International Conference on Computer Vision, ICCV (1995)

14. Rohr, K.: Landmark-based image analysis: using geometric and intensity models. Springer, Heidelberg (2001)

15. Nocedal, J., Wright, S.J.: Numerical Optimization. Springer, Heidelberg (2006)

16. Osher, S., Fedkiw, R.: Level Set Methods and Dynamic Implicit Surfaces. Springer, Heidelberg (2003)

17. Umeyama, S.: Least-squares estimation of transformation parameters between two point patterns. IEEE Trans. Pattern Anal. Mach. Intell (PAMI) 13(4), 376–380 (1991)

Continuity Order of Local Displacement in Volumetric Image Sequence

Koji Kashu[1], Yusuke Kameda[2], Masaki Narita[1],
Atsushi Imiya[3], and Tomoya Sakai[3]

[1] School of Advanced Integration Science, Chiba University
[2] JSPS/School of Advanced Integration Science, Chiba University
[3] Institute of Media and Information Technology, Chiba University
Yayoi-cho 1-33, Inage-ku, Chiba, 263-8522, Japan

Abstract. We introduce a method for volumetric cardiac motion analysis using variational optical flow computation involving the prior with the fractional order differentiations. The order of the differentiation of the prior controls the continuity class of the solution. Fractional differentiations is a typical tool for edge detection of images. As a sequel of image analysis by fractional differentiation, we apply the theory of fractional differentiation to a temporal image sequence analysis. Using the fractional order differentiations, we can estimate the orders of local continuities of optical flow vectors. Therefore, we can obtain the optical flow vector with the optimal continuity at each point.

1 Introduction

As an application of the computer vision technique to clinical biomechanical motion analysis from volumetric image sequences, we deal with spatial optical flow computation for the beating heart. In recent years, it is possible to measure a series of volumetric cardiac images dynamically using MRI, Cine X-ray CT, and Ultrasonic imaging and so on. The most important physical natures of the cardiac optical flow computation are that the motion of the beating heart is spatial dynamics and the heart wall is deformable [1,7]. For registration of temporal volumetric cardiac images, optical flow is a fundamental feature to express temporal deformation. Therefore, accurate computation of optical flow field and segmentation of optical flow fields are essential tasks for pre-processing to temporal registration of cardiac image sequence.

The prior terms of variational optical flow and variationl image registration control local continuity orders of small displacements in images of a spatiotemporal image sequence and deformation for images from an atlas image. In this paper, we introduce an estimation method for the optimal continuity order of local small displacements of image sequence. The continuity order of local displacement is computed using variational optical flow computation with the prior which involves the fractional order differentiation [2,3,4,5] of the displacement field. We

B. Fischer, B. Dawant, and C. Lorenz (Eds.): WBIR 2010, LNCS 6204, pp. 48–59, 2010.
© Springer-Verlag Berlin Heidelberg 2010

apply local continuity estimation to volumetric cardiac optical flow computation. The prior term with the first-order derivatives is a common regularizer in optical-flow computation [8]. The prior term with the second-order derivatives, of which the origin in mechanics goes back to Kirchhoff [10] on the elastic theory, is a common regularizer in boundary extraction for tracking of the object-boundary and warping [11] in computational anatomy. From the viewpoint of the order of derivatives in the regularizers for the optical-flow computation, the Horn-Schunck [9] and the deformable-model [6] constraints require that the solution is a continuous twice differentiable function and a continuous four-time differentiable function, respectively. The order of the differentiations in the prior controls the continuity class of the solution. Therefore, by selecting an appropriate order of the differentiation in the prior of variational optical flow computation, we can estimate motion boundary and classify the continuity order of the motion field.

Total variational (TV) regularization is a successful method of optical flow computation of an image sequence with discontinuity of the gray values and motion field. TV regularization uses the total variation of optical flow field as the prior, although the classical Horn-Schunck method [9] uses the L_2 norm of the gradient of flow field. TV regularization optical flow computation [22] derives a nonlinear elliptic partial differential equation as the Euler-Lagrange equation of the energy functional of the problem. The generalization of the order of differentiation in a Horn-Schunck-type prior is another modification of the original Horn-Schunck regularization, since this generalization yields a linear Euler-Lagrange equation [4,5]. There are two types of generalization of the differentiations in priors; the first one deals with higher-order differentiations, and the second one deals with fractional order differentiations. We focus on the second type of generalization, that is, we deal with the variational optical flow computation with a prior term involves a fractional order differentiation of optical flow vectors.

Recently, fractional partial differential equations have been widely used in various areas of science and engineering, because fractional differential equations describe diffusion and wave propagation in inhomogeneous media and fractal structures [18,20]. As a sequel, we propose variational optical flow computation involving the prior with fractional order differentiations on optical flow vectors. A definition of fractional differentiation is based on the Fourier transform of differential operations, which is easily implemented using the first Fourier transform and the filter theory [2]. We solve the spatially fractional partial differential equation using the Fourier transform method to compute fractional derivatives. Since fractional differentiations[1] are linear operations, the fractional order regularization for optical flow computation [22] derives a linear fractional order elliptic partial differential equation as the Euler-Lagrange equation of the

---

[1] The definitions of fractional derivative are

$$\frac{d^\alpha}{dx^\alpha} f(x) = \frac{1}{\Gamma(n-\alpha)} \frac{d^n}{dx^n} \int_0^t (t-r)^{n-\alpha-1} f(r) dr.$$

Therefore, the relations $\frac{d^{1/2}}{dx^{1/2}} x = \frac{1}{\sqrt{2\pi}} x^{1/2}$ and $\frac{d^{1/2}}{dx^{1/2}} \frac{1}{\sqrt{2\pi}} x^{1/2} = 1$ are satisfied.

energy functional. Therefore, we can numerically solve the problem using the same strategy that is used to solve the Horn-Schunck method.

2 Fractional Optical Variational Problem

2.1 Fractional Order Differentiations

Using the Fourier transform pair

$$F(\boldsymbol{\xi}) = \frac{1}{(2\pi)^{3/2}} \int_{\mathbf{R}^3} f(\boldsymbol{x}) e^{-i(\boldsymbol{x}^\top \boldsymbol{\xi})} d\boldsymbol{x}, \tag{1}$$

$$f(\boldsymbol{x}) = \frac{1}{(2\pi)^{3/2}} \int_{\mathbf{R}^3} F(\boldsymbol{\xi}) e^{i(\boldsymbol{x}^\top \boldsymbol{\xi})} d\boldsymbol{\xi}, \tag{2}$$

for $\boldsymbol{x} = (x, y, z)^\top$ and $\boldsymbol{\xi} = (\xi, \eta, \zeta)^\top$, we define the operations Λ

$$\Lambda f(\boldsymbol{x}) = \frac{1}{(2\pi)^{3/2}} \int_{\mathbf{R}^{3/2}} |\boldsymbol{\xi}| F(\boldsymbol{\xi}) e^{i(\boldsymbol{x}^\top \boldsymbol{\xi})} d\boldsymbol{\xi}. \tag{3}$$

We have the equality

$$\int_{\mathbf{R}^3} |\nabla f|^2 d\boldsymbol{x} = \int_{\mathbf{R}^3} |\Lambda f|^2 d\boldsymbol{x}, \tag{4}$$

since

$$\int_{\mathbf{R}^3} |f|^2 d\boldsymbol{x} = \int_{\mathbf{R}^3} |F|^2 d\xi d\boldsymbol{\xi}. \tag{5}$$

2.2 Variationl Image Analysis

For the positive integer $n \geq 1$, setting the operator D^n to be

$$D^{n+1} f = \begin{pmatrix} \partial_x D^n f \\ \partial_y D^n f \\ \partial_z D^n f \end{pmatrix}, \quad Df = \nabla f = \begin{pmatrix} \partial_x f \\ \partial_y f \\ \partial_z f \end{pmatrix}, \tag{6}$$

we define the operation

$$|T^\alpha f|^2 = \begin{cases} |D^\alpha f|^2, & \text{if } \alpha \text{ is an integer,} \\ |\Lambda^\alpha f|^2, & \text{otherwise.} \end{cases} \tag{7}$$

As a generalization of the Horn-Schucnk method [9] such that

$$H(\boldsymbol{u}) = \int_{\mathbf{R}^3} \{ (\nabla f^\top \boldsymbol{u} + \partial_t f)^2 + \kappa(|\nabla u|^2 + |\nabla v|^2 + |\nabla w|^2) \} \, d\boldsymbol{x}, \tag{8}$$

we deal with the variational energy functional

$$J_\alpha(\boldsymbol{u}) = \int_{\mathbf{R}^3} \{ D(f, \boldsymbol{u})^2 + \kappa(|T^\alpha u|^2 + |T^\alpha v|^2 + |T^\alpha w|^2) \} d\boldsymbol{x}, \tag{9}$$

where $\kappa \geq 0$ and $\alpha = n + \varepsilon$ where $0 < \varepsilon < 1$ and n is a non-negative integer for $\boldsymbol{u} = (x, y, z)^{\top}$. Since $\varLambda = \varLambda^*$, the Euler-Lagrange equation and the associated diffusion equation of eq. (9) are

$$\varLambda^{2\alpha}\boldsymbol{u} + \frac{1}{\kappa}D(f, \boldsymbol{u})\nabla_{\boldsymbol{u}}D(f, \boldsymbol{u}) = 0, \tag{10}$$

$$\partial_{\tau}\boldsymbol{u} = (-\varLambda^{2\alpha})\boldsymbol{u} - \frac{1}{\kappa}D(f, \boldsymbol{u})\nabla_{\boldsymbol{u}}D(f, \boldsymbol{u}), \tag{11}$$

where $\nabla_{\boldsymbol{u}}$ is the gradient with respect to $\boldsymbol{u}$ and ∂_{τ} is the partial derivative with respect to τ. For variational optical flow computation and variational image registration, the first term of eq. (9) is

$$D(f, \boldsymbol{u}) = \nabla f^{\top}\boldsymbol{u} + f_t = f_x u + f_y v + f_z w + f_t \tag{12}$$

for a spatiotemporal image sequence $f(\boldsymbol{x}, t)$ and

$$D(f, \boldsymbol{u}) = g(\boldsymbol{x}) - f(\boldsymbol{x} + \boldsymbol{u}) \tag{13}$$

for a pair of given functions g and f, respectively. Equation (10) coincides with the Euler-Lagrange equation of the Horn-Schunck method and the deformable-model method for $\alpha = 1$ and $\alpha = 2$, respectively, if the function $D(f, \boldsymbol{u})$ in the first term of eq. (9) is given by eq. (12). Furthermore, for variational image registration, we have

$$\varLambda^{2\alpha}\boldsymbol{u} - \frac{1}{\kappa}(g(\boldsymbol{x}) - f(\boldsymbol{x} + \boldsymbol{u}))\nabla f(\boldsymbol{x} + \boldsymbol{u}) = 0. \tag{14}$$

Therefore, if $\alpha = 1$ and $\alpha = 2$, the prior term of eq. (9) is that of diffusion registration and curvature registration, respectively [15].

2.3 Selection of Order of Prior

The solution involving the lth-order prior is

$$\boldsymbol{u}(x, y, z) = \begin{pmatrix} u \\ v \\ w \end{pmatrix} = \begin{pmatrix} \sum_{i,j,k=0}^{l-1} a_{ijk} x^i y^j z^k \\ \sum_{i,j,k=0}^{l-1} b_{ijk} x^i y^j z^k \\ \sum_{i,j,k=0}^{l-1} c_{ijk} x^i y^j z^k \end{pmatrix} \tag{15}$$

for nonnegative integers k, that is, the solution is locally a $(k-1)$th-order polynomial of x and y. This property implies that the priors involving the first- and second-order differentiations derive a piecewise linear and affine optical flow, respectively.

Let $\boldsymbol{u}(x, y, t; \alpha)$ be the optical flow vector computed for fixed α. For each point $\boldsymbol{x}$, we select

$$\boldsymbol{u}^*(x, y, t; \alpha^*) = \arg\min_{\alpha} F(\boldsymbol{u}; \alpha, \kappa), \quad \alpha^*(x, y, t) = \arg\min F(\boldsymbol{u}; \alpha, \kappa) \tag{16}$$

where

$$F(\boldsymbol{u}; \alpha, \kappa) = D(f, \boldsymbol{u})^2 + \kappa(|T^\alpha u|^2 + |T^\alpha v|^2 + |T^\alpha w|^2) \tag{17}$$

for a predetermined positive parameter κ as the solution vector of point $\boldsymbol{x}$. Equation (16) estimates the local continuity order of the optical flow vector, that is, point $\boldsymbol{x}$ with the optical flow vector $\boldsymbol{u}(x, y, t; \alpha)$ is the class $(\alpha - 1)$ function of $\boldsymbol{x}$. We call $\alpha^* = \alpha(\boldsymbol{x}, t)$, which establishes the minimum of eq. (16), the α-map [21] of the optical flow field (α-map in abbreviation.).

Using α-map, we construct a two-path algorithm such that

1. Let α_0 and α_1 be a pair of constants such that $\alpha_0 < \alpha_1$. Compute optical flow for each α for $\alpha_0 \le \alpha \le \alpha_1$ and construct α-map $\alpha^*(\boldsymbol{x})$.
2. Compute displacement field $\boldsymbol{u}^{**}(\boldsymbol{x})$ for point $\boldsymbol{x}$ as the solution of the equation

$$\partial_\tau \boldsymbol{u} = -\Lambda^{2\alpha^*(\boldsymbol{x})} \boldsymbol{u} - \frac{1}{\kappa} D(f, \boldsymbol{u}) \nabla_{\boldsymbol{u}} D(f, \boldsymbol{u}). \tag{18}$$

3   Numerical Examples

3.1   Discretization of Equation

From eq. (11), we have semi-explicit discretizations such that

$$\frac{\boldsymbol{u}_{kmn}^{(l+1)} - \boldsymbol{u}_{kmn}^{(l)}}{\Delta\tau} = (-\Lambda^{2\alpha}) \boldsymbol{u}_{kmn}^{(l)} - \frac{1}{\kappa} D(f, \boldsymbol{u}_{kmn}^{(l+1)}) \nabla_{\boldsymbol{u}} D(f, \boldsymbol{u}_{kmn}^{(l+1)}), \tag{19}$$

$$\frac{\boldsymbol{u}_{kmn}^{(l+1)} - \boldsymbol{u}_{kmn}^{(l)}}{\Delta\tau} = (-\Lambda^{2\alpha}) \boldsymbol{u}_{kmn}^{(l+1)} - \frac{1}{\kappa} D(f, \boldsymbol{u}_{kmn}^{(l)}) \nabla_{\boldsymbol{u}} D(f, \boldsymbol{u}_{kmn}^{(l)}). \tag{20}$$

3.2   Numerical Computation

We evaluate numerical performances of the fractional order derivative in the prior for volumetric cardiac optical flow computation. Equation (19) derives the iteration form [14]

$$(\boldsymbol{I} + \frac{\Delta\tau}{\kappa} \boldsymbol{S}_{kmn}) \boldsymbol{u}_{kmn}^{(l+1)} = \boldsymbol{u}_{kmn}^{(l)} + \Delta\tau(-\Lambda^{2\alpha}) \boldsymbol{u}_{kmn}^{(l)} - \frac{\Delta\tau}{\kappa} \boldsymbol{c}_{kmn}, \ l \ge 0 \tag{21}$$

for the numerical computation of α optical flow, where

$$\boldsymbol{S}_{kmn} = (\nabla f)_{kmn} (\nabla f)_{kmn}^\top, \quad \boldsymbol{c}_{kmn} = (\partial_t f)_{kmn} (\nabla f)_{kmn}. \tag{22}$$

The numerical Fourier transform achieves the operation $(-\Lambda^{2\alpha} \boldsymbol{u})_{kmn}^{(l)}$ [2]. To use the FFT (the Fast Fourier Transform) with the Neumann condition $\frac{\partial \boldsymbol{u}}{\partial \boldsymbol{n}} = 0$, the function $f(x, y, z)$ defined in $0 \le x, y, \le L$ is expanded by using the relations

$$f(L+x, L+y, L+z) = f(L-x, L-y, L-z), \ f(x, y, z) = (x+2mL, y+2nL, z+2nL) \tag{23}$$

for integers k, m, and n. Setting the discrete differentiations to be

$$D_x f(x,y,z) = \frac{1}{h} f(x + \frac{1}{2}h, y, z) - f(x - \frac{1}{2}h, y, z),$$
$$D_y f(x,y,z) = \frac{1}{h} f(x, y + \frac{1}{2}h, z) - f(x, y - \frac{1}{2}h, z), \qquad (24)$$
$$D_z f(x,y,z) = \frac{1}{h} f(x, y, z + \frac{1}{2}h) - f(x, y, z - \frac{1}{2}h)$$

for unit sampling step h, the Fourier transform of $\Delta f(x,y,z)$ is

$$FT\{\Delta f(x,y)\} = -\frac{4}{h^2} \left(\sin^2 \frac{h}{2}\xi + 4\sin^2 \frac{h}{2}\eta + +4\sin^2 \frac{h}{2}\eta \right) F(\xi, \eta, \zeta), \qquad (25)$$

where FTf expresses the Fourier transform of f, since

$$FT\{D_x f(x,y,z)\} = \frac{2}{h} i \sin \frac{h}{2}\xi F(\xi, \eta, \zeta),$$
$$FT\{D_y f(x,y,z)\} = \frac{2}{h} i \sin \frac{h}{2}\eta F(\xi, \eta, \zeta), \qquad (26)$$
$$FT\{D_z f(x,y,z)\} = \frac{2}{h} i \sin \frac{h}{2}\zeta F(\xi, \eta, \zeta).$$

Therefore, we obtain the relation

$$(-\Delta)^\alpha f_{ijr} = IDFT \left\{ \left(4\sin^2 \frac{h}{2}k + 4\sin^2 \frac{h}{2}m + 4\sin^2 \frac{h}{2}n \right)^\alpha \right\} F_{kmn} \qquad (27)$$

for discrete images f_{ij} and its discrete Fourier transform F_{mn}, where $IDFT$ expresses the inverse discrete Fourier transform.

3.3 Numerical Results

Figure 1 shows three-dimensional slices on the coronal, transverse, and sagittal planes. From left to right, Fig. 1 shows the three views of the original images, the flow fields computed by the Horn-Schunck method, and the flow fields computed by the deformable model. The three-dimensional flow field vector of each point is projected onto the plane, and the projected two-dimensional flow vector is expressed in the Middlebury Color Chart expression of vector field, which expresses directions and lengths of two dimensional vectors.

Since the Horn-Schunck and deformable model methods yield the piecewise constant flow field and piecewise affine flow field, respectively, the computational results by the former and latter methods are an over-smoothed field and the field shaped on the curved boundary, respectively.

Figure 2 shows α-map $\alpha^*(\boldsymbol{x})$, the optical flow field $\boldsymbol{u}^*(\boldsymbol{x}, \alpha^*)$ which minimizes $F(\boldsymbol{u}, \alpha; \kappa)$, and the solution of the two-path algorithm $\boldsymbol{u}^{**}$ from left to right.

Fig. 1. Three-dimensional optical flow fields. From left to right images flow fields computed by the Horn-Schunck method, the deformable-model method, on the coronal, transverse, and sagittal planes.

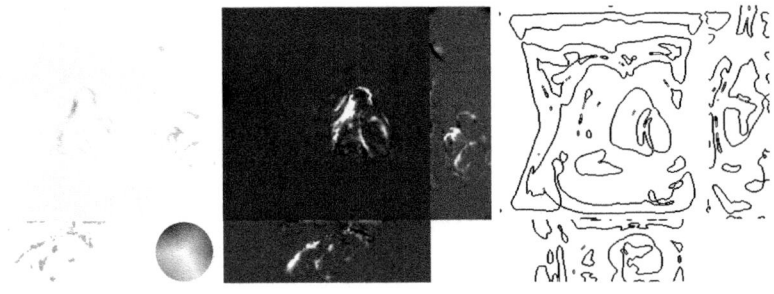

Fig. 2. Boundary surfaces on coronal, transverse, and sagittal planes. From left to right, color chart expression of optical flow field, norm of optical flow field, and the boundary surface line of the image. The boundary surface $\phi(x,y,z) = 0$ is extracted by a 3D version of Krueger's method [24]. $\phi(x,y,0) = 0$, $\phi(x,0,z) = 0$, and $\phi(0,y,z) = 0$ are illustrated.

Comparing with the boundary curves on planes,[2] our method clearly extracts the motion boundary. The result $\boldsymbol{u}^{**}$ is computed using the iteration

$$(\boldsymbol{I} + \frac{\Delta\tau}{\kappa}\boldsymbol{S}_{kmn})\boldsymbol{u}_{kmn}^{(l+1)} = \boldsymbol{u}_{kmn}^{(l)} + \Delta\tau(-\boldsymbol{\Lambda}^{2\alpha_{kmn}})\boldsymbol{u}_{kmn}^{(l)} - \frac{\Delta\tau}{\kappa}\boldsymbol{c}_{kmn}, \ l \geq 0, \quad (28)$$

where α_{mn} is estimated as

$$\alpha_{kmn} = \min arg\{(\nabla f^{\top}\boldsymbol{u} + \partial_t f)^2 + \kappa(|T^{\alpha}u|^2 + |T^{\alpha}v|^2 + |T^{\alpha}w|^2)\} \quad (29)$$

---

[2] Setting f_G to be the convolution of the Gaussian with an appropriate variance and f, the segment boundary is the collection of points which satisfy $\nabla f_G^{\top}\boldsymbol{H}_G\nabla f_G = 0$ where $\boldsymbol{H}_G$ is the Hessian of f. For the boundary surface $\phi(x,y,z) = 0$, the boundary curves on the coronal, transverse, and sagittal planes are $\phi(x,y,0) = 0$, $\phi(x,0,z) = 0$, and $\phi(0,y,z) = 0$, respectively.

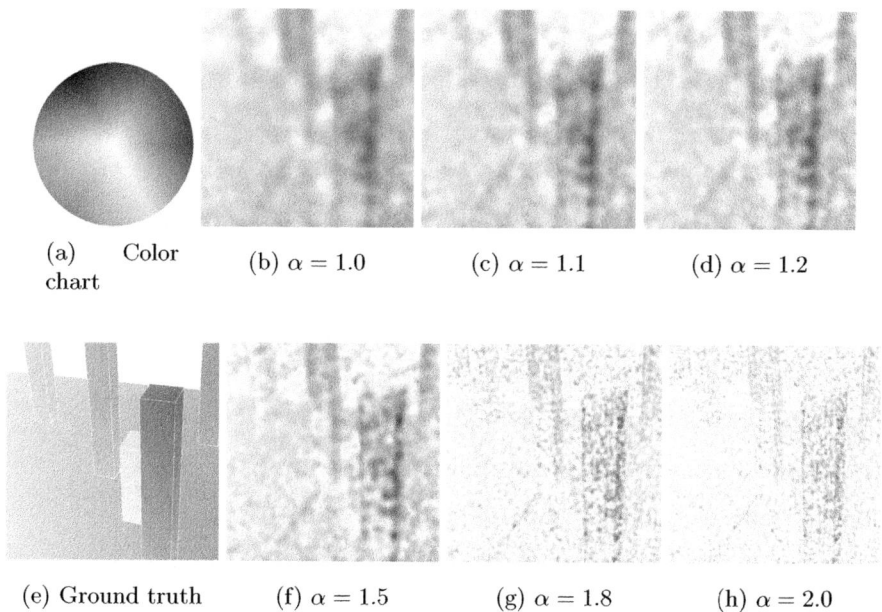

(a)   Color   (b) $\alpha = 1.0$ (c) $\alpha = 1.1$ (d) $\alpha = 1.2$
chart

(e) Ground truth   (f) $\alpha = 1.5$ (g) $\alpha = 1.8$ (h) $\alpha = 2.0$

Fig. 3. Computational results for λ = max $|f|$. Results for α = $1.0, 1.1, 1.2, 1.5, 1.8,$ and 2.0.

in the first step of the algorithm. These results show that the solution of the two-path algorithm detects the motion discontinuity caused on the motion boundary using the operation $\Lambda^{\alpha^*(\boldsymbol{x})}$.

Since we have no ground truth for the heart image sequence, we show the performance evaluation of the boundary detection using a two-dimensional image sequence with the ground truth.

Figure 3 shows the effect of the fractional order derivatives in the prior of the Horn-Schunck method. For $1 \leq \alpha \leq 2$, the method clearly detects the motion boundary.

Figures 4(d) and (h) are the results obtained by our method using the α-maps in Figs. 4(b) and (f). Setting $\boldsymbol{u}_T$ to be the ground truth fields, α_{true} is computed as

$$\alpha_{\text{true}} = \min arg\{(\nabla f^\top \boldsymbol{u}_T + \partial_t f)^2 + \kappa(|T^\alpha u|^2 + |T^\alpha v|^2 + |T^\alpha w|^2)\}. \quad (30)$$

Figures 4(b) and (f) show that the values of α-map on the motion boundaries are large, since for the description of motion fields on the motion boundaries, we are required to use higher order terms of eq. (15).

For the two-pass method, the results of the Horn-Schunck method are used as the initial estimation of the iteration algorithm. Figures 4(d) and (h) show that the boundaries of the sphere and blocks on the images are sharply extracted, since on the boundary, both the gray value of the image and the optical

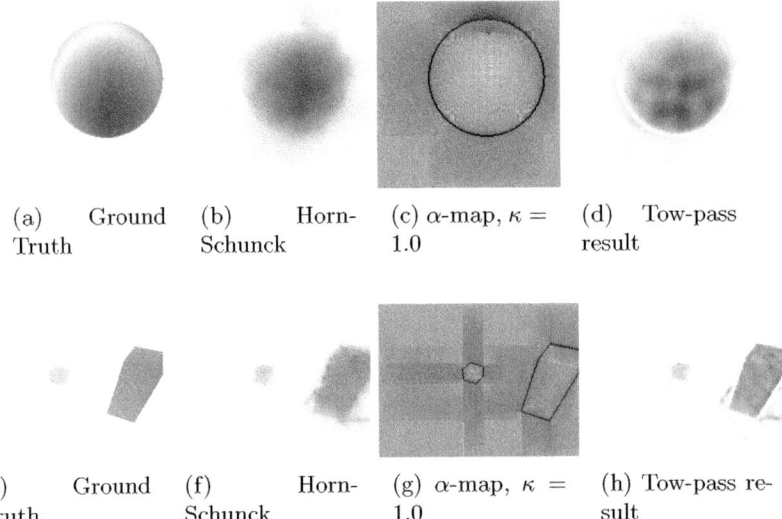

(a)   Ground   (b)   Horn-   (c) α-map, $\kappa =$ (d)   Tow-pass
Truth   Schunck   1.0   result

(e)   Ground   (f)   Horn-   (g) α-map, $\kappa =$ (h) Tow-pass re-
Truth   Schunck   1.0   sult

Fig. 4. Results: Rotating sphere and New marbled block. From left to right, motion field, α-map, the results of Horn-Schunck method, and results of the two-pass method. For the two-pass method, the results of the Horn-Schunck method are used as the initial estimation of the iteration algorithm.

flow process discontinuity in the gray-value topography and motion field, respectively. For both examples, the motion discontinuity on the segment boundaries is extracted by the fractional order optical flow.

3.4   Discussion

Setting $\{\boldsymbol{x}_k = (x_k, y_k, z_k)^\top\}_{k=1}^n$ and $\{t_k\}_{k=1}^n$ to be sets of sample points and sample values, respectively, the minimization of

$$J(f) = \sum_{k=1}^{n} (f(\boldsymbol{x}_k) - t_k)^2 + \kappa \int_\Omega |\Lambda^\alpha f|^2 d\boldsymbol{x} \tag{31}$$

where Ω is the define domain of the function $f(\boldsymbol{x})$, is a generalization [25] of the variational then-plate spline approximation. Here, the order α controls the continuity orders of the reconstructed function $f(x)$. We applied this property for the computation of volumetric cardiac optical flow field [6,7,1,25].

The result in Fig. 3 shows the flow fields which minimize

$$D(\boldsymbol{u}) = \int_{\mathbf{R}^2} (\nabla f^\top \boldsymbol{u} + f_t)^2 dxdy + \kappa E_2(\boldsymbol{u})$$

$$E_2(\boldsymbol{u}) = \int\int_{\mathbf{R}^2} (|D^2 u|^2 + |D^2 v|^2 + |D^2 w|) dxdy, \tag{32}$$

where

$$D^2 f = (f_{xx}, f_{xy}, f_{xz}, f_{xy}, f_{yy}, f_{yz}, f_{zx}, f_{zy}, f_{zz})^\top. \tag{33}$$

From the results in Figs 4 and 3, we observe the following properties on the boundary motion.

Observation 1. *If the motion of points in the neighborhood of the boundary is locally stationary, for instance, the motion is pure translation in a region, the projection of the ridge boundary moves elastically on the image. Therefore, the prior (regularizer) $E_2(\boldsymbol{u})$ of eq. (32) is suitable to detect the moving boundary.*

Observation 2. *If the motion of points in the neighborhood of the boundary on the image is nonstationary because of motion delay in the neighborhood, for instance, the delay in the global translation caused by local rotation, the projection of the ridge boundary moves viscoelastically on the image. Motion delay is expressed as a phase delay of the propagation of motion front. Therefore, the prior (regularizer)*

$$V(\boldsymbol{u}) = \int \int_{\mathbf{R}^3} (|\Lambda^{n+\varepsilon} u|^2 + |\Lambda^{n+\varepsilon} v|^2 + |\Lambda^{n+\varepsilon} w|^2) dx dy \tag{34}$$

for $0 < \varepsilon < 1$ is suitable to detect moving boundary.

For $\alpha = n + \varepsilon$ such that $0 < \varepsilon < 1$, the fractional order Laplacian is decomposed into the harmonic operation $(-\Delta)$ and fractional Laplacian $\Lambda^{2\varepsilon} = (-\Delta)^\varepsilon$. This decomposition can be read that $\Lambda^{2\alpha} f$ is achieved by applying the harmonic operation $(-\Delta)^n$ to $g = (-\Delta)^\varepsilon f$, which is achieved by convolution between the function f and the Riesz potential [23]. Numerical filtering of the operation $(-\Delta)^\varepsilon$ derived in eq.(27) possesses a smoothing effect to the optical flow field $\boldsymbol{u}^{(l)}$ in each step of iteration. Therefore, our numerical scheme generates a smoothed optical flow before applying the harmonic operation. This presmoothing property of the numerical scheme yields a better performance for $\alpha = n + \varepsilon$ such that $0 < \varepsilon < 1$.

Our method estimates the continuity order of the optical flow field. Furthermore, as shown in the results, our method also extracts a higher order optical flow if the gray-value distribution of an image is discontinuous. The results mathematically provide a method to estimate the local continuity order of the optical flow field, and theoretically shows that for motion boundary extraction and tracking, the prior with higher order differentiation is preferable. For the tracking of the image of an elastic boundary of a ridged object in space, the order of the differentiation is two. If the optimal order of the points is between 1 and 2, the points are viscoelastically moving [16,17] on an image. The results lead to the conclusion that using the local continuity order, it is possible to extract the motion boundary and separate moving segments from the background.

4   Concluding Remarks

The order of differentiation in the prior decides the continuity order of the optical flow field. Therefore, our results show that orders between one and two are preferable to detect discontinuity optical flow vectors, which appear on the motion boundary. Although TV regularization [12,13] accurately and stably computes an optical flow field and extracts moving segments from the background, the operation is nonlinear. The results leads to the conclusion that using the local continuity order, it is possible to extract the motion boundary and separate moving segments from the background.

This research was supported by "Computational anatomy for computer-aided diagnosis and therapy: Frontiers of medical image sciences" funded by Grant-in-Aid for Scientific Research on Innovative Areas, MEXT, Japan, Grants-in-Aid for Scientific Research founded by Japan Society of the Promotion of Sciences, Research Fellowship for Young Scientist founded by Japan Society of the Promotion of Sciences, and Research Associate Program of Chiba University. Y. Kameda is supported as a Research Fellow of the Japan Society for the Promotion of Science, The heart image sequence is provided from Robarts Research Institute at the University of Western Ontario through Prof. John Barron.

References

1. Sorzano, C.Ó.S., Thévenaz, P., Unser, M.: Elastic registration of biological images using vector-spline regularization. IEEE Tr. Biomedical Engineering 52, 652–663 (2005)
2. Davis, J.A., Smith, D.A., McNamara, D.E., Cottrell, D.M., Campos, J.: Fractional derivatives-analysis and experimental implementation. Applied Optics 32, 5943–5948 (2001)
3. Zhang, J., Wei, Z.-H.: Fractional variational model and algorithm for image denoising. In: Proceedings of 4th International Conference on Natural Computation, vol. 5, pp. 524–528 (2008)
4. Oldham, K.B., Spanier, J.: The Fractional Calculus: Theory And Applications of Differentiation and Integration to Arbitrary Order, Dover Books on Mathematics. Dover, New York (2004)
5. Podlubny, I.: Fractional Differential Equations. An Introduction to Fractional Derivatives, Fractional Differential Equations, Some Methods of Their Solution and Some of Their Applications. Academic Press, London (1999)
6. Suter, D.: Motion estimation and vector spline. In: Proceedings of CVPR 1994, pp. 939–942 (1994)
7. Suter, D., Chen, F.: Left ventricular motion reconstruction based on elastic vector splines. IEEE Tr. Medical Imaging, 295–305 (2000)
8. Nagel, H.-H., Enkelmann, W.: An investigation of smoothness constraint for the estimation of displacement vector fields from image sequences. IEEE Trans. on PAMI 8, 565–593 (1986)
9. Horn, B.K.P., Schunck, B.G.: Determining optical flow. Artificial Intelligence 17, 185–204 (1981)
10. Timoshenko, S.P.: History of Strength of Materials. Dover, New York (1983)
11. Grenander, U., Miller, M.: Computational anatomy: An emerging discipline. Quarterly of Applied Mathematics 4, 617–694 (1998)
12. Papenberg, N., Bruhn, A., Brox, T., Didas, S., Weickert, J.: Highly accurate optic flow computation with theoretically justified warping. IJCV 67, 141–158 (2006)

13. Yin, W., Goldfarb, D., Osher, S.: A comparison of three total variation based texture extraction models. J. Visual Communication and Image Representation 18, 240–252 (2007)
14. Eckstein, J., Bertsekas, D.P.: On the Douglas-Rachford splitting method and the proximal point algorithm for maximal monotone operators. Mathematical Programming 55, 293–318 (1992)
15. Modersitzki, J.: Numerical Methods for Image Registration. Oxford Univ. Pr., Oxford (2004)
16. Momani, S., Odibat, Z.: Numerical comparison of methods for solving linear differential equations of fractional order. Chaos, Solitons and Fractals 31, 1248–1255 (2007)
17. Murio, D.A.: Stable numerical evaluation of Grünwald-Letnikov fractional derivatives applied to a fractional IHCP. Inverse Problems in Science and Engineering 17, 229–243 (2009)
18. Debbi, L.: Explicit solutions of some fractional partial differential equations via stable subordinators. J. of Applied Mathematics and Stochastic Analysis, Article ID 93502 2006, 1–18 (2006)
19. Debbi, L.: On some properties of a high order fractional differential operator which is not in general selfadjoint. Applied Mathematical Sciences 1, 1325–1339 (2007)
20. Chechkin, A.V., Gorenflo, R., Sokolov, I.M.: Fractional diffusion in inhomogeneous media. J. Phys. A: Math. Gen. 38, L679–L684 (2005)
21. Duits, R., Felsberg, M., Florack, L.M.J., Platel, B.: α scale spaces on a bounded domain. In: Griffin, L.D., Lillholm, M. (eds.) Scale-Space 2003. LNCS, vol. 2695, pp. 502–518. Springer, Heidelberg (2003)
22. Papenberg, N., Bruhn, A., Brox, T., Didas, S., Weickert, J.: Highly accurate optic flow computation with theoretically justified warping. IJCV 67, 141–158 (2006)
23. Ortiguera, M.D.: Riesz potential operations and inverses via fractional centred derivatives. International Journal of Mathematics and Mathematical Sciences, Article ID 48391, 1–12 (2008)
24. Krueger, W.M., Phillips, K.: The geometry of differential operator with application to image processing. PAMI 11, 1252–1264 (1989)
25. Unser, M., Blu, T.: Fractional spline and wavelets. SIAM Review 43, 43–67 (2000)

Registration of 2D Images from Fast Scanning Ophthalmic Instruments

Alfredo Dubra and Zachary Harvey

Flaum Eye Institute, University of Rochester
Rochester, NY 14642-0314, USA
adubra@cvs.rochester.edu

Abstract. Images from high-resolution scanning ophthalmic instruments
are significantly distorted due to eye movement. Accurate image registration is required to successfully image subjects who are unable to fixate due
to retinal conditions. Moreover, all scanning ophthalmic imaging modalities using adaptive optics will benefit from image registration, even in subjects with good fixation and anaesthetized animals. Transformation
functions used to map two images could in principle be very complex. Here,
we show that when the scanning in ophthalmic instruments is sufficiently
fast with respect to the speed of involuntary eye movement, these mapping functions become the addition of a linear term and a single variable
function. Then, based on experimental data on eye movement amplitude
and speed of the fixating eye, minimum sampling frequencies for these instruments are discussed. Finally, a simple method for estimating the image
transformation functions by taking advantage of the finite bandwidth of
the motion signals is presented.

1 Introduction

The development of ophthalmic adaptive optics (AO) in recent years has led
to a new generation of high-resolution retinal imaging instruments [1–11]. The
unprecedented resolution of these instruments allows for *in vivo* non-invasive
imaging of retinal cell mosaics [1, 9, 10, 12]. Within this family of instruments,
scanning devices such as the AO optical coherence tomograph (AO-OCT) [3–8]
and the AO scanning laser ophthalmoscope (AOSLO) [7, 9–11] produce images
with better signal-to-noise ratio (SNR), lateral resolution and axial sectioning
than flood-illuminated cameras [1, 2]. On the other hand, scanning instruments
are susceptible to image distortion due to eye movement. The distortion scales
with the magnification of the instrument, which is an order of magnitude greater
in AO ophthalmic instruments than in commercial clinical devices.

When using high magnification to view the retina *in vivo*, light safety standards [13] severely restrict the number of photons that can be delivered within
a certain period of time. For example, when visualizing lipofuscin in retinal pigment epithelial cells using single-photon fluorescence [10, 12] at safe light levels,
over 99% of the recorded image pixels had no signal. The resulting images, dom-
inated by photon noise, do not contain enough information for registration. This

B. Fischer, B. Dawant, and C. Lorenz (Eds.): WBIR 2010, LNCS 6204, pp. 60–71, 2010.
© Springer-Verlag Berlin Heidelberg 2010

led to the development of a dual-imaging method, in which a second imaging channel simultaneously recorded a reflectance signal with much higher SNR. The motion in the image was then estimated as a rigid translation using the normalized cross-correlation (NCC) in the reflectance image series, and compensated for in the matching fluorescence image series. This method produced fluorescence images in which sub-cellular structures could be identified after averaging > 1000 frames. The image registration using rigid translations was successful with anaesthetized animals and some human subjects. However, this method does not produce acceptable images in subjects that are unable to fixate. More importantly, the light safety limits are based on data from healthy subjects, and very little is known about how the damage thresholds change with eye disease, in particular, from the photochemical point of view. Therefore, in order to reduce the subjects' exposure to light and increase SNR, more advanced registration methods such as the one discussed here are required.

The next section presents the requirements for adequate sampling in scanning ophthalmic instruments. This is followed by the introduction of a mathematical model used for fitting the retinal motion transformation functions based on physical arguments. Section 4 details how the parameters of the model can be estimated from the image pairs, and illustrates the improvement that can be obtained from this registration with real data.

2   Eye Movements and Sampling Frequency

When subjects are being imaged in a high-magnification scanning ophthalmic instruments they suppress all voluntary eye movement by fixating onto a target. Fixation, however, does not suppress involuntary eye movements like tremor, drift and micro-saccades [15–19]. These eye movements have amplitudes comparable to or greater than the Rayleigh criterion for lateral resolution [20]. In a human eye with an 8 mm pupil diameter and a wavelength (λ) in the 0.5–1.0 μm range, the resolution limit is 16–31 arcsec. Tremor is a fast jerky random movement with amplitudes of 10–20 arcsec at frequencies of up to 200 Hz [15–17, 21]. According to the Whittaker-Nyquist-Shannon theorem, in order to reproduce tremor faithfully, the sampling rate should be at least 400 Hz. Drift is a continuous motion in a random direction, with speeds that could vary from 5–20 arcmin/s in normal subjects [18, 21], to 200 arcmin/s in subjects with diseased

Table 1. Temporal frequencies required to adequately sample retinal motion in scanning ophthalmic instruments due to involuntary movement in the fixating human eye

Eye movement	Minimum sampling frequency (Hz)
Drift (normal subjects, $\lambda = 0.5\mu$m)	150
Tremor	400
Drift (diseased retina, $\lambda = 0.5\mu$m)	1500
Micro-saccade	5000

retinas [19]. According to the resolution criterion for $\lambda = 0.5\mu m$ adequate sampling requires a minimum frequency of 150 Hz for normal subjects and 1.5 kHz for subjects with poor fixation. Microsaccades are short fast eye movements that compensate for the gaze drift, with amplitudes between 1 and 20 arcmin [21] and speeds in the order of 10 deg/s. Adequately sampling this type of eye movement would require sampling frequencies greater than 5 kHz. Note that the sampling frequencies mentioned above, and summarized in table (1), assume the absence of noise in the sampling process.

3   Transformation Function Model

The registration of 2D images requires transformation functions that map the coordinates (x, y) in a given (current) frame onto the corresponding coordinates (X, Y) in another (reference) frame. These mapping functions should be part of a mathematical model that adequately describes the imaging process,

$$X = f_x(x, y; p_1, \ldots, p_n),$$
$$Y = f_y(x, y; q_1, \ldots, q_n), \tag{1}$$

with the model parameters p_j and q_j estimated using a number of control points (x_i, y_i), (X_i, Y_i) with $i = 1, \ldots, N$.

In scanning ophthalmic instruments, the image distortion due to eye movement is minimized by scanning the retina as fast as both the technology and light safety limits allow [13]. Fast scanners (y-axis) currently used for creating 2D rectangular images are either rotating polygon mirrors or resonant galvanometric optical scanners. On the other hand, the slow scanner (x-axis) is usually a non-resonant galvanometric optical scanner. The image line capture rate along the x-axis is currently in the order of 8–16 kHz. For resonant scanners the line capture occurs in the semi-cycle of the mirror oscillation, usually referred to as the forward scanning. Thus, the line acquisition time is around 20–40 μs. According to the eye movement data from the previous section, retinal features would displace about 0.01 μm due to tremor, $0.004 - 0.04\,\mu m$ due to drift and 0.12 μm due to microsaccades during the recording of a single image line. Given that these values are an order of magnitude smaller than the resolution limit, it is reasonable to assume that the retinal motion can be neglected within each image line. If, in addition, it is assumed that involuntary eye rotations can be neglected, then the form of the transformation functions simplifies to

$$X = x + \epsilon_x(x), \tag{2}$$
$$Y = y + \epsilon_y(x). \tag{3}$$

Note that the linear terms have unit amplitude because the scanning speed does not change across frames. The functions ϵ_x and ϵ_y represent eye motion along the corresponding axes, and describe the compression and shear observed in the retinal images, respectively.

The eye is a mechanical system with inertia and therefore, the functions ϵ_x and ϵ_y can be modeled as having finite bandwidths, with an associated maximum frequency $f_{\max}$. If the sampling frequency achieved with every image line in a scanning system is greater than $2f_{\max}$, then ϵ_x and ϵ_y can be described as a sum of cosines with increasing frequencies. The amplitude of those cosines can be calculated using the discrete cosine transform II (DCT), retaining only the coefficients associated to the frequencies $f_i \leq f_{\max}$,

$$X = x + p_0 + \sqrt{2} \sum_{k=1}^{N/2} p_k \cos\left[\frac{\pi}{N} k \left(x + \frac{1}{2}\right)\right], \tag{4}$$

$$Y = y + q_0 + \sqrt{2} \sum_{k=1}^{N/2} q_k \cos\left[\frac{\pi}{N} k \left(y + \frac{1}{2}\right)\right]. \tag{5}$$

The use of the DCT implies that the N control points are equally spaced along the x-axis in the current frame.

4 Transformation Function Estimation

The parameters of the transformation functions in Eqs. (4) and (5) are estimated following a similar approach to that followed by Stevenson and Roorda [14]. A frame with minimal distortion is manually selected as the reference, while the other frame (current) is divided into strips, each of them with only a few lines along the direction of the fast scanner (y-axis). The actual number of lines on each strip must be manually selected, based on the SNR and the structure present on each data set. Then, the NCC between each strip and the reference frame is calculated, and its maximum within a certain region of interest (ROI) located. The dimensions and location of the of the ROI is determined by the maximum eye motion considered acceptable. The position of the maximum within the NCC matrix corresponds to the x- and y-shifts of the strip with respect to the reference frame. The definition of the NCC between the reference frame (R) and the current strip (S) used in this work is,

$$C_{R,S}(m, n) = \frac{\sum_{i,j} R(i,j)\, S(m+i, n+j)}{\sqrt{\sum_{i,j} R(i,j)^2 \sum_{p,q} S(p,q)^2}}, \tag{6}$$

where the sums are performed over pixels in the overlap area between the reference frame and the strip. The actual calculations are performed by taking advantage of the correlation theorem in the Fourier domain, a fast implementation of the discrete Fourier transform (DFT), and with adequate zero-padding to avoid periodization artifacts. The NCC definition in terms of the DFT can be written as

$$C_{R,S} = \frac{\text{IDFT}\left[\text{DFT}\left[R_p\right]^* \text{DFT}\left[S_p\right]\right]}{\sqrt{\text{IDFT}\left[\text{DFT}\left[P_R\right]^* \text{DFT}\left[S_p^2\right]\right] \text{IDFT}\left[\text{DFT}\left[R_p^2\right]^* \text{DFT}\left[P_S\right]\right]}}, \tag{7}$$

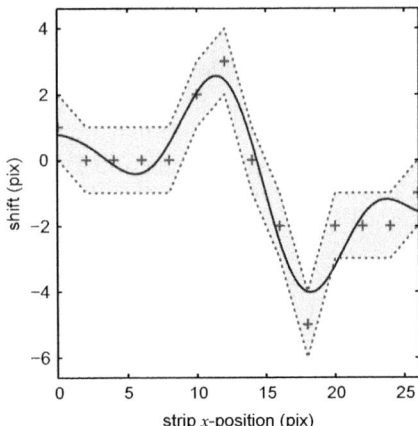

Fig. 1. Fitted ϵ_x model (blue line) of a sample set of current frame strip shifts (red crosses) using only the first $N/2$ coefficients returned by the DCT. The shaded area indicates the acceptable region, based on a shift uncertainty of 1 pixel. Note that although the fit might appear poor with respect to the data points, it is consistent with the uncertainty limits. In this example, each image strip consisted of two lines.

where IDFT denotes inverse DFT, * indicates complex conjugate and R_p and S_p are the zero-padded reference frame and strip, respectively. P_R and P_S are zero-padded templates of the reference frame and strip, with unit value over the corresponding pixels. It is worth noting that the use of the NCC does not require any prior knowledge of the structures being imaged, and it uses all information in the image, as opposed to other algorithms with lower computational complexity [22]. In addition, the normalization used here makes the shift estimation robust to overall intensity fluctuations, which are very common in ophthalmic instruments, due to subject misalignment, tear film break up, etc. The NCC was implemented using the correlation theorem (Eq. 7) and the graphic processing units of CUDA-enabled graphics cards (Nvidia Corporation, Santa Clara, California, USA). The DFT was calculated using the CuFFT function. Figure 2 shows a plot of the performance of the NCC implemented using the CuFFT using single- and double-precision, against a double-precision Matlab implementation of Eq. 7 using the FFTW package (http://www.fftw.org/). Given current frame rates in ophthalmic instruments, the achieved performance allows real-time image registration, that produces motion signals that can be fed back to the scanning mirrors, to stabilize the imaging raster in the selected retinal location. There are two sources of error inherent to the shift estimation method. First, the use of the NCC on images with a finite number of pixels, which leads to a quantization of the shift values. This error can be reduced to an arbitrary level of accuracy by increasing the pixel density through interpolation, provided that computing power and memory requirements are not a limitation. The second source of uncertainty in the shift estimation comes from distortion within each strip. This error can be reduced by decreasing the number of lines in each strip, provided the information left

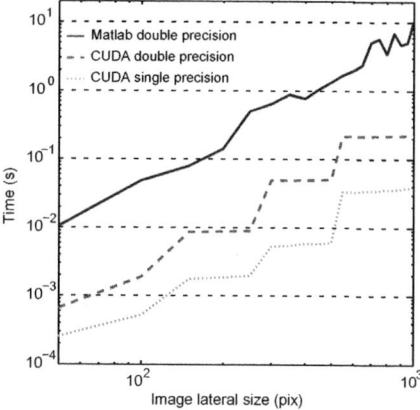

Fig. 2. Evaluation of the NCC implementation using CuFFT (CUDA) running on a GeForce GTX 285 graphics card from Nvidia for different (square) frame sizes. For reference, the performance of the FFTW in Matlab running on an Intel Xeon CPU E5430 using Microsoft Windows XP is provided.

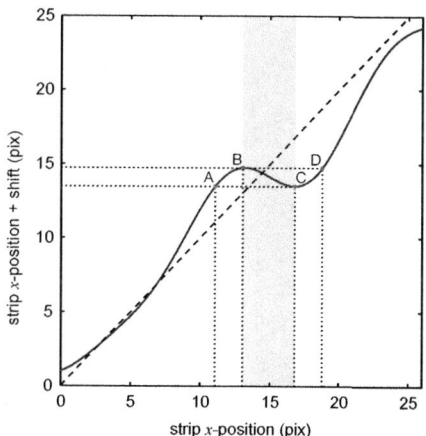

Fig. 3. Transformation model (blue line) corresponding to the ϵ_x from figure (1). The black dashed line shows the linear term of Eq. (4) that would correspond to the model in the absence of eye movement. The portion of the current frame corresponding to the decreasing part of the curve (shaded area) is not considered for the image registration.

within the strip is sufficient to correctly estimate the shifts. Once the x- and y-shifts of the (N) strips are estimated, they are used to fit the models in Eqs. (4) and (5). Note that the curve calculated using only $N/2$ cosine terms will in most cases not pass through all the control points (see figure 1). If the sample density of the strip and reference frame are not increased when calculating the

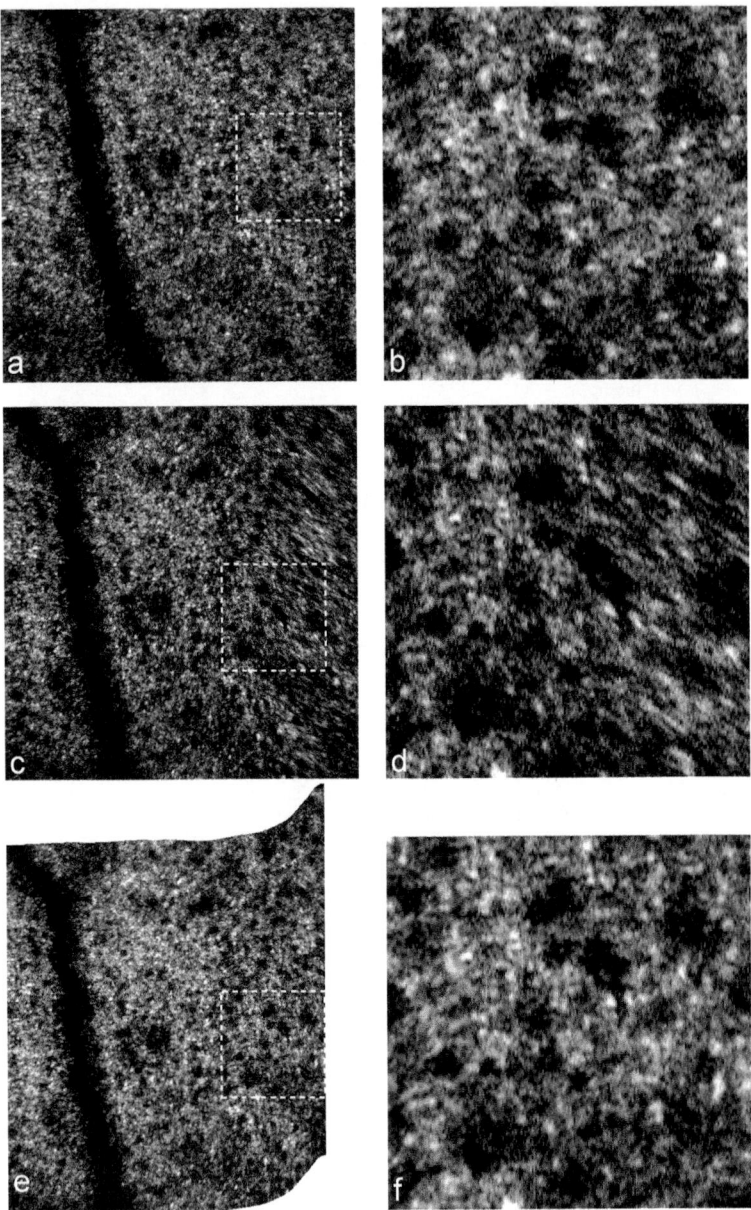

Fig. 4. Photoreceptor layer of a subject with poor fixation: (a) reference frame with minimal distortion, (c) a frame affected by eye motion and (e) the same frame after registration with the strip-based method. The images in panels (b), (d) and (f) show the regions indicated with the dashed squares in (a), (c), and (e) respectively.

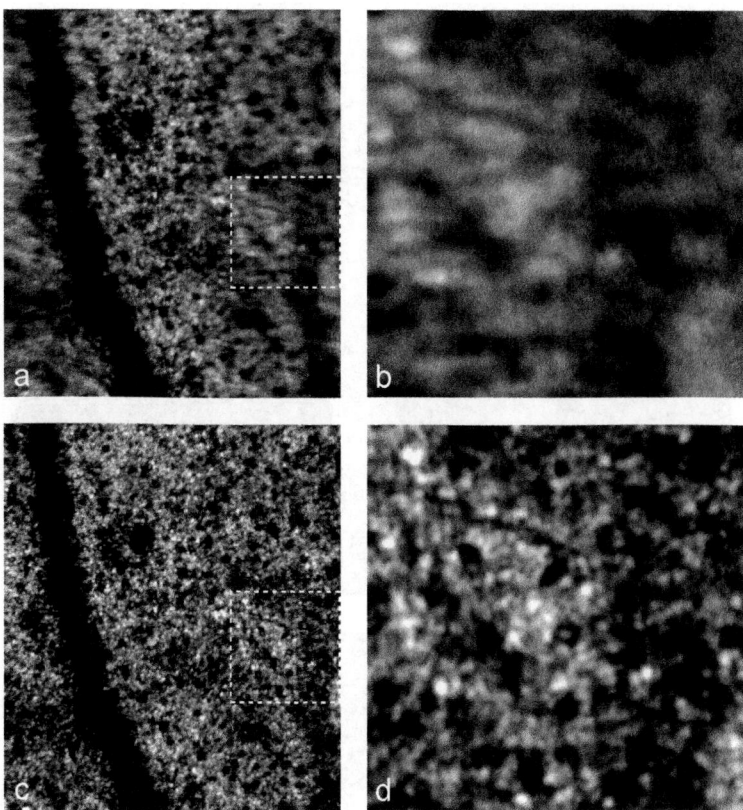

Fig. 5. Images that result from registering the sequence of 50 images that include those of Fig. 4 using: (a) the rigid registration and (b) the method proposed in this work. The latter method used 16 pixel-wide strips in a sequence of images of 708×688 pixels. The panels (b) and (d) show the regions indicated with the dashed squares in (a) and (c), respectively. Note the increased contrast and resolution achieved with the strip-based registration method, and the noise reduction with respect to figure 4.

NCC, then the minimum uncertainty is due to shift quantization into integer values (± 0.5 pixels). As mentioned before, another source of error is the image distortion within the strip. The effect of this source of error is difficult to quantify, as it varies with the structure being imaged, the amplitude, and speed of eye movement. A metric of distortion within a strip is the NCC value associated with the estimated shifts. These NCC values can be compared against a threshold in order to accept or discard strips.

Once the transformation functions are estimated from the strip shifts, the resulting curve from the x-shift has to be split into strictly monotonic intervals When the curve is not strictly increasing, the same retinal patch is imaged multiple times in a single current frame. For example, according to the curve in Fig. (3), the section of the current frame corresponding to the intervals AB, BC

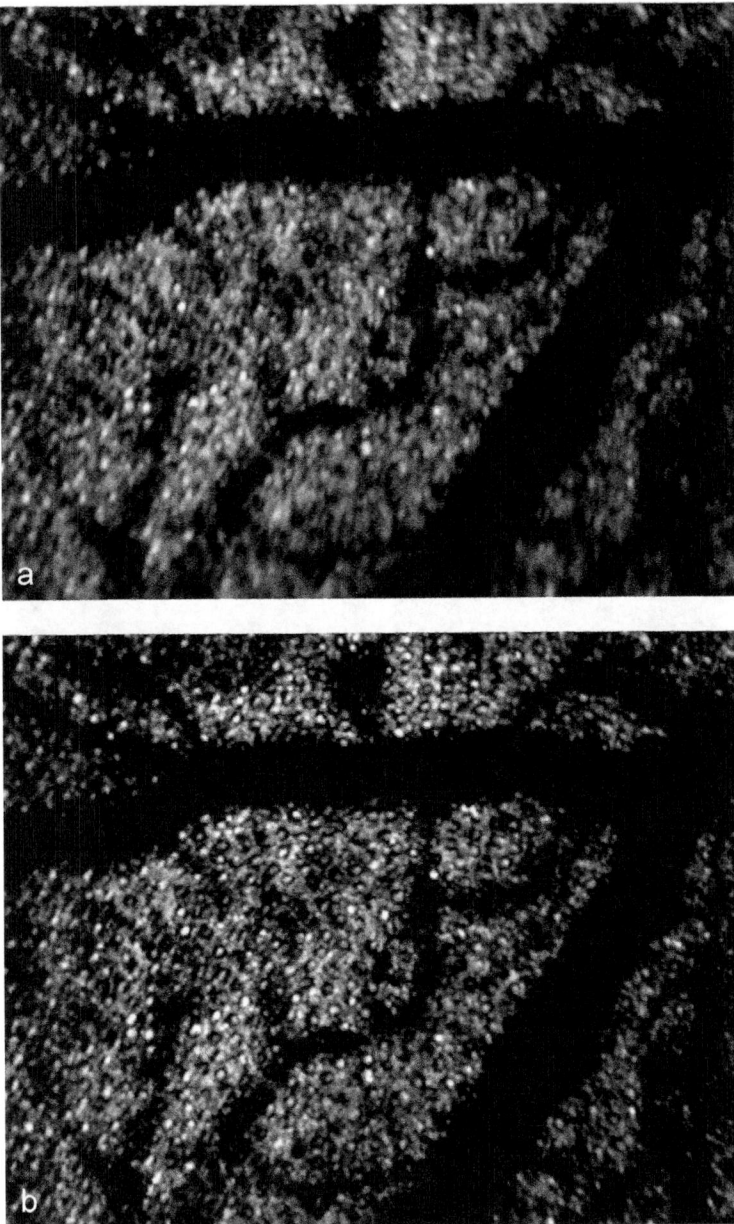

Fig. 6. Output image showing the photoreceptor mosaic of a healthy human subject with stable fixation, after registering a sequence of 500 images acquired using a reflectance AOSLO using: (a) rigid registration and (b) the method proposed in this work. Note the contrast and resolution increase achieved with the strip-based method.

and CD would all show the same retinal patch. The BC segment indicates retinal movement in the direction of the slow scanner. In practice, the corresponding portion of the image would be inverted and too distorted to be useful. There is no need to verify that the y-transformation function is monotonic because of the high speed of the fast scanner with respect to eye motion.

Finally, each monotonic interval in the x-transformation function and the corresponding interval in the y-transformation function are used to calculate the values of the registered image over the grid of pixels of the reference frame, using a bilinear interpolation. In this way, the reference and the registered images can be summed to produce images with higher SNR.

Figures 4, 5 and 6 illustrate how the proposed strip-based method works and how it performs with respect to a simple rigid translation. Figures 4, and 5 show the retina of a human subject suffering from blue cone monochromacy, a condition that results in very poor visual acuity and fixation. The panels in figure 4 are single frames taken from a sequence of 50 frames, while those in figure 5 correspond to the averaged registered sequence. For comparison, registered images from a subject with no eye conditions and good fixation are provided in Fig. 6.

5   Summary and Discussion

We have shown that when the scanning in ophthalmic instruments is sufficiently fast with respect to the speed of involuntary eye movement, the mapping functions become the addition of a linear term and a single variable function. Then, based on experimental data on eye movement amplitude and speed in the fixating eye, minimum sampling frequencies for these instruments were discussed. Assuming finite bandwidth of the involuntary eye motion, a method for estimating the transformation functions was presented. The proposed registration method can be used to improve the signal-to-noise ratio (SNR) of high-resolution reflectance, single-photon fluorescence and phase images from the live retina. Currently, the only part of the registration process that requires significant user input is the selection of the reference frame, which is also necessary for rigid registration or any other registration method. Finally, two examples illustrating the dramatic image quality improvement provided by the proposed method with respect to rigid translation were presented.

Acknowledgements

Alfredo Dubra-Suarez, Ph.D., holds a Career Award at the Scientific Interface from the Burroughs Welcome Fund. This research was partially supported by the National Institute for Health, Bethesda, Maryland through the grants BRP-EY014375 and 5 K23 EY016700.

References

1. Liang, J., Williams, D.R., Miller, D.T.: Supernormal vision and high-resolution retinal imaging through adaptive optics. J. Opt. Soc. Am. A 14(11), 2884–2892 (1997)

2. Rha, J., Jonnal, R.S., Thorn, K.E., Qu, J., Zhang, Y., Miller, D.T.: Adaptive optics flood-illumination camera for high speed retinal imaging. Opt. Exp. 14(10), 4552–4569 (2006)
3. Hermann, B., Fernandez, E.J., Unterhuber, A., Sattmann, H., Fercher, A.F., Drexler, W., Prieto, P.M., Artal, P.: Adaptive-optics ultrahigh-resolution optical coherence tomography. Opt. Lett. 29(18), 2142–2144 (2004)
4. Zawadzki, R., Jones, S., Olivier, S., Zhao, M., Bower, B., Izatt, J., Choi, S., Laut, S., Werner, J.: Adaptive-optics optical coherence tomography for high-resolution and high-speed 3D retinal in vivo imaging. Opt. Exp. 13(21), 8532–8546 (2005)
5. Fernandez, E.J., Povazay, B., Hermann, B., Unterhuber, A., Sattmann, H., Prieto, P.M., Leitgeb, R., Ahnelt, P., Artal, P., Drexler, W.: Three-dimensional adaptive optics ultrahigh-resolution optical coherence tomography using a liquid crystal spatial light modulator. Vision Res. 14(20), 8900–8917 (2006)
6. Zhang, Y., Rha, J., Jonnal, R., Miller, D.: Adaptive optics parallel spectral domain optical coherence tomography for imaging the living retina. Opt. Exp. 13(12), 4792–4811 (2005)
7. Merino, D., Dainty, C., Bradu, A., Podoleanu, A.G.: Adaptive optics enhanced simultaneous en-face optical coherence tomography and scanning laser ophthalmoscopy. Opt. Exp. 14(8), 3345–3353 (2006)
8. Bigelow, C.E., Iftimia, N.V., Ferguson, R.D., Ustun, T.E., Bloom, B., Hammer, D.X.: Compact multimodal adaptive-optics spectral-domain optical coherence tomography instrument for retinal imaging. J. Opt. Soc. Am. A 24(5), 1327–1336 (2007)
9. Roorda, A., Romero-Borja, F., Donnelly III, W.J., Queener, H., Hebert, T.J., Campbell, M.C.W.: Adaptive optics scanning laser ophthalmoscopy. Opt. Exp. 10(9), 405–412 (2002)
10. Gray, D.C., Merigan, W., Wolfing, J.I., Gee, B.P., Porter, J., Dubra, A., Twietmeyer, T.H., Ahamd, K., Tumbar, R., Reinholz, F., Williams, D.R.: In vivo fluorescence imaging of primate retinal ganglion cells and retinal pigment epithelial cells. Opt. Exp. 14(16), 7144–7158 (2006)
11. Burns, S.A., Tumbar, R., Elsner, A.E., Ferguson, D., Hammer, D.X.: Large-field-of-view, modular, stabilized, adaptive-optics-based scanning laser ophthalmoscope. J. Opt. Soc. Am. A 24(5), 1313–1326 (2007)
12. Morgan, J.I.W., Dubra, A., Wolfe, R., Merigan, W.H., Williams, D.R.: In vivo autofluorescence imaging of the human and macaque retinal pigment epithelial cell mosaic. Invest. Ophth. Vis. Sci. 50(3), 1350–1359 (2009)
13. American National Standard for safe use of lasers (ANSI Z136.1), Laser Institute of America, Orlando, Florida, USA (2007)
14. Stevenson, S.B., Roorda, A.: Correcting for miniature eye movements in high resolution scanning laser ophthalmoscopy. In: Proc. SPIE, vol. 5688A, pp. 145–151 (2005)
15. Hart Jr., W.H.: Adler's physiology of the eye: clinical application, 9th edn., Mosby-Year Book Inc., 11830 Westline Industrial Drive, St. Louis, Missouri 63146 (1992)
16. Riggs, L.A., Armington, J.C., Ratliff, F.: Motions of the retinal image during fixation. J. Opt. Soc. Am. 44(4), 315–321 (1954)
17. Eizenman, M., Hallett, P.E., Frecker, R.C.: Power spectra for ocular drift and tremor. Vision Res. 25(11), 1635–1640 (1985)

18. Ditchburn, R.W., Ginsborg, B.L.: Involuntary eye movements during fixation. J. Physiol. 119, 1–17 (1953)
19. Whittaker, S.G., Budd, J., Cummings, R.W.: Eccentric fixation with macular scotoma. Invest. Ophth. Vis. Sci. 29(2), 268–278 (1988)
20. Smith, G., Atchison, D.A.: The eye and visual optical instrumentation, 1st edn. Cambridge University Press, Cambridge (1997)
21. Charman, N.: Handbook of optics: Vision and vision optics. In: Bass, M. (ed.) Optics of the Eye, ch. 1, 3rd edn., vol. III. Mc Graw Hill, New York (2009)
22. Arathorn, D.W., Yang, Q., Vogel, C.R., Zhang, Y., Tiruveedhula, P., Roorda, A.: Retinally stabilized cone-targeted stimulus delivery. Opt. Exp. 15(21), 13731–13744 (2007)

Registration of 3D Retinal Optical Coherence Tomography Data and 2D Fundus Images

Radim Kolar and Pavel Tasevsky

Department of Biomedical Engineering,
Faculty of Electrical Engineering and Communication,
Brno University of Technology, Brno, Kolejni 4, 61200, Czech Republic
kolarr@feec.vutbr.cz

Abstract. This paper is focused on multimodal and multidimensional image data registration: the three-dimensional retinal optical coherence tomographic (OCT) data and two-dimensional color images of fundus. The registration of these two modalities is not common in retinal image processing, but it might help to remove the moving artifacts in OCT and correct the true positions of acquired OCT scans on retina. The proposed framework consists of three steps: global dataset pre-registration, preprocessing and OCT to fundus image registration. Two alternating registration criteria are used in the main step due to changing spatial image properties. Three-parametric spatial transformation (shift and scale) for each OCT scan and exhaustive search is used in this preliminarily work. The achieved results are presented on several examples.

1 Introduction

The optical coherence tomography (OCT) has found many applications in medical and biological sciences, mainly in clinical ophthalmology. On of the most important application is an early glaucoma diagnosis either based on the examination of the retinal nerve fibre layer from cross-sectional scans [1] or based on the optic disc cup and rim segmentation [2]. Another clinical application for glaucoma diagnosis uses autofluorescent images produced also by OCT devices, e.g. [3].

Nowadays devices work in the spectral domain, which enables faster acquisition of particular cross-sectional tomographic images (B-scans) of retinal structures [4]. The data set from one measurement is therefore three dimensional (3D). Although the data acquisition is fast, eye movement, including fast microsaccades, can cause misalignments of neighboring B-scans [5]. The advanced eye-tracking technology can help to minimize these artifacts but misalignments can still occur and can disturb the process of data processing and analysis.

Furthermore, the eye-tracker aligns these B-scans with respect to the image obtained by scanning laser (SL) method, which can also suffer from motion artifacts, because of the scanning acquisition. These drawbacks lead to idea to use the retinal images, acquired by digital fundus camera, for misalignments correction. The main advantage of digital fundus cameras is that, they acquire retinal image at once, without scanning. These cameras are also cheap and became

B. Fischer, B. Dawant, and C. Lorenz (Eds.): WBIR 2010, LNCS 6204, pp. 72–82, 2010.

a standard examination tool in ophthalmology clinics. The registration of this two different modalities open a new possibilities of image fusion/visualization and qualitative and quantitative comparison of these two modalities. Example of retinal image registration and fusion is for example in [6].

This paper describes part of our ongoing research dealing with registration, visualization and analysis of OCT image sets and 2D fundus photographes. In this preliminary study we are mainly studying the appropriate criteria for registration on several test image set. The results are summarized in the following sections.

2   Image Data

The image data were acquired by two different imaging devices: OCT device (Spectralis OCT, Heidelberg Engineering) and digital color fundus camera (Canon CR-1). One color image taken by this color camera is shown in Fig.1a and images from the same eye taken by OCT are shown in Fig. 1b,c. The SL image is a gray scale image taken by laser scanning technique. (Fig. 1b). One typical B-scan image (cross-sectional image) acquired through the retinal tissue across the optic disc is in Fig. 1c, where several retinal layers can be recognized.

3   Registration Method

The main aim of this preliminary study is to find an appropriate framework for fundus image and B-scan image registration. This registration task consists of three main steps:

1. Global pre-registration: global correction of rotation and selection of region of interest.
2. OCT and fundus data preprocessing.
3. B-scan to fundus image registration.

3.1   Global Pre-registration

A FFT-based technique of phase correlation is a method for image registration, which can cover several spatial transformations - shift, rotation and scaling. This method is based on the Fourier shift theorem. Let $f_1(x, y)$ and $f_2(x, y)$ be two functions, which differs only by displacement x_0 and y_0, i.e. [7]

$$f_2(x, y) = f_1(x - x_0, y - y_0).$$ (1)

The corresponding Fourier transforms are, in this case, related as

$$F_2(u, v) = F_1(u, v)e^{-j(ux_0 + vy_0)}.$$ (2)

Then, the normalized cross power spectrum is given by

$$\frac{F_2(u, v)F_1(u, v)^*}{|F_2(u, v)F_1(u, v)^*|} = e^{-j(ux_0 + vy_0)}.$$ (3)

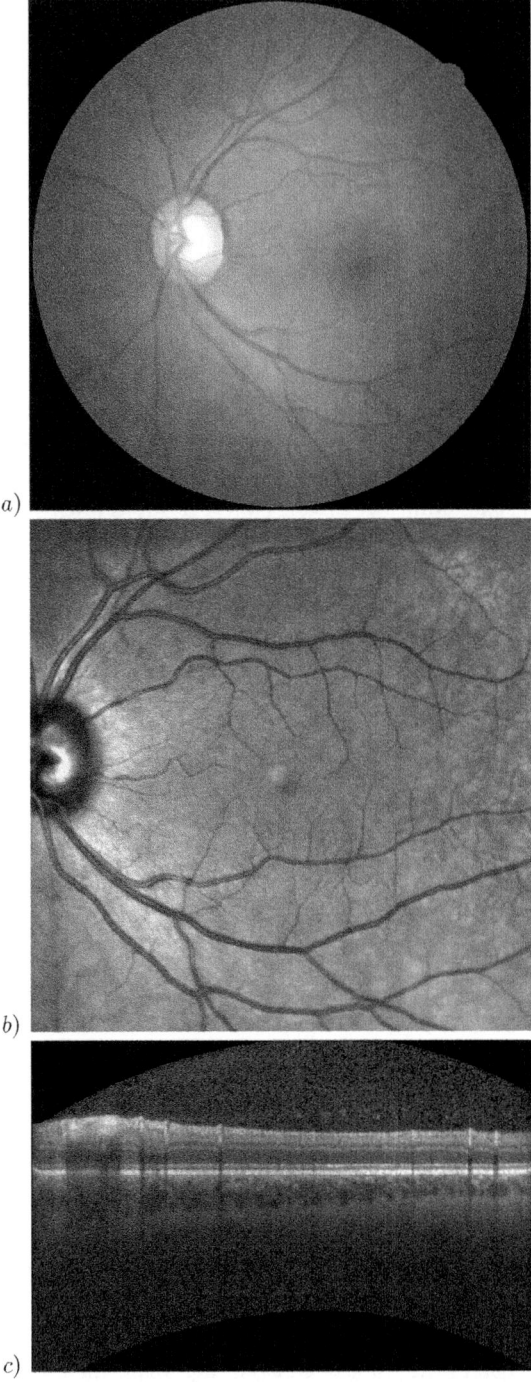

Fig. 1. a) Image from the fundus camera; b) Scanning laser image from OCT; c) One B-scan from OCT

Taking the inverse Fourier transform of right hand side term leads to Dirac function $\delta(x - x_0, y - y_0)$ at coordinates (x_0, y_0) defining the spatial shift [8]. This approach can be also extended to spatial rotation, which leads to the Fourier-Mellin transform. According to Fourier transform properties, the image rotation and shift:

$$f_2(x, y) = f_1(x \cos \theta_0 + y \sin \theta_0 - x_0, -x \sin \theta_0 + y \cos \theta_0 - y_0) \qquad (4)$$

is related in the spectral Fourier domain as:

$$F_2(u, v) = e^{-j(ux_0 + vy_0)} F_1(u \cos \theta_0 + v \sin \theta_0, -u \sin \theta_0 + v \cos \theta_0). \qquad (5)$$

Therefore, the magnitude spectra are the same, but one of these is rotated replica of the other. The rotation can be recovered by representing the spectra in polar coordinates, where rotation becomes shift, which can be easily estimated by phase correlation (3).

It is also possible to estimate the scale of two images. If $f_1(x, y)$ is a scaled replica of $f_2(x, y)$ with the scale factor s (the same factor for horizontal and vertical directions). The Fourier spectra are related as:

$$F_2(u, v) = \frac{1}{|s^2|} F_1(u/s, v/s). \qquad (6)$$

This formula can be utilized by converting axes to logarithmic scale. More details are given for example in [7].

Several practical steps should be considered for implementation. First, the Discrete version of Fourier transform (DFT) has to be used and 2D window function (e.g. Hanning or Hamming window) has to be applied before taking these transforms, due to periodicity of DFT. Second, when dealing with the retinal images, the circle defining the field of view (see Fig.1a) must be eliminated by smoothing kernel. Third, we can roughly match the resolution of fundus and OCT data using *a priori* determined scaling factor obtained from resolution of both devices. The fundus image was decimated with factor 2 in both axis in our case.

The result obtained by this phase correlation approach for registration of Fig. 1a and Fig. 1b is shown in Fig. 2. This pre-registration step must be applied in order to compensate rotation of the SL image with respect to the fundus image and to define the region of interest (ROI).

The next section describes the preprocessing of OCT scans and color fundus images.

3.2   Preprocessing

The preprocessing is a crucial step because of multimodality and 3D-to-2D matching. The flowchart of preprocessing is shown in Fig. 3. The RGB color fundus image is converted into grayscale image as a mean of the green and blue channel, because light reflections from the corresponding wavelengths carry information about the main retinal structures (blood-vessels, macula, optic disc and retinal nerve fibres) [9]. Red channel is ignored. The preprocessing of this

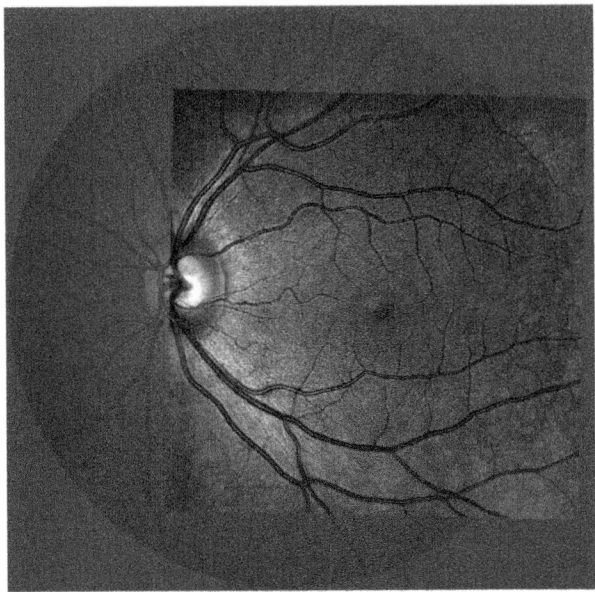

Fig. 2. Result of global pre-registration using phase correlation. The SL image was translated, rotated and scaled to match the color fundus image.

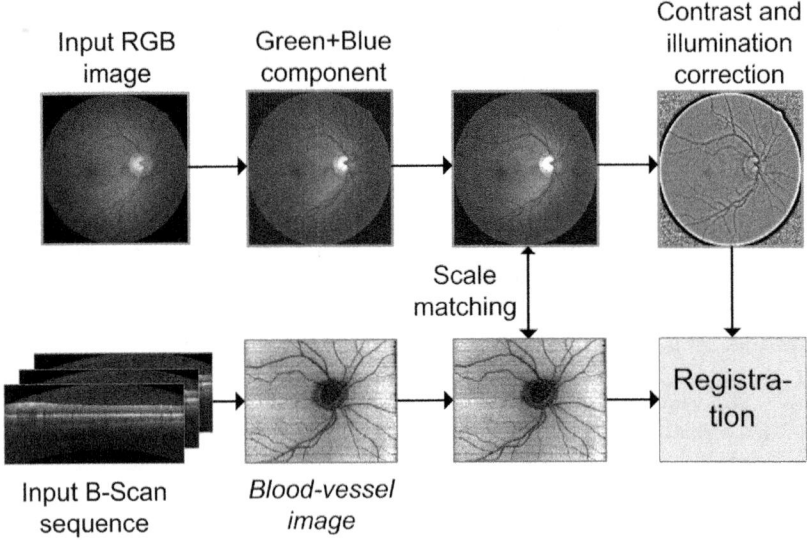

Fig. 3. Flowchart of preprocessing method

fundus image ends with correction of the non-uniform illumination and contrast enhancement. The method is based on a simple additive-multiplication illumination model [10]. To estimate this nonuniform illumination function an averaging large kernel is used for filtering. The mask size is 51×51 pixels, which is large enough with respect to the maximum blood-vessel diameter (about 20 pixels). From this filtered fundus image, the normalized correction coefficients are computed:

$$r_{ij} = \frac{\max f_{ij}^{aver}}{f_{ij}^{aver}}, \tag{7}$$

where f_{ij}^{aver} is the spatially averaged fundus image. These coefficients are used for image correction as:

$$f_{ij}^{corr} = (f_{ij} - f_{ij}^{aver})r_{ij} + c, \tag{8}$$

where c is a constant to make the mean value of corrected image approximately equal to 128 and f_{ij} is the measured image. To eliminate to border effect, the intensity values in this image are cropped into range 0 and 255.

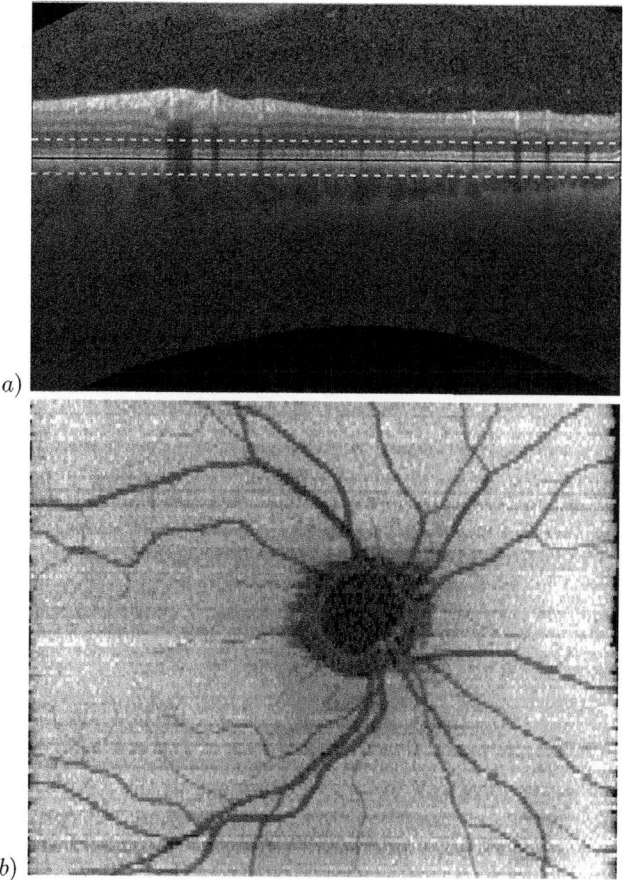

Fig. 4. a) One B-scan with automatically determined region containing the RPE (dashed lines) and the row with the highest contrast (black line) located approximately between the dashed lines. b) The reconstructed 2D *blood-vessel image.*

The 3D OCT data are also preprocessed starting with conversion to 2D using only one row from each B-scan. It can be seen from Fig. 1c, that blood vessels create shadows. This influences the pixel values below the blood vessels, mainly in the retinal pigment epithelium (RPE). The RPE is the brightest layer in the deeper retinal layers and can be relatively easily identified computing the B-scan profile through the columns [11]. The automatically determined RPE position including fixed predefined row range is presented in Fig. 4a by the dashed lines. The black line in this figure depicts the row with the highest contrast (*blood-vessel row*). This row selection is performed for each B-scan in measured set to reconstruct a new 2D image (*blood-vessel image*, see Fig.4b).

3.3   Registration Algorithm

The registration starts with one manually determined corresponding point in the fundus image and *blood-vessel image*. These corresponding positions can slightly differ, because they are used as a rough starting estimation for whole registration, which will be refined. Usually the center of the optic disc has been marked, but other starting points can be used (e.g. blood-vessels bifurcations or crossings). This step determines the correspondence between I^{th} row from the *blood-vessel image* (OCT_I) and J^{th} row from fundus image. Thereafter the iterative registration runs in the following steps, starting with $i = I$, $j = J$:

1. Select i^{th} row from the *blood-vessel image*, OCT_i.
2. Select range of rows R_j in the scanning direction from j^{th} row (see Fig. 5).
3. Search for the optimal parameters of the spatial transformation

$$max_{\alpha_i}\{\, C(\, R_j,\, T_{\alpha_i}(OCT_i)\,)\,\}, \tag{9}$$

where C is the criterium and T_{α_i} is spatial transformation with vector of parameters α_i.
4. Set $j = J_{optimal}$, where $J_{optimal}$ is an optimal row computed from optimization results.
5. Increase/decrease i, according to the scanning direction.

These steps are performed for each row from *blood-vessel image*. The selection of criterion C and spatial transformation T_α is discussed below.

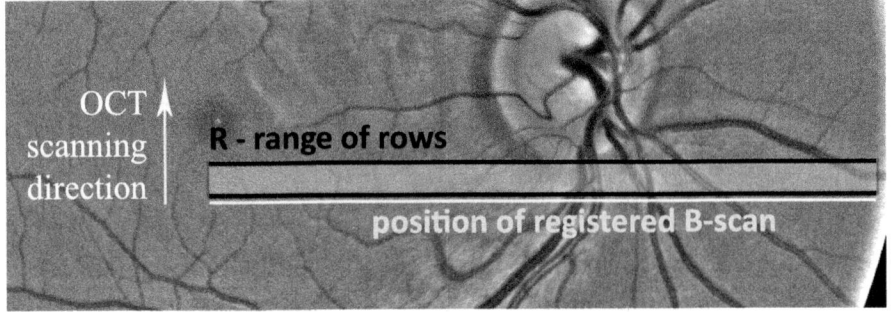

Fig. 5. Illustration of the registration process. See *registration steps* in Section 3.3.

Spatial Transformation. Three parameters are optimized during registration for each row from the *blood-vessel image* in the fundus image: its translations in x, y axis and its scaling in x axis (for horizontal scanning). Although the image scales were roughly matched during preprocessing, precise scaling will be found for each row separately.

Criterion. Several criteria were tested with respect to the multimodality and image properties. It can be seen that the blood-vessels are darker than background in both images (preprocessed fundus image and *blood-vessel image*), which leads to correlation criterion r:

$$r = \frac{\sum_{i=1}^{N}(x_i - \overline{x})(y_i - \overline{y})}{\sqrt{\sum_{i=1}^{N}(x_i - \overline{x})^2 \sum_{i=1}^{N}(y_i - \overline{y})^2}} \tag{10}$$

for two overlapping rows x_i, y_i with length N and corresponding means $\overline{x}, \overline{y}$. This has been successfully tested on the main part of the image. Nevertheless, the optic disc is darker than the background in the *blood-vessel image* and brighter in fundus image and therefore negative correlation must be considered. But we have found that this negative value gives false position of the correlation maxima. Therefore, mutual information has been also studied to cope with this problem. We have used the normalized version, defined via marginal and joint (Shannon) entropies $H(x)$, $H(y)$ and $H(x, y)$, respectively [12]:

$$MI = 2 - 2\,\frac{H(x, y)}{H(x) + H(y)}. \tag{11}$$

It has been observed that the results were comparable or worse in comparison to correlation metric up to B-scans crossing the optic disc. Therefore an alternating

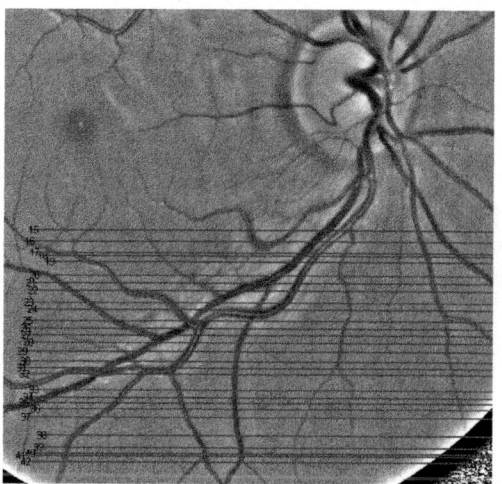 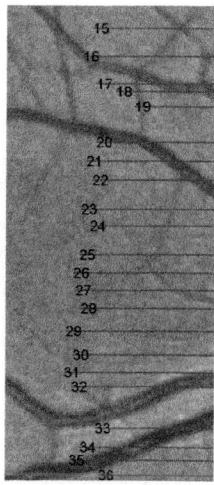

Fig. 6. Left: The lines depict the positions of B-scans within the fundus image. Right: The detail image showing the numbers of B-scans and their spatial variations.

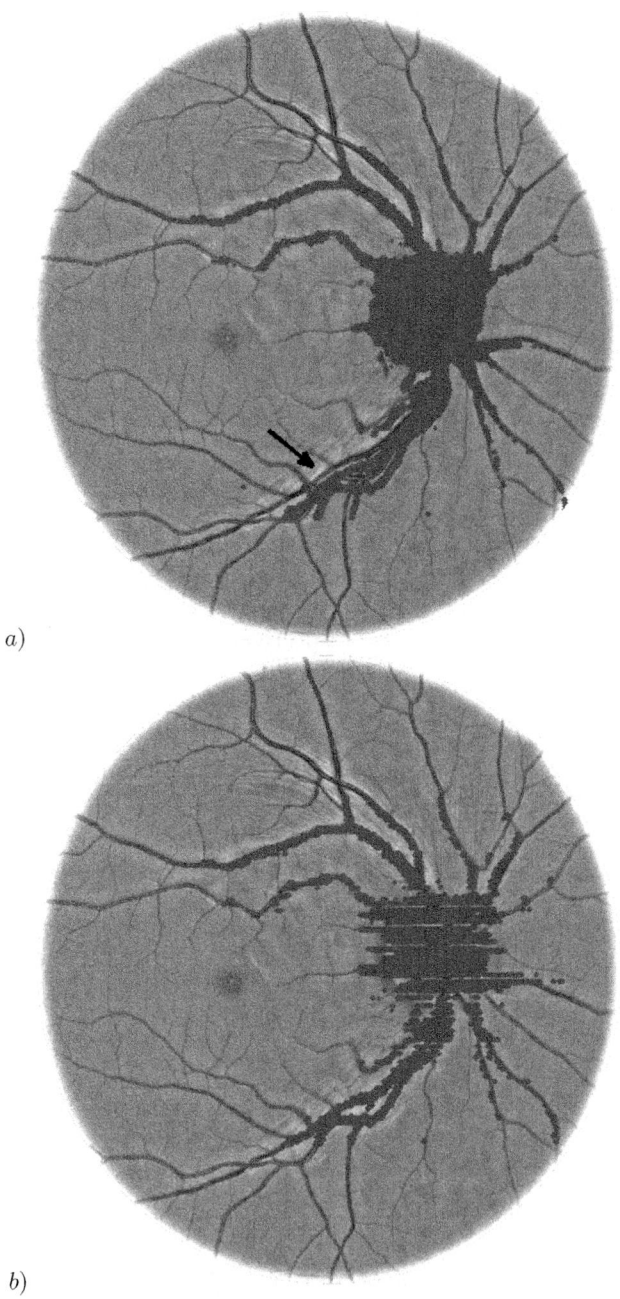

a)

b)

Fig. 7. The positions of the blood-vessels segmented in *blood-vessel image* are depicted in fundus image as gray dots: a) before registration, b) after registration

criteria approach has been proposed: if the correlation coefficient was positive, the corresponding optimal transformation parameters α_i has been used; if the the correlation was negative, we switched to mutual information criterion. This approach gives satisfactory results (see Section 4) than using only single criterion.

Searching Strategy. In this testing phase, the method has been implemented without optimization to ensure, that global maximum will be always found. This leads to exhaustive computation in 3D parametric space, but it can be easily parallelize when searching for the optimal position of B-scan within the fundus image. Matlab parallel computing toolbox was used for implementation.

4   Results and Discussion

The proposed approach was tested and results were evaluated on semi-subjective level. The positions of registered B-scans were visualized in the fundus image to analyze the correct location. This is shown in Fig. 6. It can be seen, that the scanning across the rows is not uniform and the shifts of B-scans beginning are also different for each B-scan. This probably implies small uncorrected eye movements during scanning.

The registration was also evaluated on less subjective visualization method. The dark areas (blood-vessels and optic disc) were roughly segmented in the *blood-vessel image* and these positions were visualized in the fundus image before and after registration. The visualization before registration was performed using manually selected corresponding points. The result for one data set is shown in Fig. 7. Improvement along all blood-vessels can be seen, particularly below optic disc.

5   Conclusion

We proposed new approach for registration of fundus and OCT images with possibility of easy parallelization. Due to several simplifications in this preliminary study, the framework will be extended in future to be more robust. These extending steps will include rotation correction and modification of the B-scan spatial transformation to cover possible rotation separately. Another issue is the use an optimization approach to speed up the computation. The last step will cover automatization of registration process by detection of one or more corresponding points via segmentation of optic disc and blood-vessels.

Acknowledgment

This work has been supported by the project of Czech Science Foundation no GA102/09/1600 and two projects sponsored by the Ministry of Education of the Czech Republic: the national research center DAR (Data, Algorithms and Decision making) project no. 1M0572 coordinated by the Institute of Information

Theory and Automation, Academy of Science and partly also by the institutional research frame no. MSM 0021630513. The authors highly acknowledge the cooperation with the Eye Clinic of MUDr. Kubena (T. Kubena and P. Cernosek), Zlin, Czech Republic, University Eye Hospital Erlangen-Nurnberg (R. Tornow and R. Laemmer), Erlangen, Germany and Chair of Computer Science 5 (Pattern Recognition), University of Erlangen-Nurnmberg (M. Mayer and J. Hornegger).

References

1. Trip, S.A., Schlottmann, P.G., Jones, S.J., Altmann, D.R., Garway-Heath, D.F., Thompson, A.J., Plant, G.T., Miller, D.H.: Retinal nerve fiber layer axonal loss and visual dysfunction in optic neuritis. Am. J. Ophthalmol. 140(6), 1173–1179 (2005)
2. Lee, K., Niemeijer, M., Garvin, M.K., Kwon, Y.H., Sonka, M., Abramoff, M.D.: Segmentation of the optic disc in 3-d oct scans of the optic nerve head. IEEE T. Med. Imaging 29(1), 159–168 (2010)
3. Kolar, R., Laemmer, R., Jan, J., Mardin, C.Y.: The segmentation of zones with increased autofluorescence in the junctional zone of parapapillary atrophy. Physiol. Meas. 30(5), 505–516 (2009)
4. Drexler, W., Fujimoto, J.G.: Optical Coherence Tomography. Springer, Heidelberg (2008)
5. Ricco, S., Chen, M., Ishikawa, H., Wollstein, G., Schuman, J.: Correcting motion artifacts in retinal spectral domain optical coherence tomography via image registration. In: Yang, G.-Z., Hawkes, D., Rueckert, D., Noble, A., Taylor, C. (eds.) MICCAI 2009. LNCS, vol. 5761, pp. 100–107. Springer, Heidelberg (2009)
6. Kolar, R., Kubecka, L., Jan, J.: Registration and Fusion of the Autofluorescent and Infrared Retinal Images. International Journal of Biomedical Imaging, 11 (2008), doi:10.1155/2008/513478
7. Reddy, B.S., Chatterji, B.N.: An FFT-based technique for translation, rotation, and scale-invariant image registration. IEEE T. Image Process. 5(8), 1266–1271 (1996)
8. Balci, M., Foroosh, H.: Subpixel registration directly from the phase difference. EURASIP J. Appl. Si. Pr. 2006, 231 (2006)
9. Kolar, R., Jan, J.: Detection of glaucomatous eye via color fundus images using fractal dimensions. Radioengineering 17(3), 109–114 (2008)
10. Niemann, H., Chrastek, R., Lausen, B., Kubecka, L., Jan, J., Mardin, C.Y., Michelson, G.: Towards automated diagnostic evaluation of retina images. Pattern Recogn. Image Anal. 16(4), 671–676 (2006)
11. Koozekanani, D., Boyer, K., Roberts, C.: Retinal thickness measurements from optical coherence tomography using a markov boundary model. IEEE T. Med. Imaging 20(9), 900–916 (2001)
12. Studholme, C., Hill, D.L.G., Hawkes, D.J.: An overlap invariant entropy measure of 3d medical image alignment. Pattern Recogn. 32(1), 71–86 (1999)

A Computational White Matter Atlas for Aging with Surface-Based Representation of Fasciculi

Hui Zhang[1], Paul A. Yushkevich[1], Daniel Rueckert[2], and James C. Gee[1]

[1] Penn Image Computing and Science Laboratory (PICSL),
Department of Radiology, University of Pennsylvania, Philadelphia, USA
[2] Department of Computing, Imperial College, London, UK

Abstract. Voxel-based analysis, either whole-brain or tract-specific, is a widely used approach for localizing white matter (WM) differences across populations using diffusion tensor imaging (DTI). A prerequisite to this approach is to spatially normalize all the subjects to a common template. The accuracy of spatial normalization can be improved by using a population-specific template that is, morphologically, most similar to the subjects in the population of interest. Here, we report the development of a population-specific DTI template for the elderly using the publicly available IXI brain database. The template captures the average shape and diffusion properties of the aging population and contains segmentations of major WM fasciculi parcellated via fiber tractography. Furthermore, the segmentations are modeled using surface-based representation to support the tract-specific analysis recently proposed by Yushkevich et al. The utility of the template is demonstrated in an examination of WM changes in Amyotrophic Lateral Sclerosis.

1 Introduction

Diffusion tensor imaging (DTI) depicts *in vivo* the intricate architecture of white matter (WM) [1] and has become an indispensable tool for studying WM both in normal populations and in populations with brain disorders. To localize WM differences across populations using DTI, both whole-brain and tract-specific analyses are commonly used [2,3]. A prerequisite to such analyses is spatial normalization which establishes anatomical correspondence among all the subjects in a study, by registering them to some template.

To spatially normalize DTI data, a DTI template is required to leverage recent advances in tensor-based image registration algorithms shown to improve the quality of spatial alignment [4]. Mori et al. has recently developed such a template, known as the ICBM-DTI-81 template [5], which defines the same stereotactic space as the widely used ICBM-152 anatomical template and contains manually-delineated WM regions. The ICBM-DTI-81 template is destined to become an important neuroimaging resource. However, because it is built with healthy controls between 18 and 59 years old, this template does not capture significant morphological changes in brain anatomy for the elderly population (65 years or older). As a result, its application to the aging population may adversely affect the quality of spatial normalization.

B. Fischer, B. Dawant, and C. Lorenz (Eds.): WBIR 2010, LNCS 6204, pp. 83–90, 2010.
© Springer-Verlag Berlin Heidelberg 2010

In this paper, we report the construction of a population-specific DTI template appropriate for the aging population which, to the best of our knowledge, does not yet exist. To accomodate large morphological variation in anatomy of this population, the template was constructed using a high-dimensional tensor-based image registration method rather than the affine registration method used for creating the ICBM-DTI-81 template. The template construction algorithm also captures simultaneously the average shape and diffusion properties of the population. In addition, a large set of major WM tracts were parcellated using fiber tractography and modeled with the skeleton surface representation to support the tract specific analysis recently developed by Yushkevich et al. [3]. We demonstrated the utility of the template in a study of WM changes in Amyotrophic Lateral Sclerosis (ALS), a devastating, usually fatal, disease of motor neuron degeneration.

The rest of the paper is organized as follows: Sec. 2 gives the imaging and demographic details of the dataset used for building the template, describes the method of template construction, WM tract parcellation and modeling, and discusses the application of the template in ALS. Sec. 3 illustrates the resulting template and the associated skeleton surface models and reports the results from the ALS study. Finally, the paper is summarized in Sec. 4.

2   Materials and Methods

2.1   Subjects and Data Acquisition

The subjects used to construct the proposed aging template are extracted from the IXI brain database (http://www.ixi.org.uk) developed jointly by Imperial College of Science Technology & Medicine and University College London. The IXI database consists of brain MR images from 550 normal subjects between the age of 20 and 80 years that are freely available for downloads. The inclusion criteria for this template construction are 1) subjects are of age 65 years or older; 2) DT-MR images are available and of sufficient quality (i.e., no significant motion or suscepitibility-induced artifacts). A total of 51 subjects, currently determined to meet the selection criteria, have been included in the current paper. The additional qualified subjects will be added in the future. The demographics of the included subjects are age 65-83, mean age and standard deviation 70.4±4.0; 21 males and 30 females. DT-MR data was collected at two sites (Guy's Hospital and Hammersmith Hospital, London, UK) with two different scanners (Philips 1.5 T and 3.0 T) with a single-shot echo-planar diffusion-weighted sequence with 15 non-collinear gradient directions @ b = 1000 s/mm^2 with a SENSE factor of 2. The imaging matrix was 128 x 128 with a field of view 224 x 224 mm^2, resulting in in-plane resolution of 1.75 x 1.75 mm^2. The slice thicknesses are 2.35 mm and 2.0 mm for the two sites, respectively.

2.2   Construction of the Population-Averaged DTI Template

The population-averaged DTI template was constructed using the DT-MR images of all the chosen subjects. We chose the template construction algorithm described in [4] because the algorithm has been tailored for handling DT-MR images. Briefly, the initial average image is computed as a log-Euclidean mean [6] of the input DT-MR images. The average is then iteratively refined by repeating the following procedure: register the subject images to the current average, then compute a refined average for the next iteration as the mean of the normalized images. This procedure is repeated until the average image converges. The resulting template is unbiased towards any single subject and captures the average diffusion properties of the population at each voxel with a diffusion tensor. Subsequently, the template is "shape-corrected" to ensure that it also represents the average shape of the population, using the strategy proposed by Guimond et al. [7]. This is achieved by first computing an average of the deformation fields that warp each subject into alignment with the template, then warping the template with the inverse of the average deformation field.

In contrast to the ICBM-DTI-81 template that was constructed via affine registration of scalar images derived from diffusion data, the registration algorithm [8] used in the current template construction captures high-dimensional spatial deformations and matches DT-MR images directly. By computing image similarity on the basis of full tensor images, rather than scalar features, the algorithm incorporates local fiber orientations as features to drive the alignment of individual WM tracts. When measuring similarity between tensor images, it is essential to take into account the fact that when a transformation is applied to a tensor field, the orientation of the tensors is changed [9]. A unique property of this registration algorithm is the ability to model the effect of deformation on tensor orientation as an analytic function of the Jacobian matrix of the deformation field. By using full tensor information in the similarity metric, the method aligns WM regions better than scalar-based registration methods, as demonstrated in a task-driven evaluation study [4].

2.3   White Matter Parcellation of the DTI Template

We followed the approach described in [3] and parcellated the DTI template into individual WM tracts using an established protocol by Wakana et al. [10], which is based on fiber tracking. The validity of tracking in a population-averaged DTI template has recently been demonstrated by Lawes et al. [11] in a comparison to classic postmortem dissection. We delineated six major tracts that includes: corpus callosum (CC), corticospinal tracts (CST), inferior fronto-occipital tracts (IFO), inferior longitudinal tracts (ILF), superior longitudinal tracts (SLF), and uncinates (UNC). A common property of these tracts is that all have a major portion that is sheet-like and can be modeled using the surface-based representation as described in Sec. 2.4. White matter tracts that are more appropriately represented by tubular models, such as the tapetum of the CC, the cingulum, the fornix and the optic tract were not segmented. Fasciculi in the cerebellum and brain stem were not considered either. These tubular structures will be included in the future. Only the arcuate portion of the SLF, which can be tracked consistently, was segmented. Binary 3D segmentations of individual tracts were generated by labeling voxels in the DTI template through which at least one fiber passed. The binary segmentations were further edited using ITK-SNAP [12] to remove extraneous connections.

2.4 Surface-Based Geometric Modeling of WM Tracts

Geometrical modeling of the WM tracts was achieved with the algorithm proposed by Yushkevich et al. [3], which involves fitting deformable medial models (cm-reps) to the binary segmentations derived in Sec. 2.3. The cm-reps are models that describe the skeleton and the boundary of a geometrical object as parametric digital surfaces with predefined topology. The models describe the geometrical relationship between the skeleton and the boundary, such that, during fitting, deformations applied to the model's skeleton can be propagated to the model's boundary.

A key feature of medial models is their ability to parametrize the entire interior of the model using a shape-based coordinate system. This is due to the fact that in medial geometry every point on the skeleton surface is associated with a sphere that is tangent to the boundary surface at a pair of points (which may coincide at edges of the skeleton). The line segments connecting the sphere's center to the points of tangency are called "spokes" and are orthogonal to the boundary. Furthermore, no two spokes intersect inside the model. This allows us to define a coordinate system for interior of the object based entirely on the shape of the object, where two of the coordinate values parametrize the skeleton surface and the third gives the position of a point on the spokes. As shown in [3], in the context of modeling sheet-like WM tracts, this coordinate system affords us the ability to reduce the dimensionality of the problem by projecting data onto the skeleton along the arguably "less interesting" thickness dimension. From the point of view of statistical analysis, this may result in improved sensitivity without much loss in spatial specificity.

2.5 Application to Identify WM Changes in ALS

To demonstrate the utility of the proposed DTI template with surface-based WM modeling, we employed the template to identify WM changes in ALS. The structure-specific statistical mapping described in [3] was used for our analysis, which takes advantage of the surface-based WM models developed as part of our template. Because of the existing hypothesis that ALS strongly affects the motor pathway, only the left and right CSTs were included in the analysis. Briefly, for each subject, its DT-MR image was first registered to the DTI template using the algorithm [8] and warped into the template space. The fitted cm-rep models of the CSTs parcellated in the template were then used to sample the diffusion data in the shape-based coordinate systems established by these models. Specifically, for each location on the skeleton surfaces of the CSTs, the average fractional anisotropy (FA) along its two associated spokes was computed, resulting in an average FA map associated with the skeleton surfaces. After repeating this process for each subject, the original volumetric dataset was dimensionality reduced into a surface dataset. Permutation-based non-parametric suprathreshold cluster analysis was then applied to identify WM differences between the two groups and the statistics on both CSTs were pooled. The cluster-defining threshold was set at uncorrected p-value $= 0.01$ and the clusters with FWE-corrected p-value < 0.05 were deemed significant.

The dataset that we chose to analyze were from an earlier ALS study that we have studied [omitted]. It consists of 8 healthy controls and 8 ALS patients. The DT-MR data for these subjects were collected using a 12-direction diffusion imaging protocol on a 3 T Siemens scanner without parallel imaging. In our previous study, we applied the same analysis as here but using a population-specific template built from the subject data alone. We leveraged this earlier result and compared it to the current finding to provide a qualitative assessment of the feasibility of using our proposed template for datasets acquired on different scanners and with different sequences.

3   Results

The population-averaged DTI template is shown in Fig. 1 in terms of its fiber orientation map. Compared to the ICBM-DTI-81 template [5], which is constructed using affine registration, our template has considerably sharper edge features as well as much richer details in the cortical regions. Furthermore, the additional shape-correction step allows our template to capture the average shape of the WM anatomy in the aging population. In particular, observe the distinct asymmetry in the size and shape of the left and right SLFs, with the left SLF (image right) being significantly larger than the right. This is consistent with the known observation that the SLF is larger in the left hemisphere, likely a result of language lateralization [13].

The surface-based geometric modeling of WM tracts is illustrated with Fig. 2 using the left CST as an example. The cm-rep model of the left CST is shown in Panel (c), which consists of a smooth surface patch represented as a triangular mesh and the associated radius function map, which encodes the radius of the sphere at each vertex of the mesh. The boundary surface computed from this model is shown in Panel (d), which is very similar to the binary segmentation of the tract shown in Panel (b), the fitting target. The high-quality of fitting was confirmed quantitatively. Except for the ILF, the Dice overlaps between the binary segmentations and the fitted cm-rep models range from 90% to 95%. The Dice overlap for the ILF is slightly less, around 85%. This is consistent with the results reported in [3], which observed that the poorer fitting of the ILFs is due to the branching near the posterior end of ILF.

The skeleton surfaces of the cm-rep models fitted to all the parcellated tracts are shown in Fig. 3. For the tracts that exist bilaterally, their left and right copies were individually fitted to their corresponding cm-rep models. Hence, the resulting skeleton surfaces reflect the underlying asymmetry in antomy. The asymmetry in the SLFs observed above is evident here as well. Another apparent asymmetry is in the ILFs. However, we believe that this is a result of the intrinsic ambiguity in separating the posterior portion of the ILFs and the IFOs rather than true anatomical ambiguity.

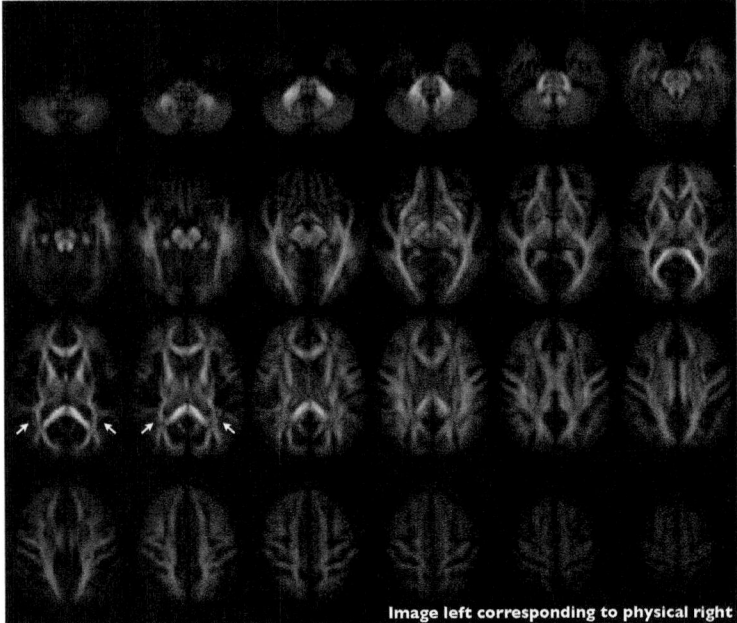

Fig. 1. Axial slices of the fiber orientation map of the constructed DTI template. The fiber orientations are visualized with the standard RGB encoding: red for left-right, green for anterior-posterior and blue for inferior-superior. The two pairs of white arrows highlight the visually distinct asymmetry in the left and right SLFs.

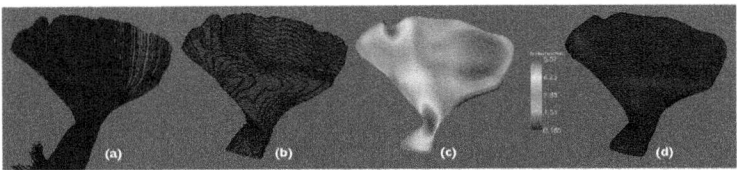

Fig. 2. The surface-based geometric modeling of the left CST. Panel (a): The results from fiber tractography. Panel (b): The binary segmentation computed from the fiber tracking results. Panel (c): The skeleton surface of the cm-rep model fitted to the binary segmenation overlaid with the corresponding radius function. Panel (d): The boundary surface corresponding to the fitted cm-rep model.

The result of applying the surface-based tract models to identify WM changes in ALS is shown in Fig. 4. Under the stringent significance level described in Sec. 2.5, we found three significant clusters of reduced FA in ALS compared to healthy controls. This finding is highly consistent with that of our previous analysis of this dataset using the same analysis [omitted]. The previous analysis reported two significant clusters, one on each CST, in the similar location as the

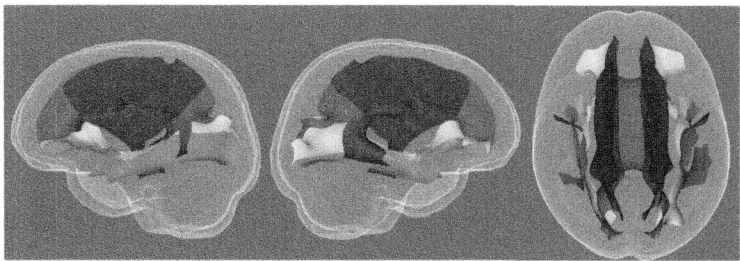

Fig. 3. The skeleton surfaces of the cm-rep models fitted to all the tracts. The skeleton surface of CC is colored in red. The surfaces of left and right CSTs, IFOs, ILFs, SLFs and UNCs are colored in blue, yellow, green and cyan, respectively. The brain mask is also shown as a translucent mesh for anatomical guidance. From left to right are the views of the skeleton surfaces from left (physical right), right (physical left), and top.

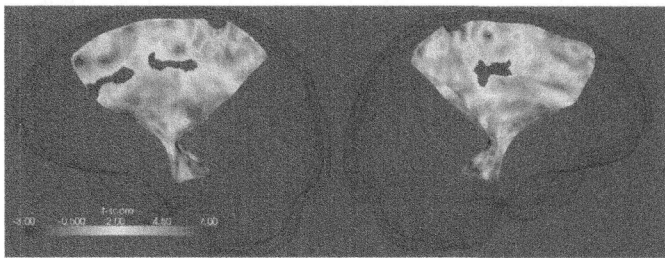

Fig. 4. The significant clusters of reduced FA in ALS compared to healthy controls (in red) overlaid on the skeleton surfaces of the CSTs. From left to right are the right and left CSTs.

ones identified here. The cluster on the right CST covers the combined area of the two clusters on the right CST found here.

4 Discussion

In this paper, we described the construction of a population-specific DTI template for the aging population. The template will enable standard whole-brain analyses, such as the popular TBSS method [2], to leverage advanced tensor-based spatial normalization techniques. Equipped with the parcellation of a large set of major WM tracts and their corresponding skeleton surface models, it will also support the recent development in tract-specific analysis by Yushkevich et al. [3]. We demonstrated qualitatively the feasibility of using the template for analyzing data acquired with different scanners or diffusion protocols, which should encourage its adoption as a useful public resource for the broad neuroimaging community studying aging and aging-related diseases.

Acknowledgment. The authors gratefully acknowledge support of this work by the NIH via grants AG027785 (PY), DA022807 (JG), EB006266 (JG), EB009321 (JG), NS061111 (PY), and NS065347 (JG).

References

1. Pierpaoli, C., Jezzard, P., Basser, P.J., Barnett, A., Chiro, G.D.: Diffusion tensor MR imaging of the human brain. Radiology 201 (1996)
2. Smith, S.M., Jenkinson, M., Johansen-Berg, H., Rueckert, D., Nichols, T.E., Mackay, C.E., Watkins, K.E., Ciccarelli, O., Cader, M.Z., Matthews, P.M., Behrens, T.E.J.: Tract-based spatial statistics: Voxelwise analysis of multi-subject diffusion data. NeuroImage 31 (2006)
3. Yushkevich, P.A., Zhang, H., Simon, T.J., Gee, J.C.: Structure-specific statistical mapping of white matter tracts. NeuroImage 41, 448–461 (2008)
4. Zhang, H., Avants, B.B., Yushkevich, P.A., Woo, J.H., Wang, S., McCluskey, L.F., Elman, L.B., Melhem, E.R., Gee, J.C.: High-dimensional spatial normalization of diffusion tensor images improves the detection of white matter differences in amyotrophic lateral sclerosis. TMI 26, 1585–1597 (2007)
5. Mori, S., Oishi, K., Jiang, H., Jiang, L., Li, X., Akhter, K., Hua, K., Faria, A.V., Mahmood, A., Woods, R., Toga, A.W., Pike, G.B., Neto, P.R., Evans, A., Zhang, J., Huang, H., Miller, M.I., van Zijl, P., Mazziotta, J.: Stereotaxic white matter atlas based on diffusion tensor imaging in an icbm template. NeuroImage 40, 570–582 (2008)
6. Arsigny, V., Fillard, P., Pennec, X., Ayache, N.: Log-Euclidean metrics for fast and simple calculus on diffusion tensors. MRM 56, 411–421 (2006)
7. Guimond, A., Meunier, J., Thirion, J.P.: Average brain models: a convergence study. CVIU 77, 192–210 (2000)
8. Zhang, H., Yushkevich, P.A., Alexander, D.C., Gee, J.C.: Deformable registration of diffusion tensor MR images with explicit orientation optimization. MIA 10 (2006)
9. Alexander, D.C., Pierpaoli, C., Basser, P.J., Gee, J.C.: Spatial transformations of diffusion tensor magnetic resonance images. TMI 20 (2001)
10. Wakana, S., Jiang, H., Nagae-Poetscher, L.M., van Zijl, P.C., Mori, S.: Fiber tract-based atlas of human white matter anatomy. Radiology 230 (2004)
11. Lawes, I.N., Barrick, T.R., Murugam, V., Spierings, N., Evans, D.R., Song, M., Clark, C.A.: Atlas-based segmentation of white matter tracts of the human brain using diffusion tensor tractography and comparison with classical dissection. NeuroImage 39 (2008)
12. Yushkevich, P.A., Piven, J., Hazlett, H.C., Smith, R.G., Ho, S., Gee, J.C., Gerig, G.: User-guided 3D active contour segmentation of anatomical structures: significantly improved efficiency and reliability. NeuroImage 31, 1116–1128 (2006)
13. Lazar, M., Field, A.S., Lee, J., Alexander, A.L.: Lateral asymmetry of superior longitudinal fasciculus: a white matter tractography study. In: ISMRM (2004)

Anatomical Landmark Based Registration of Contrast Enhanced T1-Weighted MR Images

Ali Demir[1], Gozde Unal[1,⋆], and Kutlay Karaman[2]

[1] Sabanci University, Istanbul, Turkey
ademir@sabanciuniv.edu, gozdeunal@sabanciuniv.edu
[2] Anadolu Medical Center, Kocaeli, Turkey

Abstract. In many problems involving multiple image analysis, an image registration step is required. One such problem appears in brain tumor imaging, where baseline and follow-up image volumes from a tumor patient are often to-be compared. Nature of the registration for a change detection problem in brain tumor growth analysis is usually rigid or affine. Contrast enhanced T1-weighted MR images are widely used in clinical practice for monitoring brain tumors. Over this modality, contours of the active tumor cells and whole tumor borders and margins are visually enhanced. In this study, a new technique to register serial contrast enhanced T1 weighted MR images is presented. The proposed fully-automated method is based on five anatomical landmarks: eye balls, nose, confluence of sagittal sinus, and apex of superior sagittal sinus. After extraction of anatomical landmarks from fixed and moving volumes, an affine transformation is estimated by minimizing the sum of squared distances between the landmark coordinates. Final result is refined with a surface registration, which is based on head masks confined to the surface of the scalp, as well as to a plane constructed from three of the extracted features. The overall registration is not intensity based, and it depends only on the invariant structures. Validation studies using both synthetically transformed MRI data, and real MRI scans, which included several markers over the head of the patient were performed. In addition, comparison studies against manual landmarks marked by a radiologist, as well as against the results obtained from a typical mutual information based method were carried out to demonstrate the effectiveness of the proposed method.

1   Introduction

Image registration refers to the problem of finding a geometric transformation, which is optimal in a certain sense, between two or more corresponding images. Nature of the correspondence problem describes the type of necessary geometric transformation [1]. Registration is a major problem in many medical imaging applications such as image guided neurosurgery, surgical planning, radiotherapy planning, patient population analysis, and monitoring tumor growth.

⋆ This work was partially supported by Tubitak Grant No:108E126, and EU FP7 Grant No: PIRG03-GA-2008-231052.

B. Fischer, B. Dawant, and C. Lorenz (Eds.): WBIR 2010, LNCS 6204, pp. 91–103, 2010.

In this study we focused on the registration of serial Magnetic Resonance (MR) images intended for the change detection problem in tumor monitoring [5,6]. General methods and strategies for image registration are reviewed in [2,3,4]. Registration problem for change detection in brain can be classified as a rigid body motion of invariant brain structures. Therefore, the most challenging part of the change detection is to overlay invariant structures accurately. Ettinger et al. used intracranial cavity (ICC) as an invariant structure to register serial images. Their strategy involves computation of dense point correspondences based on segmented ICC [7]. Anatomical landmark localization on Talairach space is also a popular approach for registration [13,15,14]. Chui et al. extracted the outer cortical surface and major sulcal ribbons to register brain MR images [8]. Geometrical features such as curves, lines, curvatures, corners, and so on, are also used extensively in image registration problems. Davatzikos et al. uses the curves and boundaries in regions to preregister the volumes for elastic registration [9,10]. Geometric landmarks make the registration procedure automatic and robust [11,12,16]. On the other hand, intensity similarity based methods are also widely utilized in most of the registration problems [17,18,19]. Duffau et al. [5] in their review, reported that the image intensity is not a reliable measure in the presence of growing tumors, which introduce additional challenges for registration algorithms. Therefore, detection of invariant landmarks in serial images is expected to perform better than an intensity similarity based optimization approach.

Registration is inherently an ill-posed problem, therefore usually no unique solution is available. Often, constraints are introduced, particularly for a deformable registration problem, constraints on a deformation field can be defined. On the other hand, depending on the domain and application of the problem, specific intensity similarity measures or different feature-based approaches are proposed [1]. In this paper, for the clinical problem of brain tumor monitoring, where anatomical features can be extracted from the contrast enhanced T1-weighted MRI (contrast T1-MRI), we present a new method where strong anatomical features drive the registration without depending on intensity similarity measures, which can become problematic in presence of significant tumor change over time [5]. Another advantage of this approach is that it is invariant due to an intra-patient registration scenario, i.e. the same anatomical landmarks can be found in the follow-up images. Following a first anatomic landmark based registration, an extracted surface, which is constrained by the available anatomical landmarks obtained in the first phase of the method, drives the second phase of the registration. This is a surface registration step that propagates the solution towards matching of the important features over a consistent part of the scalp for a better and extensive fit over the head surface for a refinement of the final affine transformation. Apart from its use in tumor follow-up studies, the proposed rigid/affine registration method can be used as a pre-processing before generic deformable registration applications, which require an initial rigid alignment phase.

The organization of the paper is as follows. In Section 2, the specific anatomical landmarks used in our algorithm and their extraction is described. The proposed registration method based on anatomical landmarks is presented in Section 3. The results are demonstrated in Section 4 with consistency tests and validation studies, followed by conclusion and discussion in Section 5.

2   Extraction of Anatomical Landmarks

The first step of the proposed registration algorithm involves extraction of anatomical brain landmarks on given contrast T1-MRI volumes. Thus, a patient-specific coordinate system, which can be invariably found on all human brain images, is obtained based on five selected anatomical landmarks: nasal bone tip, center of two eyeballs, confluence of sinus, and apex of superior sagittal sinus. The landmark selection process, i.e. determining brain landmarks that can be reliably observed and computationally extracted, was carried out jointly with the radiologists in the team.

2.1   Nasal Bone from Nose

The anatomic landmark extraction step starts with detection of a binary head mask. It is obtained on dilated canny edge map through region growing seeded from the outside at the grid boundaries. This connects the boundary components and complement of this result is eroded with the same size of dilation mask, forming the head mask. Anterior tip point of each axial slice is the nearest point of mask to the top most row of the slice. It is detected with a linear search in rows starting from the top most row. Another geometric definition derived from head mask is the symmetry line estimate which is defined as the line passing through the anterior tip point and center of mass (1st order image moments) of the slice. Noting that this is not necessarily symmetry line of brain, it will be defined after the nose tip points are located. Figure 1-a depicts four geometric

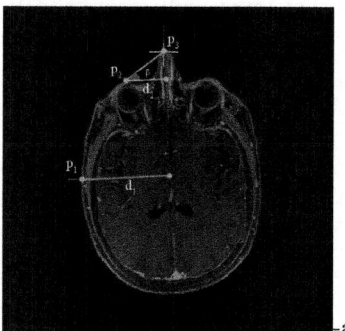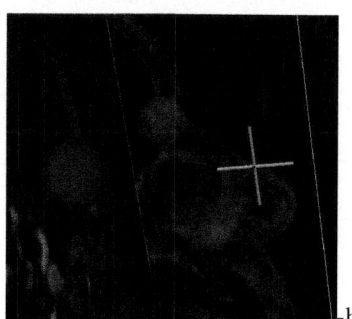

Fig. 1. a)Geometric features (Symmetry line, p_1, p_2, p_3,d_1, and d_2, and the angle β) used to find the nose tip points. b)Detected nose landmark.

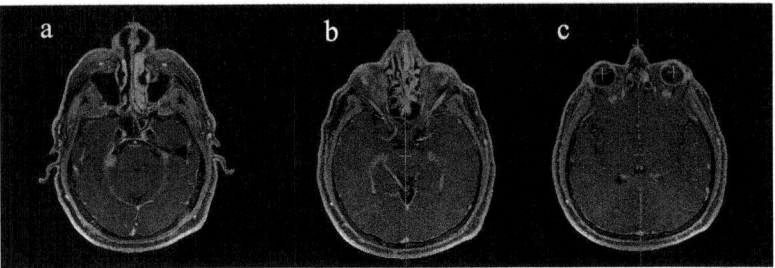

Fig. 2. Sample slices with nose tip points detected: (a) Bottom nose slice, (b) Middle nose slice, c) Top nose slice

features utilized in finding the nasal bone anatomic feature: p_1, the point with the maximum distance to the symmetry line, p_2, the most anterior point of eye balls, and d_1 and d_2 are minimum distances from p_1 and p_2, to the symmetry line. The ratio of $d_2/d_1 := c$ is found to be almost biometric constant with a mean and variance 0.42 ± 0.01, which was measured over 20 MRI scans. Using this constant, for each slice we find p_1 and d_1, then estimate the point p_2, where $d_2 = cd_1$. We also define the angle β between lines of p_2 to anterior tip point (p_3) and p_2 to the corresponding point on symmetry line. Tip points of the slices with high values of $\tan\beta$ are marked as nose tip points. Figure 2 depicts a few sample slices with nose tip points marked. Finally, a single nose landmark is marked at the center of selected nose tip points, which is located at the end point of nasal bone (see Figure 1-b).

2.2   Eye Balls

An eye ball is segmented using a sphere model, which is initiated at a seed point based on the nose feature. Two seed coordinates for the left and right eye balls are first estimated on the top most slice of the nose, e.g. see Figure 2-c, then given d_1, the maximum distance to symmetry axis, d_2 is calculated using the ratio c (Section 2.1). Using an anatomical fact that an eyeball is roughly 10 mm in radius, the seed is initialized 10 mm away from p_2 towards the symmetry

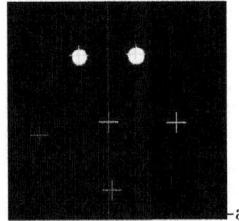
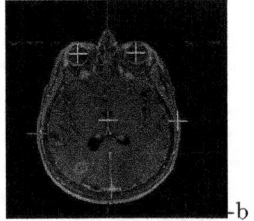

Fig. 3. (a) A slice from the obtained 3D binary eyeball masks; (b) T1-MRI slice marked with estimated seed points on eyeballs

axis to ensure that the seed point falls in the eye ball region. Initialized sphere parameters, the center and the radius, are evolved until convergence with ordinary differential equations derived to maximize the difference between the mean intensity statistics inside and outside the sphere within a band around its surface. A sample slice from 3D eye mask and estimated eyeball seeds are shown in Figure 3.

2.3   Confluence of Sinus

Confluence of sinus is the conjunction point of the superior sagittal sinus, straight sinus, and occipital sinus. A distinguishing feature of the confluence of sinus is that it is located where the superior sagittal sinus bifurcates as depicted in Figure 5-a.

Confluence of sinus (CoS) detection starts by locating a seed point on the superior sagittal sinus. As depicted in Figure 4, the seed point is selected on the axial slice which is 30 mm above the center of eyeballs. It is searched on the symmetry axis, and below the center of mass of the slice within a finite width, with respect to a maximum brightness criterion.

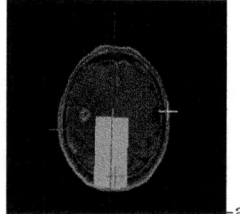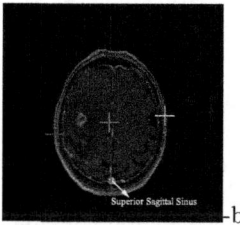

-a   -b

Fig. 4. Seed point search region over a T1-MRI slice for sinus map extraction

After the seed is initialized over the sagittal sinus (Figure 4-b marked with a +), mean μ and standard deviation σ values over a small window are calculated, and a 3D region growing is performed with an initial downward motion and a growing criterion of pixel intensities greater than $\mu - \sigma$. The result of segmentation by region growing produces a sinus map, as visualized in Figure 5 with a height map overlay.

Next, the segmented sinus map is analyzed using region moments of axial slices. In this study, we defined the confluence of sinus at the slice, which has the maximum variance in the left-right direction. This is performed using a covariance matrix formed by second order central moments of the sinus map over each slice: $[\mu_{20}, \mu_{11}; \mu_{11}, \mu_{02}]$. This matrix is then decomposed into its eigenvector and diagonal eigenvalue matrices using singular value decomposition. The ratio between the two eigenvalues is used to select the slice of CoS and successfully discriminates the desired slice (Z coordinate). Axial (X and Y) coordinate of CoS is calculated using the average center of mass of the sinus map over five upper slices. Figures 5-b and 5-c depict a detected CoS landmark shown with an axis bar widget.

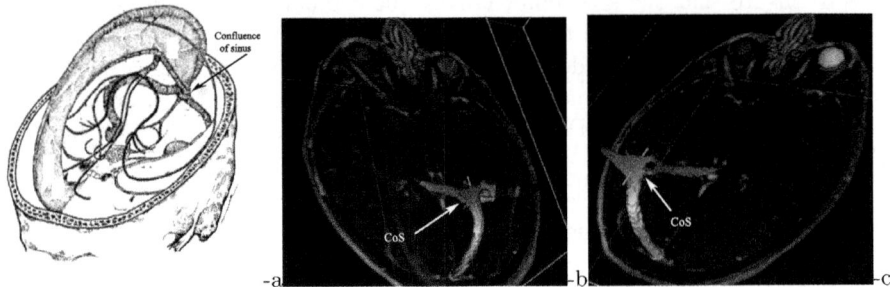

Fig. 5. (a) Cerebral venous system (figure adapted from Osborn A. Diagnostic neuroradiology. St. Louis: Mosby, 1994.) (b,c)Sinus map and CoS are shown from two different viewpoints with a height map overlaid over the surface.

2.4   Apex of Superior Sagittal Sinus

For an even sampling of landmarks over the brain, a final anatomical landmark is selected at the apex of the superior sagittal sinus. Similar to extraction of CoS, superior sagittal sinus (SSS) surface is delineated by region growing constrained by an initial upward motion. A sample SSS extracted from a contrast T1-MRI volume is shown in Figure 7. We define a plane constructed from the three anatomical landmarks: CoS, and the two eye ball centroids, as in Figure 6. This plane is called CoS-Eyeballs plane, and the point on superior sagittal sinus having a maximum distance to this plane is marked. For robustness, the center of a cloud of points with distances greater than 98% of the maximum distance is defined as the apex of superior sagittal sinus (Figure 7).

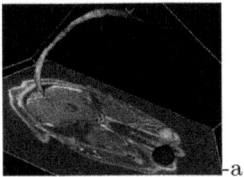
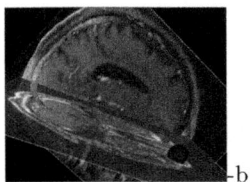

Fig. 6. CoS-Eyeballs planes from two different viewpoints

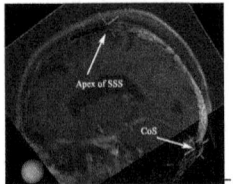
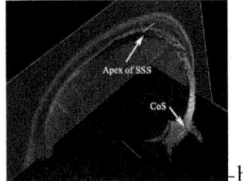

Fig. 7. Apex of Superior Sagittal Sinus is marked with axis bar widget

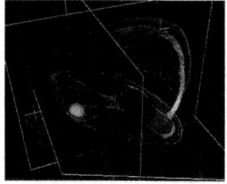
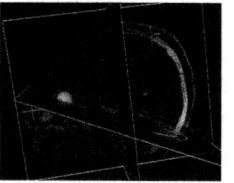

Fig. 8. All five extracted anatomical landmarks visualized together

Finally, all five anatomical extracted landmarks are visualized in Figure 8 from two different viewpoints for a sample patient contrast T1-MRI scan.

3   Registration Method

3.1   Anatomic Landmark-Based Registration

In the specific problem of registering serial MR images, a fixed reference volume, which is usually the baseline MRI scan, is to be rigidly aligned with a moving volume, which is a follow-up MRI scan. For a landmark based approach, a 3D affine transformation ($T = A_{3\times3}, t_{3\times1}$) is estimated by minimizing the sum of squared distances between the extracted anatomic landmark coordinates of the fixed volume and the moving volume. $A \in GL(3)$, the general linear group, i.e. A is an invertible 3×3 matrix. Coordinates are all in world coordinates and the centroid of the landmarks is chosen as the reference point for each MR volume. Translation component t of T is directly obtained from the difference of the centroids of the five landmarks that belong to the fixed and the moving volumes. Let $X_f = [x_f, y_f, z_f]^T$ be a fixed landmark coordinate, $X_m = [x_m, y_m, z_m]^T$ be its corresponding moving landmark coordinate, and A is the affine transformation between the two. Then, A can be obtained as the solution of the least squares estimation problem: $A = \arg\min \sum_{i=1}^{n=5} \|X_f^i - A X_m^i\|^2$. After taking the derivative with respect to the unknown A, equating to zero, and re-arranging the terms yields:

$$N = \begin{bmatrix} M & 0 & 0 \\ 0 & M & 0 \\ 0 & 0 & M \end{bmatrix}, \quad N a = b \tag{1}$$

where 0 is a 3×3 all zeros matrix, and

$$M = \begin{bmatrix} \sum_i^n x_m^2 & \sum_i^n x_m y_m & \sum_i^n x_m z_m \\ \sum_i^n y_m x_m & \sum_i^n y_m^2 & \sum_i^n y_m z_m \\ \sum_i^n z_m x_m & \sum_i^n z_m y_m & \sum_i^n z_m^2 \end{bmatrix} \tag{2}$$

and

$$b = \left[\sum_i^n x_f x_m, \Sigma x_f y_m, \sum_i^n x_f z_m, \sum_i^n y_f x_m, \Sigma y_f y_m, \sum_i^n y_f z_m, \sum_i^n z_f x_m, \Sigma z_f y_m, \sum_i^n z_f z_m \right]^T. \tag{3}$$

The parameter vector $a = [a_{11}, a_{12}, a_{13}, a_{21}, a_{22}, a_{23}, a_{31}, a_{32}, a_{33}]^T$ of the matrix A is calculated as $a = N^{-1}b$. Final affine solution is projected to an orthogonal matrix space using a polar decomposition: $A = QS$, where Q is the closest possible orthogonal matrix to A in the sense of Frobenius norm, and S is a positive-definite symmetric matrix. The factor Q can be calculated using a singular value decomposition of $A = UKV^T$, where $Q = UV^T$ [22].

3.2 Refining Surface Registration

The result of landmark based registration is further refined for an improved extensive fit of the head/scalp surface of the moving image to that of the fixed image. The binary head masks of fixed and moving volumes confined by the CoS-Eyeballs plane (Figure 6), defined in Section 2.4, are represented as the zero-level sets of two signed distance functions Φ^f and Φ^m, respectively. The sum of squared differences between the two signed distance functions:

$$E(g) = \int_{\Omega} [\Phi^f(X) - \Phi^m(g(X))]^2 dX \tag{4}$$

where Ω is the domain of the image volume, is minimized to estimate a rigid transform $g(X) = RX + t$. The 3D rotation R, and 3D translation t parameters: $g_i, \ i = 1, ..., 6$, are obtained as the steady-state solution of the ordinary differential equations:

$$\frac{\partial g_i}{\partial t} = \int_{\Omega} [\Phi^f(X) - \Phi^m(g(X))] < \nabla \Phi^m(gX), \frac{\partial g(X)}{\partial g_i} > dX \tag{5}$$

where $< \cdot, \cdot >$ denotes the Euclidean inner product in R^3, and ∇ denotes a gradient operator. We utilized the exponential coordinate representation for the 3D rotation (e.g. see [23]). The initial conditions were set to translation and rotation matrix obtained from section 3.1.

4 Results

The experiments were carried out over 9 follow-up MRI scans obtained from our clinical partner hospital (anonymized for blind review). The study was approved by the IRB of the hospital for an ongoing research project. The proposed method is validated in various ways: over synthetically transformed MRI scans, real MRI baseline and follow-up scans, a manually expert marked data set, and a data set with non-invasive fiducial landmarks attached to a patient's head. Contrast enhanced T1-weighted MRI volumes with 1mm slice thickness and axial resolution of 0.5mm are acquired from a Siemens 1.5 Tesla MR system. The proposed registration method is fully implemented in C++ environment, using Qt and VTK libraries for visualization. The parameters of the algorithm are fixed over all experiments as follows: The threshold of $\tan\beta$ is 0.40 in Section 2.1, the width of CoS seed search bounding box is 25mm, and the window size for region growing parameter calculation is 7×7 in Section 2.3.

4.1   Consistency Tests

Consistency testing method proposed by Jenkinsen et al. [21] provides a quantitative synthetic validation procedure for our method. In this test, new images are created using several pre-determined transformations with rotation and translation. All transformed images are then registered to the reference image. If the method is consistent, prescribed and calculated transformations should be the same. Performance of the proposed method is tested with a consistency dataset containing 8 contrast enhanced T1-MR and their artificially transformed MR volumes with a known transformation matrix constructed by 5 degrees of rotation about Z axis, 5 degrees of rotation about Y axis, and translated by [2,4,-2] mm in this case. Registration is carried out using anatomical landmarks described in Section 3.1, and followed by a surface based refinement procedure described in Section 3.2. In an ideal case, prescribed and calculated transformation matrices should be identical. In this study we report the Frobenius norm $\|S\| = \sqrt{trace(S^T * S)}$, where S is the difference of the prescribed and calculated rotation part of transformation matrices. The error in translation is interpreted as distance in milimeters.

The proposed method is compared to one of the widely adopted standard rigid registration methods based on maximization of a global mutual information criterion (MI) [17]. Observed rotation and translation errors are interpreted as mean ± standard deviation as shown in Table 1. Both methods have similar error results for rotation (less variance with the proposed method), and the proposed method is more consistent in terms of the translation. Furthermore, the proposed method takes typically 5-10 minutes of processing time on a personal computer with 3.16 GHz processor, whereas the MI method takes typically 30 minutes of processing time for our datasets. Therefore, the landmark-based method is more efficient in terms of computation times.

Table 1. Transformation error measures of consistency dataset

	Mutual Information Based	Anatomical Landmark Based with Surface Refinement
Rotation Error	0.015 ± 0.014	0.019 ± 0.008
Translation Error (mm)	1.53 ± 0.56	0.53 ± 0.20

4.2   Validation Studies on T1-MRI

Validation Studies on a Dataset with Fiducial Landmarks. For a validation study on a real MRI data, fish oil tablets are used as fiducial landmarks and 6 tablets are positioned with an unbiased sampling over the surface of the head of a patient. Two contrast enhanced T1-MRI scans are performed: the first scan in a regular patient position, and the second scan performed after the patient head is gently tilted about the axial axis. For both scans, fiducial landmarks are segmented and a rigid transformation matrix is calculated using the method mentioned in Section 3.1. These parameters are used as the "ground truth" transformation parameters in this experiment. Fiducial landmarks are then removed from both of the volumes, and anatomical landmarks are automatically extracted, and registration is performed as described in Section 3. The two fiducially marked volumes are also aligned using the mutual information based registration algorithm. Differences between the estimated transformation parameters and the "ground truth" parameters are reported in Table 2. The parameters estimated by the proposed registration method were closer to the "ground truth" parameters than those of the mutual information based method for the fiducially marked volumes.

Table 2. Transformation error measures for fiducial landmark data. Rotation error is reported in the sense of Frobenius norm between the two rotation matrices.

Registration Method	Rotation Error	Translation Error (mm)
Landmark based	0.013	0.54
Landmark based with surface refinement	0.016	0.45
Mutual Information based	0.496	8.18

Studies on Follow-up contrast T1-MRI. In order to show the effect of the surface registration step (Section 3.2) in our algorithm, an intensity based measure, which is the sum of squared intensity differences (SSID) is utilized:

$$SSID = \int_{\Omega} [I(\boldsymbol{X}_f) - I'(\boldsymbol{T}(\boldsymbol{X}_m))]^2 \, d\Omega \qquad (6)$$

where I is the fixed intensity image and I' is the registered intensity image. Follow-up MRI scans from 8 patients were registered to their baseline scans and the mean SSID results are presented in Table 3. It can be observed that adding the surface refinement process after landmark-based registration reduces the intensity match error in the registration of follow-up scans to their baseline scans, and in general improves the registration performance.

Table 3. SSID error measures over registration of T1-MRI baseline and follow-up datasets

Registration Method	Error
Landmark based	2.34E+07
Landmark based with surface refinement	2.05E+07

Validation Studies with manual expert guided registration. For comparison of our automatic landmark extraction to an expert's manual landmark extraction, one radiologist in our team manually marked 6 landmarks, which are not necessarily the computationally extracted landmarks (since for instance it is

Table 4. SSID error measure in comparison tests with expert guided manual landmarks

Registration Method	Error
Landmark based	2.12246E+07
Landmark based with surface refinement	2.29632E+07
Expert guided manual landmark based	2.34145E+07

not possible to visually mark the 3D centroid of eyeballs), in two baseline and corresponding follow-up contrast T1-MRI volumes. Registration is performed using these expert guided manual anatomical landmarks, and also using the proposed method (both with and without surface refinement step). SSID measures are given in Table 4, and as can be observed the expert guided registration produced larger errors after registration. This indicates that the consistency of manual landmark localization is lower when compared to our automatic landmark extraction algorithm.

Qualitative Results. We show sample image registration results for qualitative evaluation of the proposed method. Figure 9 shows image slices from two different patients having tumors appearing in various locations of the brain. The follow-up scan, which was performed several months later, was aligned with the

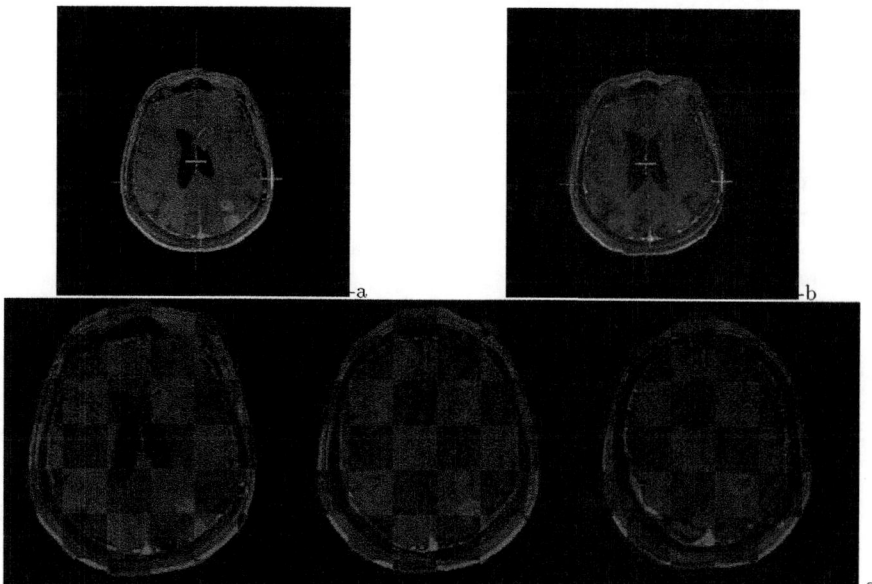

Fig. 9. Qualitative evaluation of a sample case with 3 months follow-up volume registration results: a)Baseline slice, b)Registered Follow-up slice, c)Checker board view with baseline image slices (green patches) and registered follow-up slices (red patches).

baseline scan using the proposed rigid registration method. As can be observed in the checker board view, the proposed method successfully registered the two contrast T1-MRI volumes, which are routinely used in monitoring tumor progress and response to therapy. In both cases, after treatment, the tumors regressed significantly, with reduced margins as observed in the follow-ups.

5   Conclusions and Discussions

We presented a new rigid registration method which is based on original anatomical features extracted from brain contrast-MRI scans, and a landmark-based registration refined with a surface-based registration for an improved alignment of the brain surfaces. One main application is the registration of follow-up MRI volumes in brain tumor patients, where the image intensity characteristics will vary due to tumor growth and possible different contrast characteristics depending on the scan acquisition time of the contrast enhanced MRI scans. The presented landmark-based registration method, is relatively more robust against such changes, as it is not directly based on an intensity-based optimization procedure, and is only prone to errors at the anatomic landmark extraction stage. Various validation studies demonstrated the performance of the proposed method to be as accurate as the state-of-the-art (e.g. mutual information based registration), and more efficient in terms of computation times of the algorithm, and it successfully registers contrast enhanced T1-MRI volumes. Future directions of our work includes improvement of the robustness of feature extraction, implementation of the algorithm in a multi-resolution framework, and use of the proposed method in quantification of tumor change in serial MRI sequences.

References

1. Modersitzki, J.: Numerical methods for image registration. Oxford University Press, Oxford (2004)
2. Zitova, B., Flusser, J.: Image registration methods: a survey. Image and Vision Computing 21, 977–1000 (2003)
3. Fischer, B., Modersitzki, J.: Ill-posed medicine–an introduction to image registration. Inverse Problems 24, 1–16 (2008)
4. Maintz, J., Viergever, M.: A survey of medical image registration. Medical Image Analysis 2, 1–36 (1998)
5. Angelini, E., Clatz, O., Mandonnet, E., Konukoglu, E., Capelle, L., Duffau, H.: Glioma Dynamics and Computational Models: A Review of Segmentation, Registration, and In Silico Growth Algorithms and their Clinical Applications. Current Medical Imaging Reviews 3, 176–262 (2007)
6. Patriarche, J., Erickson, B.: A Review of the Automated Detection of Change in Serial Imaging Studies of the Brain. J. Digit. Imaging 17, 158–174 (2004)
7. Ettinger, G.J., Grimson, W.E.L., Lozano-Perez, T., Wells III, W.M., White, S.J., Kikinis, R.: Automatic registration for multiple sclerosis change detection. In: IEEE Workshop on Biomedical Image Analysis, Los Alamitos, CA, pp. 297–306 (1994)

8. Chui, H., Win, L., Schultz, R., Duncan, J.S., Rangarajan, A.: A unified non-rigid feature registration method for brain mapping. Med. Image. Anal. 7(2), 113–130 (2003)
9. Davatzikos, C., Prince, J.L.: Brain image registration based on curve mapping. In: IEEE Workshop on Biomedical Image Analysis, Los Alamitos, CA, pp. 245–254 (1994)
10. Davatzikos, C., Prince, J.L., Bryan, R.N.: Image registration based on boundary mapping. IEEE Transactions on Medical Imaging 15(1), 112–115 (1996)
11. Douglas, N.G., Bruce, F.: Accurate and robust brain image alignment using boundary-based registration. Neuroimage (2009)
12. Christensen, G.E.: Inverse consistent registration with object boundary constraints. In: IEEE International Symposium on Biomedical Imaging, vol. 1, pp. 591–594 (2004)
13. Talairach, J., Tournoux, P.: Co-planar stereotaxic Atlas of the Human Brain. Thieme Medical Publishers (1988)
14. Verard, L., Allain, P., Travere, J.M., Baron, J.C., Bloyet, D.: Fully Automatic Identification of AC and PC Landmarks on Brain MRI Using Scene Analysis. IEEE Transactions on Medical Imaging 16(5), 610–616 (1997)
15. Rohr, K., Stiehl, H., Sprengel, R., Buzug, T., Weese, J., Kuhn, M.: Landmark-based elastic registration using approximating thin-plate splines. IEEE Trans. Med. Img. 20(6), 526–534 (2001)
16. Thirion, J.P.: New feature points based on geometric invariants for 3d image registration. Int. J. of Computer Vision 18(2), 121–137 (1996)
17. Viola, P.A., Wells, W.M.: Alignment by maximization of mutual information. International Journal of Computer Vision 24(2), 137–154 (1997)
18. Penney, G.P., Weese, J., Little, J.A., Desmedt, P., Hill, D.L.G., Hawkes, D.J.: A comparison of similarity measures for use in 2-D-3-D medical image registration. IEEE Trans. on Med. Imaging 17, 586–594 (1998)
19. Pluim, J., Maintz, J., Viergever, M.: Image registration by maximization of combined mutual information and gradient information. IEEE Trans. on Med. Imaging 19(8), 809–814 (2000)
20. Fitzpatrick, J.M., West, J.B., Maurer, C.R.J.: Predicting error in rigid-body point-based registration. IEEE Trans. Med. Imaging 17, 694–702 (1998)
21. Jenkinson, M., Smith, S.: A global optimisation method for robust affine registration of brain images. Med. Image. Anal. 5(2), 143–156 (2001)
22. Golub, G.H., Van Loan, C.F.: Matrix Computations. JHU Press (1996)
23. Murray, R.M., Li, Z., Sastry, S.: A Mathematical Introduction to Robotic Manipulation. CRC Press, Boca Raton (1994)

Bayesian Estimation of Deformation and Elastic Parameters in Non-rigid Registration

Petter Risholm[1,2], Eigil Samset[2], and William Wells III[1]

[1] Harvard Medical School, Brigham and Women's Hospital
[2] Center of Mathematics for Applications, University of Oslo
pettri@ifi.uio.no

Abstract. Elastic deformation models are frequently used when solving non-rigid registration problems that are associated with neurosurgical image guidance, however, establishing precise values for the material parameters of brain tissue remains challenging. In this work we include elastography in the registration process by formulating these parameters as unknown random variables with associated priors that may be broad or sharp, depending on the situation.

A Bayesian registration model is introduced where the deformation probability is formulated by way of Boltzmann's equation and the linear elastic deformation and similarity energies. The full joint posterior on deformation and elastic random variables is characterized with a Markov Chain Monte Carlo method and can provide useful information beyond the usual "point estimates"; e.g. deformation uncertainty. Hard deformation constraints are easily accommodated in this framework which allows us to constrain the deformation of the brain to the intra-cranial space.

We describe preliminary experiments with synthetic 3D brain images for which ground truth is known for the elastic and deformation parameters. We compare a model with separate elastic parameters for three compartments (white matter, gray matter, and CSF), to a single compartment model, and show convergence, improved deformation estimates for the three compartment model and that plausible posteriors on the elastic parameters are obtained from the elastography process.

1   Introduction

Many surgical procedures induce tissue deformations such that image information acquired before surgery might not match the anatomy seen during surgery. In this paper we focus on deformations occurring during neurosurgery, however, the applicability of the framework we present is not restricted to the neurosurgical case. Opening of the dura leads to a gravitational shift of the brain tissue mainly due to the disappearance of pressure forces at the brain and ventricular boundaries[1]. This shift is commonly called brain-shift and has been reported to be ranging up to 24mm[2]. The "brain" consists of four main compartments, or tissue materials; skull (SK), gray matter (GM), white matter (WM) and cerebrospinal fluid (CSF). These compartments will deform differently during

B. Fischer, B. Dawant, and C. Lorenz (Eds.): WBIR 2010, LNCS 6204, pp. 104–115, 2010.

surgery because different tissues have different material properties. In particular, we may see a partial collapse of the ventricular areas due to CSF leakage[3]. A substantial uncertainty is involved in determining exact values for the material properties of brain tissue, and consequently the reported estimates of material parameters are quite divergent[4]. In addition, medication, radiation, or other factors related to the surgical procedure may significantly change the material parameters.

Many non-physical models have been proposed to recover tissue deformation, e.g. B-splines[5] and the Demons method[6]. However, these methods are not directly connected to the actual physical behavior of the tissue and do not explicitly model any material parameters. The most successful intra-operative registration methods use biomechanical models[7,8] which accommodates specifying separate elastic parameter values for different tissue types, but because the literature reports divergent values for the material parameters, most authors avoid the issue of varying tissue parameters and use fixed uniform material parameters for the whole registered anatomy. In [9], Ou et. al. introduced an interesting approach to elastography using a biomechanical model to estimate tissue parameters from two images that are deformed versions of each other. A disadvantage to their method is that the initial boundary conditions, i.e. the movement of boundary nodes in the biomechanical model, are not estimated in the method but needs to be specified.

In contrast to [9], we propose to integrate an elastography process in a Bayesian registration framework and thereby estimate both the boundary conditions as well as the elastic parameters simultaneously. A Markov Chain Monte Carlo sampling technique is applied to characterize the posterior distributions over deformation and elastic parameters. The sampling approach also effectively facilitates adding hard deformation constraints, for instance to constrain the deformation to the intra-cranial space.

2 Elastic Image Registration

Let $\mathbf{f}(\mathbf{x})$ and $\mathbf{m}(\mathbf{x})$, $\mathbf{x} \in \Omega$ be a pre- and intra-operative image of the brain respectively. They are defined over the d-dimensional image region $\Omega \subset \mathbb{R}^d$. We assume there exists a segmentation of $\mathbf{f}$ into disjoint anatomical regions $\Omega = \cup_{l \in \{CSF,GM,WM\}} \Omega_l$, and require a segmentation of the skull region Ω_{SK}.

We assume there exists a displacement field $\mathbf{u}(\mathbf{x})$, $\mathbf{x} \in \Omega$ such that $\mathbf{m}(\mathbf{u}(\mathbf{x}) + \mathbf{x})$ is similar to $\mathbf{f}$. We measure the similarity between two images using an energy (similarity) function $E_s(\mathbf{u}; \mathbf{f}, \mathbf{m})$. Many types of similarity measures have been proposed in the literature. Any choice of similarity measure would be applicable in the proposed framework. However, in this work we restrict ourselves to the popular sum of squared differences

$$E_s(\mathbf{u}; \mathbf{f}, \mathbf{m}) = \int_\Omega (\mathbf{f}(\mathbf{x}) - \mathbf{m}(\mathbf{u}(\mathbf{x}) + \mathbf{x}))^2 d\mathbf{x} \qquad (1)$$

It is common to restrict the deformations to model some physical meaningful process. Perhaps the most common model used in intra-subject registration is to model brain tissue as a linear elastic material. This mechanism, which may be viewed as a regularizer, is defined in terms of an energy function

$$E_r(\mathbf{u}; \boldsymbol{\mu}, \boldsymbol{\lambda}) = \int_\Omega \frac{\mu(\mathbf{x})}{4} \sum_{j,k=1}^d (\partial_{x_j} u_k + \partial_{x_k} u_j)^2 + \frac{\lambda(\mathbf{x})}{2} (\mathrm{div}\ \mathbf{u}(\mathbf{x}))^2 \mathrm{dx} \ , \qquad (2)$$

where $\mu, \lambda \in \mathbb{R}^+$ are the Lamé parameters. A subscript on $\mathbf{x}$ and $\mathbf{u}$ denotes a specific component of the 3D vector. Notice that we model the elastic parameters as functions of $\mathbf{x}$. In a traditional energy minimization registration method[10], we generally solve: $\underset{\mathbf{u}}{\mathrm{argmin}}\ E(\mathbf{u}; \mathbf{f}, \mathbf{m}, \boldsymbol{\mu}, \boldsymbol{\lambda}) = E_s(\mathbf{u}; \mathbf{f}, \mathbf{m}) + \alpha E_r(\mathbf{u}; \boldsymbol{\lambda}, \boldsymbol{\mu})$, where α is a weighting parameter.

2.1   Linear Elastic Finite Element Model

The Finite Element (FE) method is a powerful and versatile computational framework that is frequently used in the context of linear elastic problems over non-uniform domains. It provides a fast way of computing both E_r and E_s. FE-calculations are performed on a mesh that covers the region of interest. In this work we used a non-uniform tetrahedral mesh where the tetrahedral elements coarsely conform to the tissue boundaries delineated by Ω (GM, WM and CSF). The number of nodes and elements in the mesh is denoted N_e and N_n respectively.

In a FE setting we often work with the strain energy instead of the elastic potential in Eq. (2) (we refer to [11] for a detailed description of linear elastic FE-methods):

$$E_r = \frac{1}{2} \int_\Omega \epsilon^T \sigma \mathrm{dx} \ . \qquad (3)$$

Let the displacement vector be $\mathbf{u} = [u, v, w]^T$, the strain vector is then defined as:

$$\epsilon = \left[\frac{\partial u}{\partial x}, \frac{\partial v}{\partial y}, \frac{\partial w}{\partial z}, \frac{\partial u}{\partial y} + \frac{\partial v}{\partial x}, \frac{\partial u}{\partial z} + \frac{\partial w}{\partial x}, \frac{\partial v}{\partial z} + \frac{\partial w}{\partial y} \right]^T . \qquad (4)$$

We can rewrite this as $\epsilon = \mathbf{B}\mathbf{u}$ where:

$$\mathbf{B} = \begin{bmatrix} \frac{\partial}{\partial x} & 0 & 0 & \frac{\partial}{\partial y} & \frac{\partial}{\partial z} & 0 \\ 0 & \frac{\partial}{\partial y} & 0 & \frac{\partial}{\partial x} & 0 & \frac{\partial}{\partial z} \\ 0 & 0 & \frac{\partial}{\partial z} & 0 & \frac{\partial}{\partial x} & \frac{\partial}{\partial y} \end{bmatrix}^T .$$

The stress vector $\boldsymbol{\sigma}$ is related to the strain vector through Hooke's law, $\boldsymbol{\sigma} = \mathbf{C}\boldsymbol{\epsilon}$, where $\mathbf{C}$ is the material matrix. For an isotropic material this matrix is defined by the two Lamé material constants λ and μ:

$$\mathbf{C} = \begin{bmatrix} \lambda + 2\mu & \lambda & \lambda & 0 & 0 & 0 \\ \lambda & \lambda + 2\mu & \lambda & 0 & 0 & 0 \\ \lambda & \lambda & \lambda + 2\mu & 0 & 0 & 0 \\ 0 & 0 & 0 & \mu & 0 & 0 \\ 0 & 0 & 0 & 0 & \mu & 0 \\ 0 & 0 & 0 & 0 & 0 & \mu \end{bmatrix} . \qquad (5)$$

Using these relations, adding work done by internal forces, $\mathbf{f}$, and minimizing with regards to $\mathbf{u}$, we end up with a linear matrix equation for each element:

$$\mathbf{K}_e\mathbf{u}_e = V_e\mathbf{B}_e^T\mathbf{C}_e\mathbf{B}_e\mathbf{u}_e = \mathbf{f}_e \ , \tag{6}$$

where $\mathbf{K}_e$ is called the element stiffness matrix and V_e is the volume of the element. By assembling the contributions for each element into a square global stiffness matrix, $\mathbf{K}$, of size dN_n, we get a large sparse linear system:

$$\mathbf{K}\mathbf{u} = \mathbf{f} \ . \tag{7}$$

The linear system is under-determined – the solution can be seen as a mesh floating freely in space. Consequently, the positions of at least three nodes need to be specified to constrain the computations appropriately.

For a given deformation $\mathbf{u}$, the elastic energy in Eq. (3) can be computed efficiently using the FE-model. To compute the integral in Eq. (1), we use a 4-point Gaussian quadrature[11] and sum up the contributions from each element.

3   A Bayesian Framework for Elastic Image Registration

Our framework is based on a generative Bayesian probability model where the node deformations as well as the elastic material parameters can vary over the image domain.

3.1   Generative Model

We assume that the intra-operative image $\mathbf{m}$, the deformation $\mathbf{u}$, and the elastic parameters $\boldsymbol{\mu}$ and $\boldsymbol{\lambda}$ are random variables generated by the hierarchical model in Fig. 1. Notice that the pre-operative image, $\mathbf{f}$, is a model parameter. This leads to the following joint probability model:

$$p(\mathbf{m}, \mathbf{u}, \boldsymbol{\lambda}, \boldsymbol{\mu}) = p(\mathbf{m}|\mathbf{u})p(\mathbf{u}|\boldsymbol{\lambda}, \boldsymbol{\mu})p(\boldsymbol{\lambda})p(\boldsymbol{\mu}) \ . \tag{8}$$

According to the theorem of conditional probability we can write the posterior as

$$p(\mathbf{u}, \boldsymbol{\lambda}, \boldsymbol{\mu}|\mathbf{m}) = \frac{p(\mathbf{m}, \mathbf{u}, \boldsymbol{\lambda}, \boldsymbol{\mu})}{p(\mathbf{m})} = \frac{p(\mathbf{m}|\mathbf{u})p(\mathbf{u}|\boldsymbol{\lambda}, \boldsymbol{\mu})p(\boldsymbol{\lambda})p(\boldsymbol{\mu})}{p(\mathbf{m})} \ . \tag{9}$$

Since we are mainly interested in characterizing the deformation, the Lamé parameters can be seen as nuisance parameters and marginalized out:

$$p(\mathbf{u}|\mathbf{m}) = \int_\Omega \int_\Omega \frac{p(\mathbf{m}|\mathbf{u})p(\mathbf{u}|\boldsymbol{\lambda}, \boldsymbol{\mu})p(\boldsymbol{\lambda})p(\boldsymbol{\mu})}{p(\mathbf{m})}d\boldsymbol{\lambda}d\boldsymbol{\mu} \ . \tag{10}$$

We use the Boltzmann distribution to define the likelihood, often called the similarity term

$$p(\mathbf{m}|\mathbf{u}) = \frac{1}{Z_s}\exp\left(-\frac{E_s(\mathbf{u}; \mathbf{m}, \mathbf{f})}{T_s}\right), \tag{11}$$

where Z_s is a normalizing constant and T_s is the temperature parameter for the distribution. The Boltzmann distribution is similarly used to model the prior on the transformation which acts as a regularizer

$$p(\mathbf{u}|\boldsymbol{\lambda}, \boldsymbol{\mu}) = \frac{1}{Z_r} \exp\left(-\frac{E_r(\mathbf{u}; \boldsymbol{\lambda}, \boldsymbol{\mu})}{T_r}\right) . \tag{12}$$

The Lamé parameters, $\boldsymbol{\lambda}$ and $\boldsymbol{\mu}$, should be non-negative to be compatible with human tissue. There are many suitable priors that can be used to model the elastic parameters depending on the prior information that is available. We model the elastic parameter priors, $p(\boldsymbol{\lambda})$ and $p(\boldsymbol{\mu})$, by Beta distributions scaled to the region $[r1, r2]$ and assume that the parameters are independent: $p(\boldsymbol{\mu}; A_\mu, B_\mu, r_1, r_2) = \prod_{\mu_i \in \mu} Beta(\mu_i; A_\mu, B_\mu, r_1, r_2)$. The prior on $\boldsymbol{\lambda}$ is defined similarly. We have flexibility in modeling the prior – we can use separate priors for different brain compartments, or alternatively use a global prior.

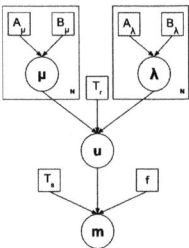

Fig. 1. A generative model of the registration problem. The deformation random variable, $\mathbf{u}$, depends on the elastic random variables, $\boldsymbol{\mu}$ and $\boldsymbol{\lambda}$. The deformation governs the image, $\mathbf{m}$, we will observe given the image $\mathbf{f}$. $A_\lambda, A_\mu, B_\lambda$ and B_μ are parameters controlling the prior (beta) distributions for the elastic random variables. The two parameters, T_s and T_r, control the temperature of the likelihood distribution and the prior distribution on the deformation respectively. The plate parameter, N, is established by the resolution we sample the elastic parameters at. It can be uniform over the image domain, per tissue compartment or per element in the FE-model.

3.2   MCMC-Optimization

We wish to characterize the posterior in Eq. (10), given images $\mathbf{f}$ and $\mathbf{m}$. Unfortunately, it is not possible to analytically compute the posterior nor feasible to draw samples directly from it. A common approach to generate samples from complicated posteriors is by way of the Metropolis-Hastings (MH) algorithm[12]. In our setting we will draw samples from $p(\mathbf{u}, \boldsymbol{\lambda}, \boldsymbol{\mu}|\mathbf{m})$ and "discard" the values for $\boldsymbol{\lambda}$ and $\boldsymbol{\mu}$ to characterize Eq. (10). However, notice that the "discarded" values can be used for characterizing the marginal posterior distributions for the elastic parameters. While deterministic optimization procedures generally requires the Euler-Lagrange equations, MCMC-optimization stochastically optimizes the posterior distribution purely based on the probability distributions defined in the previous section and thereby eliminates the need for computing any gradients of the energy equations. Algorithm 1 provides an overview of the method.

Metropolis-Hastings. In the MH-algorithm, candidate samples are drawn from a proposal distribution $q(\boldsymbol{\theta}^*|\boldsymbol{\theta}^n)$, with $\boldsymbol{\theta} = (\mathbf{u}, \boldsymbol{\lambda}, \boldsymbol{\mu})$, from which it should be easy to draw samples. For a particular step n of the algorithm, where the current state is $\boldsymbol{\theta}^n$, we draw a sample $\boldsymbol{\theta}^*$ from $q(\boldsymbol{\theta}^*|\boldsymbol{\theta}^n)$ and accept it with probability

$$A(\boldsymbol{\theta}^*, \boldsymbol{\theta}^n) = \min\left(1, \frac{p(\boldsymbol{\theta}^*|\mathbf{m})q(\boldsymbol{\theta}^n|\boldsymbol{\theta}^*)}{p(\boldsymbol{\theta}^n|\mathbf{m})q(\boldsymbol{\theta}^*|\boldsymbol{\theta}^n)}\right) . \tag{13}$$

If the sample is accepted, $\boldsymbol{\theta}^{n+1} = \boldsymbol{\theta}^*$, otherwise $\boldsymbol{\theta}^{n+1} = \boldsymbol{\theta}^n$. Notice that the evaluation of the acceptance criterion does not require knowledge of the normalizing constants Z_s, Z_r and $p(\mathbf{m})$. For symmetric proposal distributions, such as the Normal distribution, the MH algorithm reduces to the standard Metropolis criterion where the ratio of the proposal distributions equals one.

Proposal Distributions. We model the proposal distribution with three Normal *jumping kernels*[12] and assume that the parameters are independent:

$$\boldsymbol{\theta}^* \sim q(\boldsymbol{\theta}^*|\boldsymbol{\theta}^n) = N_\mathbf{u}(\mathbf{u}^*|\mathbf{u}^n, \sigma_u)N_\lambda(\boldsymbol{\lambda}^*|\boldsymbol{\lambda}^n, \sigma_\lambda)N_\mu(\boldsymbol{\mu}^*|\boldsymbol{\mu}^n, \sigma_\mu) . \tag{14}$$

By using a rejection sampler, we restrict the elastic parameters to $\mu, \lambda \in \mathbb{R}^+$ and the node positions from moving into the skull region $(\mathbf{p} + \mathbf{u}) \notin \Omega_{\mathrm{SK}}$, where $\mathbf{p}$ are the initial nodal positions. Because the proposal samplers are Normal distributions, the proposal ratio $q(\boldsymbol{\theta}^n|\boldsymbol{\theta}^*)/q(\boldsymbol{\theta}^*|\boldsymbol{\theta}^n)$ equals one.

Sampling Convergence. A problem in iterative simulations is to assess whether or not we are generating samples from the target distribution and whether we have generated enough samples to characterize it properly. A common approach of monitoring convergence is to compute the *scale reduction* for each scalar estimand using parallel Markov Chains[12]. We use three parallel Markov Chains and assume the posterior distribution has been adequately characterized when the scale reduction is less than 1.2 for all estimands.

3.3   Sampling Strategies

Deformation Sampling. We can sample deformations involving from three to all the nodes in the mesh. Calculation of Eq. (7) provides us with the nodal deformations for the nodes that are not sampled. In this work we sampled deformations for all nodes on the brain boundary, while the deformations for the inner nodes were found through the FE-calculations.

Deformation Constraints. Restricting the sampler from accepting nodal positions in Ω_{SK} avoids impossible nodal configurations. At the same time it allows the brain to slide along the skull boundary to find the minimum energy configuration.

Elasticity Sampling. We have the option of sampling the elastic parameters per element, per tissue label or uniformly over the image domain. For the present experiments we assume that the intra-tissue elastic variation is negligible and consequently sample the elastic parameters on a per-tissue basis. Hence, we sampled different λ and μ for $\Omega_{\mathrm{GM}}, \Omega_{\mathrm{WM}}$ and Ω_{CSF} so that $\boldsymbol{\lambda} = (\lambda_{\mathrm{CSF}}, \lambda_{\mathrm{GM}}, \lambda_{\mathrm{WM}})$ and $\boldsymbol{\mu} = (\mu_{\mathrm{CSF}}, \mu_{\mathrm{GM}}, \mu_{\mathrm{WM}})$.

Because no internal forces are applied in the FE-calculations, $\mathbf{f} = \mathbf{0}$, we can see from inspecting Eq. (6) that the ratios of the elastic parameters controls the tissue elasticity while the scale of $\boldsymbol{\mu}$ and $\boldsymbol{\lambda}$ will have no affect on the calculations. Hence, to avoid drifting of the parameters towards zero, we fix one of the elastic parameters and sample the rest of them. It is also worth mentioning that since nodal positions are only sampled for nodes on the boundary of the mesh, it is the sampling of the elastic parameters that effectively explores the deformation space for the internal mesh nodes.

Algorithm 1. Bayesian estimation of deformation and elastic parameters.

---

   repeat
      Sample $\mathbf{u}^* \sim N_{\mathbf{u}}(\mathbf{u}^n, \sigma_{\mathbf{u}}), (\mathbf{p} + \mathbf{u}^*) \in \Omega$.
      Sample $\boldsymbol{\lambda}^* \sim N_{\lambda}(\boldsymbol{\lambda}^* | \boldsymbol{\lambda}^n, \sigma_{\lambda}), \boldsymbol{\lambda}^* \in \mathbb{R}^+$
      Sample $\boldsymbol{\mu}^* \sim N_{\mu}(\boldsymbol{\mu}^* | \boldsymbol{\mu}^n, \sigma_{\mu}), \boldsymbol{\mu}^* \in \mathbb{R}^+$
      Compute the energies in Eqs. (1) and (3)
      Compute the MH criteria in Eq. (13).
      if Accept **then** $\theta^{n+1} = \theta^*$
      else $\theta^{n+1} = \theta^n$
      end if
   until Convergence

---

4   Results

4.1   Dataset

Preliminary validation of the framework was performed on a synthetic dataset where ground truth was established. We acquired an anatomic T1 weighted MR image together with a label map from the BrainWeb[13] database. A label-dependent tetrahedral mesh consisting of $N_e = 3807$ elements and $N_n = 801$ nodes was generated. We fixed 20 boundary mesh nodes with a deformation of $15~mm$ in the direction of the center of gravity of the brain and used the sampler to find the configuration of the remaining boundary nodes that minimized the elastic energy of the mesh. The literature[4] indicates that the elastic ratio of brain tissue should be approximately $\lambda/\mu \approx 24$. For generation of the dataset we fixed the elastic parameters to $\mu_{\mathrm{CSF}} = 10^{-6}, \mu_{\mathrm{GM}} = 1, \mu_{\mathrm{WM}} = 1, \lambda_{\mathrm{CSF}} = 10^{-6}, \lambda_{\mathrm{GM}} = 10, \lambda_{\mathrm{WM}} = 30$. The resulting dataset can be seen in Fig. 2. Even though CSF is clearly not an elastic material, we model it with small elastic values compared to GM and WM to approximate the fluid nature of CSF.

4.2 Experiments

Two separate experiments were carried out. In both experiments we sampled deformations for the 349 boundary nodes, while the deformations of the internal nodes were computed by solving Eq. (7). The elastic parameters were sampled in two different ways. In the first experiment the elastic parameters were uniformly sampled for all tissue types such that $\mu_{\mathrm{CSF}} = \mu_{\mathrm{GM}} = \mu_{\mathrm{WM}}$ and $\lambda_{\mathrm{CSF}} = \lambda_{\mathrm{GM}} = \lambda_{\mathrm{WM}}$. In the second experiment the parameters were sampled independently. We assumed no prior information on the elastic parameters and therefore used a uniform prior on them ($A_\lambda = A_\mu = B_\lambda = B_\mu = 1, r_1 = 0, r_2 = \infty$), identical deformation sampling kernels ($\sigma_u = 0.008$) and the same temperatures ($T_s = 0.05, T_r = 10\,000$) for the two experiments. These parameters resulted in a MCMC acceptance rate of approximately 25%. We used a thinning factor of 10 and generated samples until the reduction scale was less than 1.2 for all estimands. A total of 250 000 samples were generated for each of the three parallel samplers, but, after thinning, only 25 000 samples were used to characterize

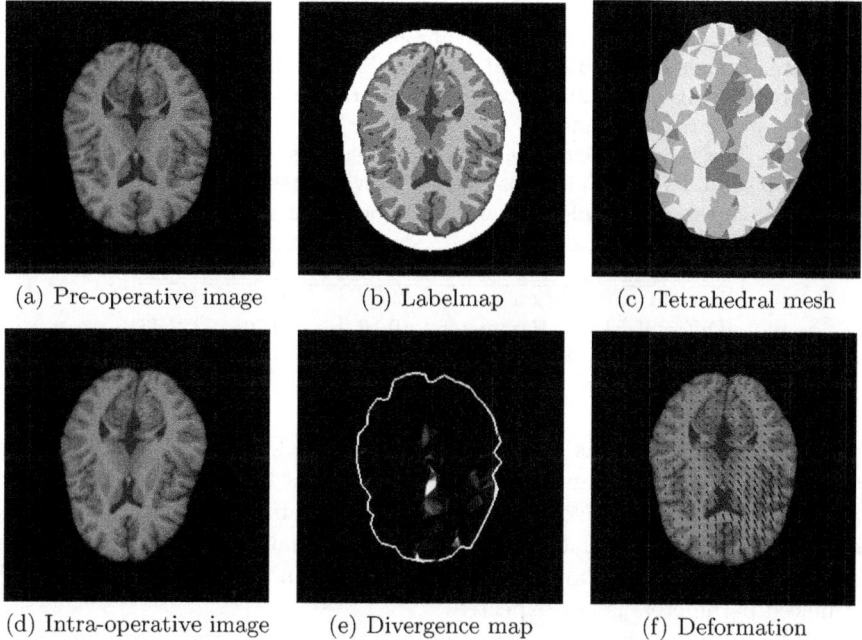

(a) Pre-operative image   (b) Labelmap   (c) Tetrahedral mesh

(d) Intra-operative image   (e) Divergence map   (f) Deformation

Fig. 2. The synthetic dataset. In (c) we show a cut through the mesh we used for the computations. CSF is colored in red, GM in green and WM in yellow. The poor correspondence between labels in (b) and (c) is a result of the coarse mesh. In (e) we show the divergence, which is governed by the λ parameter (see Eq. (2)), of the deformation field. Notice the bright areas in the divergence map, they are signs of the collapse of the ventricular areas. Also notice the skull label in (b), the sampler restricts movements of nodes into this area. Figure (f) shows the x- and y-components of the ground truth deformation field.

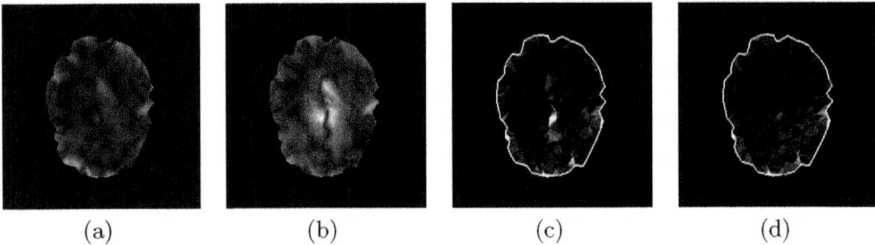

| (a) | (b) | (c) | (d) |

Fig. 3. The two images on the left shows the norm of the difference between the ground truth deformation and the estimated deformation field with varying elastic parameters (a) and with uniform elastic parameters (b). Comparing the deformation errors, it is clear that using varying elastic parameters provides a better estimate of the deformation in the interior of the brain. The collapse of the ventricles (see the divergence map in Fig. 2(e)) is better accommodated with varying elastic parameters than in the uniform case (compare the two rightmost images where (c) stems from using varying elastic parameters while (d) from uniform parameters).

Table 1. This table reports statistics on absolute error between the posterior means of the boundary node deformations and the ground truth deformations for these nodes. We also report statistics on the distance between the initial configuration of the nodes and the ground truth. From this and Tbl. 2 we can draw the conclusion that the sampler provides comparable estimates of the movements of the nodes on the boundary, while sampling different elasticity parameters provides us with a better estimate of the deformation in the interior of the brain. All values are in millimeters.

	Median	95th quantile	Max
Initial Configuration	2.56	8.24	15.08
Different Elastic Parameters	0.16	0.72	2.43
Uniform Elastic Parameters	0.18	0.83	2.40

the posterior distributions (a total of 75 000 samples). Each parallel sampler generated 5 samples per second which resulted in a total computation time of approximately 14 hours. Notice that we used the same sampling framework for generating the synthetic dataset as we used to estimate the elastic and deformation parameters. Hence, large discrepancies between the ground truth and the estimated parameters is not expected.

MCMC methods should use starting points that are crude estimates of the mode of the posterior distribution[12] that we are interested in. A simpler and faster registration method, such as the Demons method[6], can be used to find an initial configuration of the deformation parameters. We used initial deformation parameters for the boundary nodes that were in between an identity deformation and the ground truth deformation. In Tbl. 1 we report statistics on the distance between the initial configuration and the ground truth, as well as the distance between the estimated posterior means of the node deformations and the ground truth.

Table 2. In this table we report the Mean Squared Error (MSE) between the computed deformation and the ground truth deformation over different tissue types. The upper row contains results from varying the elastic parameters for each tissue type, while the results in the lower row stems from using uniform elastic parameters. It is evident that varying the elastic parameters provides a better estimate of the ground truth. All values are in millimeters squared.

	Ω	Ω_{CSF}	Ω_{GM}	Ω_{WM}
Different Elastic Parameters	0.040	0.049	0.049	0.023
Uniform Elastic Parameters	0.065	0.087	0.067	0.048

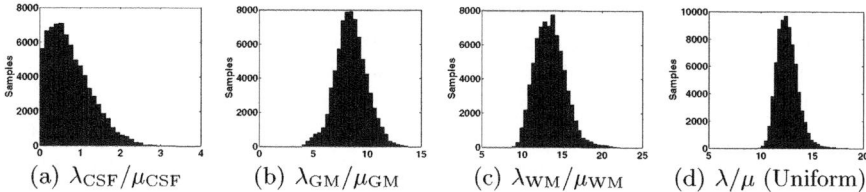

(a) $\lambda_{\mathrm{CSF}}/\mu_{\mathrm{CSF}}$ (b) $\lambda_{\mathrm{GM}}/\mu_{\mathrm{GM}}$ (c) $\lambda_{\mathrm{WM}}/\mu_{\mathrm{WM}}$ (d) λ/μ (Uniform)

Fig. 4. Marginal posteriors of the elastic ratios for each tissue compartment. The ground truth values are, $\lambda_{\mathrm{CSF}}/\mu_{\mathrm{CSF}} = 1$, $\lambda_{\mathrm{GM}}/\mu_{\mathrm{GM}} = 10$ and $\lambda_{\mathrm{WM}}/\mu_{\mathrm{WM}} = 30$. It is evident that the method is able to recover elastic parameters that distinguishes between different tissue types, but not necessarily capable of recovering the exact underlying values. It is also evident that the elastic ratios are biased towards zero. This may be explained by the drifting mentioned in Sec. 3.3 and the Boltzmann distribution of the elastic energy. The lower the temperature is set, the more regularization we apply to the registration and the more the elastic parameters will tend towards zero. WM volume is also larger than for GM, hence the ratio for WM tends more towards zero than for GM.

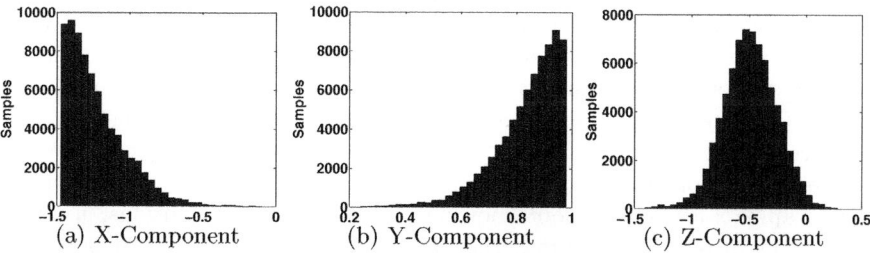

(a) X-Component   (b) Y-Component   (c) Z-Component

Fig. 5. Translations were sampled for each node on the boundary of the mesh. This figure shows the marginal posterior distributions for each translational component for one of the boundary nodes. The posterior distribution of nodes moving along the skull-brain boundary gets the truncated shape we see in (a) and (b).

Figure 3 provides qualitative results from the registrations while Tbl. 2 reports quantitative Mean Squared Error (MSE) results from comparing the final deformation field with the ground truth deformation. It is evident that sampling the elastic parameters per compartment provides better results in the brain interior, while the estimated deformations on the brain boundary (see Tbl. 1) are comparable. In Fig. 4 we plot posterior distributions of the elastic ratios. The experiments show that we are able to distinguish between tissue types and that we recover plausible elastic ratios, however the ratios are biased towards zero. Figure 5 shows the posterior distribution of one of the boundary nodes. Notice how the rejection of samples that fall in the skull region have truncated the posterior distributions for this particular node.

5 Discussion

In this paper we presented a Bayesian framework for simultaneous estimation of deformation and material parameters. One advantage of our approach is the characterization of marginal posteriors instead of point estimates for the registration parameters – not only can we find the most likely configuration of the deformation field given two images, but from the posterior distribution we can also quantify deformation uncertainty. Another novelty of the method is the ability for elastography without first determining the initial boundary conditions. Prior information on the material parameters is seamlessly included in the framework through the prior distributions on them. The MCMC sampler facilitates inclusion of hard deformation constraints; for example if a segmentation of the skull is available, brain movements can be restricted to the intra-cranial space.

Unfortunately, high-dimensional problems solved with MCMC methods require a large number of samples to adequately characterize the posterior distribution. Hence, it is a computationally intensive method that might not be suitable for intra-operative use in the near term. However, the use of parallel samplers on large computer clusters can reduce the computational time considerably. Because the method is highly computationally intensive, a coarse brain mesh was applied for the experiments to make it computationally tractable. Future work should study the sensitivity of the method to the tissue segmentation and the coarseness of the mesh. Notice that the need for a tissue segmentation can be eliminated by sampling the elastic parameters per element instead of per tissue compartment.

Three main conclusions can be drawn from the preliminary experiments: 1) elastography is feasible without knowing initial boundary conditions, and plausible marginal posteriors on material parameters are obtained, 2) it is possible to characterize posterior distributions on deformations and 3) improved registration results are achieved with finer elastic sampling resolution. Hence, this registration framework is particularly useful whenever it is difficult to establish precise values for the elastic parameters.

Acknowledgments. We are grateful to Prof. Hal Stern, University of California, Irvine, for his helpful advice. This research was supported by NIH grants R01CA138419 and U41RR019703.

References

1. Ferrant, M., Nabavi, A., Macq, B., Black, P., Jolesz, F., Kikinis, R., Warfield, S.: Serial registration of intraoperative mr images of the brain. Medical Image Analysis 6(4), 337–359 (2002)
2. Hastreiter, P., Rezk-Salama, C., Soza, G., Greiner, G., Fahlbusch, R., Ganslandt, O., Nimsky, C.: Strategies for Brain Shift Evaluation. Medical Image Analysis 8(4), 447–464 (2004)
3. Hartkens, T., Hill, D.L.G., Castellano-Smith, A.D., Hawkes, D.J., Maurer, C.R., Martin, A.J., Hall, W.A., Liu, H., Truwit, C.L.: Measurement and analysis of brain deformation during neurosurgery. IEEE Trans. Med. Imaging 22(1), 82–92 (2003)
4. Hagemann, A., Rohr, K., Stiehl, H., Spetzger, U., Gilsbach, J.: Biomechanical modeling of the human head for physically based. Nonrigid Image Registration 18(10), 875–884 (1999)
5. Rueckert, D., Sonoda, L., Hayes, I., Hill, D., Leach, M., Hawkes, D.: Nonrigid registration using free-form deformations: Application to breast mr images. IEEE Trans. Med. Imaging 18(8), 712–721 (1999)
6. Thirion, J.P.: Image matching as a diffusion process: an analogy with Maxwell's demons. Medical Image Analysis 2(3), 243–260 (1998)
7. Clatz, O., Delingette, H., Talos, I.F., Golby, A.J., Kikinis, R., Jolesz, F.A., Ayache, N., Warfield, S.K.: Robust nonrigid registration to capture brain shift from intraoperative MRI. IEEE Trans. Med. Imaging 24(11), 1417–1427 (2005)
8. Miga, M.I., Roberts, D.W., Kennedy, F.E., Platenik, L.A., Hartov, A., Lunn, K.E., Paulsen, K.D.: Modeling of retraction and resection for intraoperative updating of images. Neurosurgery 49(1), 75–85 (2001)
9. Ou, J.J., Ong, R.E., Yankeelov, T.E., Miga, M.I.: Evaluation of 3d modality-independent elastography for breast imaging: a simulation study. Physics in Medicine and Biology 53(1), 147–163 (2008)
10. Modersitzki, J.: Numerical Methods for Image Registration. Oxford University Press, Oxford (2004)
11. Zienkiewicz, O.C., Taylor, R.L.: The Finite Element Method, 5th edn. Butterworth-Heinemann, Butterworths (2000)
12. Gelman, A., Carlin, J.B., Stern, H.S., Rubin, D.B.: Bayesian Data Analysis, 2nd edn. Texts in Statistical Science. Chapman & Hall/CRC (July 2003)
13. Collins, D.L., Zijdenbos, A.P., Kollokian, V., Sled, J.G., Kabani, N.J., Holmes, C.J., Evans, A.C.: Design and construction of a realistic digital brain phantom. IEEE Trans. Med. Imaging 17(3), 463–468 (1998)

Functional Non-rigid Registration Validation: A CT Phantom Study

Sven Kabus[1], Tobias Klinder[2], Jens von Berg[1], and Cristian Lorenz[1]

[1] Philips Research Europe – Hamburg, 22335 Hamburg, Germany
sven.kabus@philips.com
[2] Philips Research North America, Briarcliff Manor, NY 10510, USA

Abstract. Validation of respiratory motion estimation is indispensable for a variety of clinical applications. For CT lung registration, current approaches employ manually defined landmark sets or contours and compute a target registration error (TRE) to quantify registration accuracy. Preferably, the landmark set is well-dispersed to reflect for lung anatomy with its varying degrees of stiffness. A recent comparison study, however, revealed that the TRE is not sufficient for functional lung analysis.

On the basis of a compressible CT phantom functional lung analysis is addressed. Non-plausible expansion patterns as they occur for CT lung data are analyzed. Motivated by the relation of Hounsfield value and local volume change, local stiffness is incorporated into registration such that an improved functional lung analysis is achieved.

1 Introduction

Respiratory motion estimation is a topic receiving high attention in medical imaging. For clinical applications such as diagnosis as well as better planning, delivery, and assessment of therapy for lung diseases, estimation of and compensation for motion is indispensable. Motion compensation requires the non-rigid registration of CT lung data typically acquired in a dynamic protocol as for respiratory-gated 4D scans. In each case, the voxel-wise computation of respiratory motion at different respiratory states is required.

The accuracy of respiratory motion estimation has direct impact on the success of any clinical application mentioned above. While rigid registration is well suited for validation [1] and has come to a maturity state in clinical applications, for non-rigid registration there is a discrepancy between its maturity in the image processing community and its dissemination in clinical workstations indicating a lack of acceptance.

A necessary criterion for a successful registration is the alignment of visible image structures, often converted into an inspection of the residuum (i.e., the subtraction of the aligned data) where mis-aligned image structures show up. However, the absence of any structure in the residuum image does not guarantee a successful non-rigid registration since the residuum is invariant to the deformation of image regions with homogeneous intensities.

B. Fischer, B. Dawant, and C. Lorenz (Eds.): WBIR 2010, LNCS 6204, pp. 116–127, 2010.

Validation of non-rigid registration is primarily based on corresponding anatomical features such as landmarks or contours. For lung data the features are located on lung structures with adequate image contrast such as vessel bifurcations or the tumor boundary. After applying the registration result, a target registration error (TRE) is computed to measure registration accuracy quantitatively. However, number and distribution of the features as well as their meaningfulness for functional lung analysis need to be discussed.

A couple of research groups contributed to landmark validation, either by increasing the number of correspondences (e.g. [2,3]) or by distributing them equally throughout the lungs [4]. The latter is reported to provide a more realistic accuracy estimation since also low-contrast lung regions near to pleura or diaphragm are covered where registration accuracy is typically worse [5]. However, it is worth to point out that landmark correspondences can – unlike for affine registration – only *estimate* the accuracy of non-rigid registrations schemes. Beside the well-disperseness of the landmark set, the number of correspondences has impact on the estimation error. For illustration, a lung with a volume of 4 l and a set of 100 defined landmarks is considered. In this example, each cube with edge length 34 mm contains one landmark on average. Taking into account the distinctive non-homogeneity of lung parenchyma, it is questionable if such a sparse setting yields a robust estimation. Even for a set of about 1500 landmarks [3] the distribution remains sparse with one position per cube of edge length 14 mm on average.

Functional lung analysis on the basis of 4D-CT was recently addressed [6,7,8] for the purpose of lung diagnosis or adaptive radiotherapy planning. From a physiological point, the lungs in a healthy state either contract (during exhalation) *or* expand (during inhalation). Following [9] the magnitude of contraction or expansion, thus the lung ventilation, is typically highest near the diaphragm. A simultaneous mixture of local expansion and contraction, however, is very unlikely for normal breathing. This is in conflict with a recent comparison study [5] where three out of six registration schemes were reported to show individual contraction-expansion patterns but resulted in similar TREs. Therefore TRE appears to be not suitable for validation on a functional level. Similar to the residuum, it can serve as necessary criterion for registration accuracy but not as a sufficient one.

In this work validation of non-rigid registration is investigated on both a landmark level and a functional level. On the basis of a compressible CT phantom, registration of structures similar to lung parenchyma is addressed (Sect. 2). A variety of registration experiments is carried out to investigate lung registration validation thoroughly (Sect. 3). In the final part of this work reliable validation criteria are discussed.

2   Materials and Methods

In CT imaging, the lungs are shown with predominantly low densities complemented by filigree structures of higher density. The low densities can be assigned to lung parenchyma consisting of alveoli and capillary vessels, the higher densities result from bronchial walls or larger vessels. In fact, due to the partial

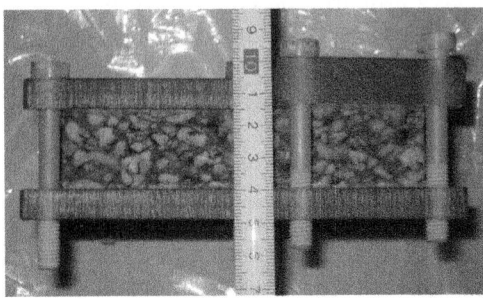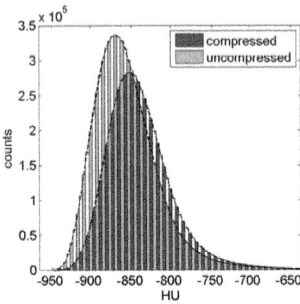

Fig. 1. Composite foam phantom ("axial" view) mounted between two plates in compressed state (left) together with an intensity histogram after CT acquisition (right)

volume effect almost all voxels represent a mixture of both types. During breathing, air can inflate or deflate the lungs, thus leading to a change in volume of lung parenchyma indicated by a change in local density. Generally the change is proportional to the fraction of air. A change in volume of a certain structure, however, requires the structure to be elastic. Thus, elasticity is proportional to the fraction of air as well. Larger vessels and upper parts of the bronchial tree (potentially attached with cartilage) are stiffer than smaller structures. A suitable CT lung phantom should therefore comprise a range from stiff to elastic structures. Compared to data from human lungs a phantom is free of artifacts induced by heart or respiratory motion. In addition, it can be acquired with high resolution since dose is not an issue.

2.1   Composite Foam Phantom

For this work, a rectangular object made of composite foam is chosen. It is composed of foam pieces with size ranging from about 1 mm to more than 10 mm. A sensory analysis reveals the single pieces to be of individual elasticity. The composite foam is mounted between two plates of acrylic glass with the upper plate splitted into two parts. Screws are used to fix the upper plate parts to the lower plate (see Fig. 1, left, for a picture of the phantom). The phantom is scanned twice using a Philips Mx8000 IDT (512x512x320 voxels, 0.33x0.33x0.45 mm^3 resolution, 168x168x144 mm^3 FOV), once in the uncompressed state and once in a compressed state by tightening the screws from 29 mm plate distance to 23–27 mm resulting in an overall volume reduction by 13.5%. To study different compressions and to make the following registration task more challenging, the two parts of the upper plate have been compressed independently (causing a step in-between) and also the screws of each part are tighten differently (see Fig. 2 for exemplary slices). A histogram analysis (Fig. 1, right) reveals that, as for the lungs, the density in the compressed state is higher than in the uncompressed state. Manual segmentation of the phantom in both scans allows for computing the relative compression relC as the reduction in plate distance divided by the plate distance in the uncompressed state (computed for each voxel column in

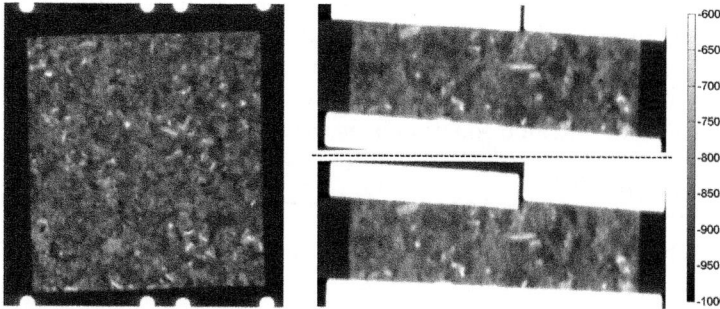

Fig. 2. Zoomed example slices of CT phantom: mid coronal slice in uncompressed state (left), mid axial slice in uncompressed (top right) and compressed state (bottom right)

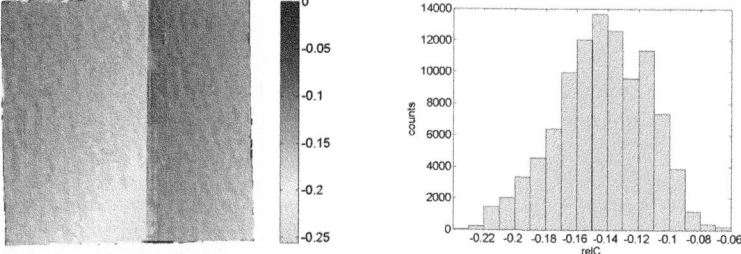

Fig. 3. Relative compression relC of phantom shown as color-coding (left; same view as in Fig. 2, left) and histogram (right). The left plot nicely demonstrates (a) the discontinuity in compression due to the splitted upper plate and (b) varying compression within each upper plate part due to the screws tightened differently.

coronal direction, see Fig. 3). For validation purposes, a software tool [4] is used to automatically define 50 landmarks in the uncompressed scan and to semi-automatically propagate these to the compressed scan. The maximum distance of a voxel position to the closest landmark position is 26.3 mm. Compared to the ideal well-dispersed distribution with a theoretically achievable maximum distance of 17.0 mm, the landmark set can be considered as being well-dispersed. The distance between corresponding landmarks in the uncompressed scan and the compressed scan was found to be 3.4±1.5 mm in the mean and 5.9 mm at maximum.

2.2   Elastic Registration

For convenience, let the uncompressed scan be the reference image R and the compressed scan the template image T. Both T, R are interpreted as mappings from $\Omega \subset \mathbb{R}^3$ to $\mathbb{R}$. The registration scheme aims at finding a deformation vector field (DVF) $u : \Omega \to \mathbb{R}^3$ such, that the displaced template image is aligned with the reference image. In this work a non-parametric approach [10] is chosen to minimize simultaneously a similarity measure $\mathcal{D}$ and a regularizing term $\mathcal{S}$. Due to the added regularizing term the registration problem is well-posed. For $\mathcal{D}$ the popular sum of squared differences is chosen while for $\mathcal{S}$ an elastic regularizer based on the Navier-Lamé equation is employed,

$$\overbrace{\int_\Omega (R(x) - T_u(x))^2 dx}^{\mathcal{D}[R,T_u]} + \overbrace{\int_\Omega E(x) \sum_{i,j=1}^{3} (\partial_{x_j} u_i(x) + \partial_{x_i} u_j(x))^2 dx}^{\mathcal{S}[u,E]} \overset{u}{\to} \min , \quad (1)$$

with T_u corresponding to the displaced template image. The elastic regularizer assumes that the underlying images can be characterized as an elastic and compressible material. Its properties are modeled by the so-called Lamé parameters which, for the special case of zero Poisson's ratio, can be translated into a single parameter: the elastic modulus E describes the amount of deformation given a constant force, it is thus linked to the material stiffness. As common to registration problems, E cannot be assigned an absolute value from the literature since its choice depends on the scale of T, R, on the chosen similarity measure, as well as on implementation issues. Therefore, in this work E is understood as $E = cE_0$ with E_0 having the unit [Pa]. As indicated in (1), the elastic modulus $E(x)$ is allowed to vary spatially [11].

3   Results

In this section the experiments and their results are described. For the elastic registration scheme as described in Sect. 2.2, two images T, R as well as the elastic modulus E are required. The elasticity can be modeled to be either constant throughout the image or spatially varying. The registration scheme results in a deformation vector field u. From the determinant of the Jacobian of u the local volume change can be computed for each voxel position as $V(x) := |\nabla u(x)| - 1$.

3.1   Standard Elastic Registration

Experiment Design: Let R be given as the uncompressed scan and T as the compressed scan, thus for u an overall contraction is expected. The elastic modulus is chosen to be constant throughout the image domain with values of (a) $62.5E_0$, (b) $250E_0$, and (c) $1000E_0$, respectively.

Findings: From a computation of the residuum (the subtraction of reference image and deformed template image) in all three cases the registration is judged as successful. A closer inspection reveals less remaining residual structures for smaller values of E demonstrating the impact of regularization on a registration scheme: a larger choice of E and thus a larger weight on the regularizer privileges a smooth deformation whereas a smaller weight allows for better adaptation to local anatomy. Regarding the alignment of the landmark positions, in all three

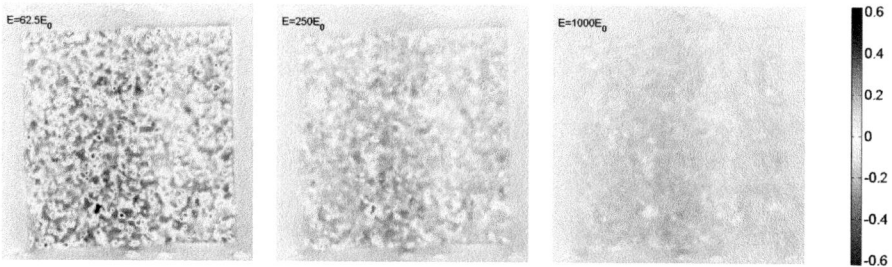

Fig. 4. Local volume change V (same coronal slice as in Fig. 2) when choosing constant values for the elastic modulus: $62.5E_0$ (left), $250E_0$ (center), and $1000E_0$ (right)

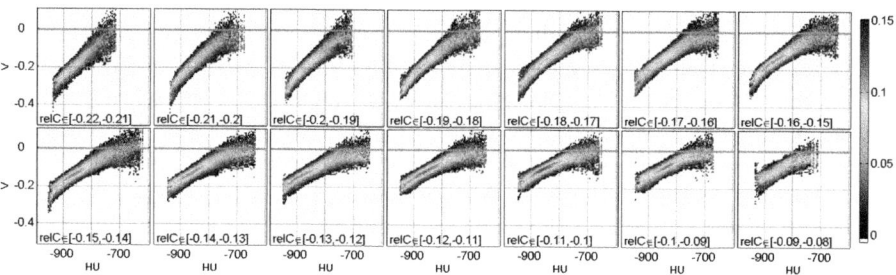

Fig. 5. Normalized joint histogram of local volume change V vs. Hounsfield values (HU) for setting (b), sorted according to relative compression relC. Note that smaller values of relC correspond to smaller plate distance and thus to higher phantom compression.

settings subvoxel accuracy is achieved. The TRE (mean±std (max) [mm]) is computed as (a) $0.27\pm0.14(0.75)$, (b) $0.28\pm0.13(0.72)$, and (c) $0.30\pm0.13(0.72)$, thus slightly better results are achieved for smaller values of E. The local volume change V, however, reveals expanding regions for (a) and (b) as depicted in Fig. 4. Recalling that the phantom was exposed to overall contraction, expanding regions would be physically unrealistic.

For closer inspection the relation of V and the Hounsfield values (HU) is analyzed[1] by means of a joint histogram: since a low (high) HU corresponds to low (high) density equivalent to a large (small) fraction of air, an impact of HU on V is reasonable. Certainly, this relationship depends on the applied force, thus on the relative compression relC. Based on relC for every percent interval with at least 1000 counts (see Fig. 3) a joint histogram of V vs. HU is computed. Normalization for each HU allows for investigating the suspected V/HU relationship (Fig. 5). To combine the information from the different compression levels, from each normalized joint histogram a graph is extracted by determing the row position for which the accumulated column values reaches 0.5. The collection

---

[1] Since u points from the reference image onto the template image, and therefore V is defined in the domain of the reference image, for the HU the uncompressed state is taken as reference image.

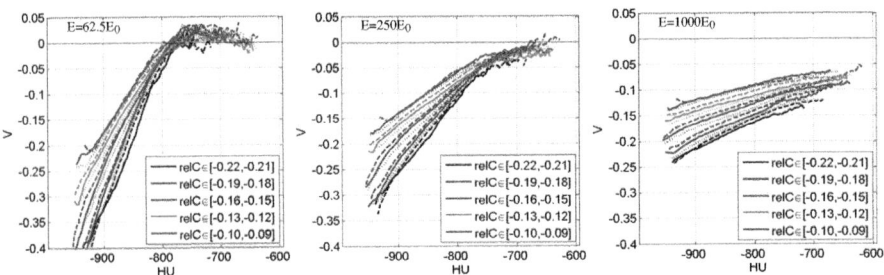

Fig. 6. Ensemble plots derived from normalized joint histograms (see text for explanation) for elasticity settings (a), (b), and (c) as in Fig. 4

of graphs shown in an ensemble plot (Fig. 6) now describes the reaction of a material of a given HU to individually applied forces. A comparison of setting (b) to the settings (a) and (c) (shown center, left, and right, respectively) underlines the impact of the regularizer on the registration result: a small or medium elastic modulus results in a graph ensemble with larger slope accompanied by non-plausible positive values of V for voxels with higher intensity. The positive values are directly linked to the expanding regions visible in Fig. 4. On the contrary, a larger value for E yields a graph ensemble with smaller slope which asymptotically converges to a negative value of V. Here, the deformation field is protected from non-plausible expansions but, at the same time, non-contracting regions are forced to contract. In view of a lung CT this effect can cause parts of bronchial or vessel tree to erroneously contract during exhalation.

Finally, the occurrence of non-plausible expansions is investigated in light of the TRE. For every landmark position the value of V is computed and plotted against the TRE in Fig. 7. Since for settings (a) and (b) the majority of landmark positions shows a TRE between 0.1 mm and 0.35 mm as well as a local expansion ($V > 0$), a possible correlation of local expansion and TRE is ruled out. Also, it is ensured that landmarks are placed both in contracting and expanding regions. Therefore, the TRE cannot be used to determine the registration accuracy on a functional level.

3.2   Synthetic Example

The following experiment investigates the paradoxical expansion of image regions with higher density as observed for settings (a) and (b) in Sect. 3.1.

Experiment Design: Let R, T consist of an identical sphere around the image center surrounded by a shell of reduced intensity which is spherical in R but ellipsoidal in T (see Fig. 8, left). This synthetic example is designed to model the overall contraction of a composite object with a less stiff material in its shell and a stiff material in its center region. To reflect the properties of the CT phantom, intensity values are chosen as -700, -900, and -1000 for the center region, the shell, and the background, respectively. The elastic modulus is set

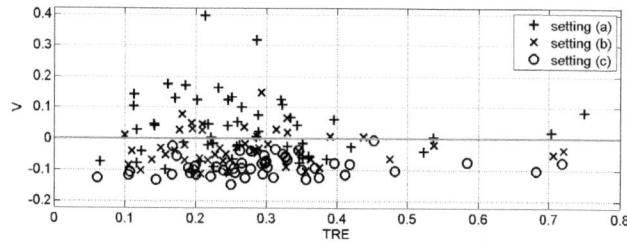

Fig. 7. Comparison of TRE with volume change V at landmark position for settings (a)-(c)

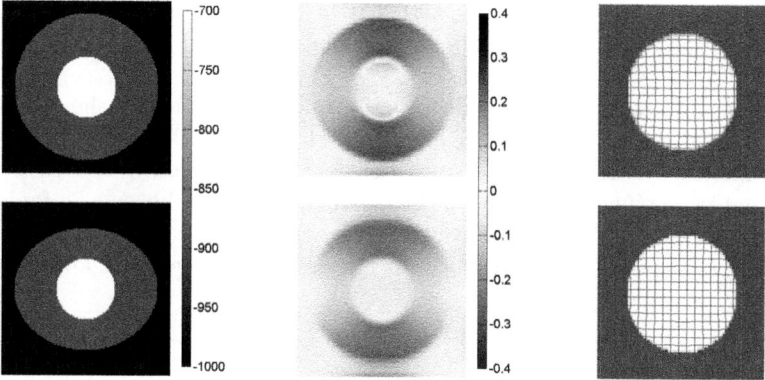

Fig. 8. Axial slices of R (top left) and T (bottom left) for a 3D synthetic phantom. The center column displays the local volume change V after registration with a constant elastic modulus (top) and with a spatially variable one (bottom). For both settings, the right column visualizes the resulting DVFs (zoomed for the center region).

either constantly to $E = 100E_0$ or spatially varying with $E_{center} = 10000E_0$ and $E_{shell} = E_{background} = 100E_0$.

Findings: Regarding the transition from center region to shell and from shell to background, both the constant and the variable setting result in a perfect registration, thus the residuum is the same for both settings. An inspection of the local volume change V, however, reveals local expansions within the center region (Fig. 8, top center). Since the integral of V over the center region is zero, the correct alignment of the center-shell interface is confirmed. To investigate the paradox, the DVF is applied to an orthogonal grid and visualized in Fig. 8, top right (zoomed and overlayed onto center region): even though the center region in R, T is untouched, deformation within this region occur. The explanation can be found in the role of the regularizer. At first, deformation in the shell region is necessary to allow for its contraction. Then, due to the regularizer, continuation of this deformation ("smooth vectorfield") into the center region is privileged unless the similarity of deformed template and reference image is worsened. If, however, the center region remains undeformed, the similarity measure was unchanged but a higher gradient of the DVF at the center-shell interface would cause increased penalization by the regularizer.

The second setting with a higher elastic modulus in the center region takes up the balance of similarity measure and regularizer. By increasing the stiffness of the center region, non-plausible expansion is prohibited (see Fig. 8, bottom center and bottom right).

3.3   Local Elastic Registration

Based on the experiences with the synthetic example the CT phantom is re-investigated, now with a spatially varying elastic modulus. Existing work addressing spatial variability assigns high elastic modulus values to bone structures to prevent these from implausible deformations [12,13].

Experiment Design: Let R, T denote the uncompressed and the compressed scan as in the first experiment. Since the elastic modulus is proportional to the stiffness of a structure and since the density measured by CT is also proportional to a structure's stiffness, the elastic modulus is chosen as a function of the local Hounsfield values. Motivated by the very high elastic modulus of a stiff structure such as a main bronchus (which is assigned a density of approximately

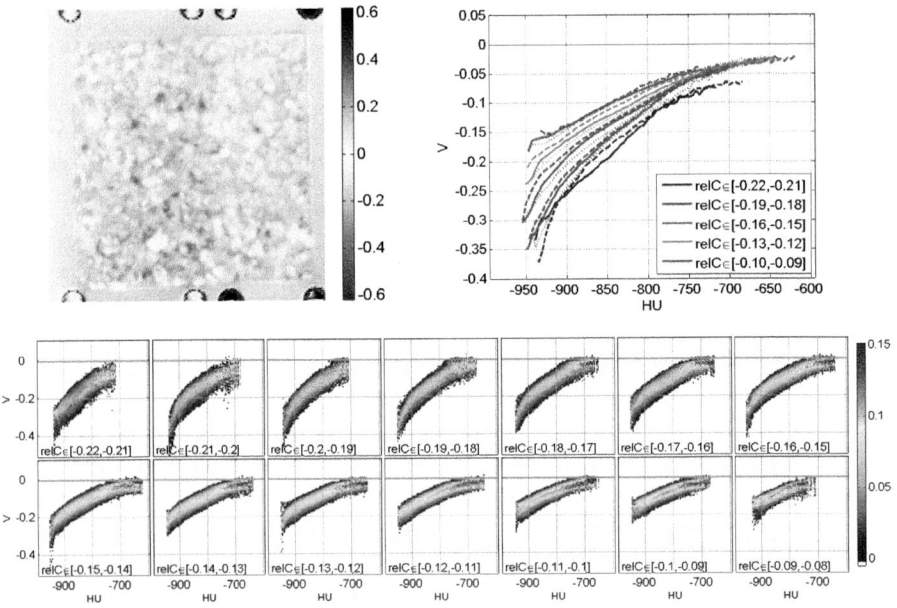

Fig. 9. Top left: local volume change V shown for same coronal slice as in Figs. 2,4; bottom: normalized joint histogram of V vs. Hounsfield values sorted according to relative compression relC; top right: ensemble plot derived from normalized joint histograms

1) and the low elastic modulus of a lung compartment containing mainly air, it is reasonable to model the transfer function as an exponential function of type $t(x) = t_0 + c^{x+1000}$ mapping the Hounsfield scale to the positive real numbers. For the choice of base c and offset t_0, settings from the first experiment are considered: a transfer function with $t_0 = 37E_0$ and $c = 1.02$ assigns the elastic modulus values from setting (b) to the histogram peak for the uncompressed state and setting (c) to its 90% quantile (see Fig. 1, right).

Findings: From the resulting DVF the residuum, the TRE as well as the local volume change are computed. While the residuum resembles the residua of settings (b),(c) from the first experiment, the TRE is increased to $0.33 \pm 0.14(0.76)$ but still within subvoxel accuracy. The local volume change reflects the spatially varying elastic modulus as visible from Fig. 9: no part of the phantom has been expanded while, at the same time, contractions up to -0.5 occur. The ensemble plot summarizes the joint histograms and can be directly compared to the results achieved with constant elastic modulus (see Fig. 6).

4   Discussion

An elastic registration scheme is applied to a compressible CT phantom with the elastic modulus chosen either constantly (Sect. 3.1) or spatially varying (Sect.3.3) and to a synthetic phantom with one or two elasticity regions (Sect. 3.2).

Applying a constant elastic modulus E to the entire image region, the registration result can vary between a homogeneous and a locally adapted deformation, depending on the value of E. For three different stiffness settings investigated, however, standard validation criteria such as the residuum or the TRE do not allow for clear distinction since all settings are registered with subvoxel accuracy. Computation of the local volume change on the one hand allows for a clear distinction and on the other hand reveals non-plausible local expansion for certain settings. The smaller the elastic modulus is, the more distinct the local expansions are. Correlation of local volume change and TRE at all landmark positions verifies that the TRE fails to detect non-plausible deformations.

From the CT phantom construction it is obvious that, given the compression of the plates, any region of the phantom must either contract or preserve its volume. Since, in addition, image regions with low Hounsfield value (HU) and thus a large fraction of air are more compressible than regions with high HU, the local volume change V of a certain structure is expected to be inverse proportional to its HU which is confirmed by a joint histogram of V and HU. The necessity for all regions to either contract or be volume-preserved (i.e. $V \leq 0$), however, is violated if the elastic modulus is chosen too small (see the ensemble plots in Fig. 6). There are four ways to circumvent the violation: (1) increase of the elastic modulus, (2) addition of constraint to the registration scheme such that $V \leq 0$ is forced everywhere, (3) spatially varying choice of the elastic modulus, (4) incorporate the compression-induced change in density into the similarity measure [14]. While (1) is demonstrated to fail (Figs. 4,6, right) since an increased elastic modulus forces all image regions to homogeneously contract, and

(2) is not optimal since it would result in an ensemble plot with the single graphs just upper clamped to zero, (3) is shown to solve the problem. (4) has the potential to solve the problem by modifying the similarity measure rather than the regularizer. However, robustness against noise needs to be investigated.

The use of a spatially varying elastic modulus to prevent non-contracting regions from contraction is analyzed for a synthetic phantom. The effect of local expansions can be traced back to the balance of similarity measure and regularizer in case of image regions with homogeneous intensity. Since most non-rigid registration schemes can be interpreted as a combination of similarity measure and regularizer (otherwise the registration problem would not be well-posed), the finding is of general relevance.

For applying a spatially varying elastic modulus to the CT phantom a transfer function is defined to automatically translate the HUs of the reference image into values for the elastic modulus. The exponential type of the transfer function can be justified by physics since the elastic modulus relates the amount of deformation to a given force. So far, the specific choice of the exponential function is motivated only by the intensity histogram of the underlying image and previous experiments (Sect. 3.1) and needs for detailed investigation. The result as shown in Fig. 9, however, demonstrates its applicability. Not only no part of the CT phantom undergoes non-plausible expansion, but also the volume change of regions with low density nicely reflects the different compression levels. The relation of local volume change and CT density can even be extended to an automatic tool for local estimation of registration accuracy.

A first application to CT lung data acquired in inhale and exhale state showed a similar relation of local volume change and CT density compared to the CT phantom. Given the complicated dynamics of lungs, however, further investigation is needed.

5   Conclusion

Motivated by inconsistent estimations for CT lung registration accuracy using (a) landmark correspondences as a point-based measure and (b) lung ventilation as a functional measure, a CT phantom with a comparable range of stiffness properties is chosen for deeper investigation. The CT phantom benefits from the controlled compression and the absence of any motion artifacts as they are likely to occur in CT lung data. Registration of the phantom showed that an elastic registration scheme with global uniform elasticity is unable to align the uncompressed and the compressed state in a way which is both plausible *and* adapted to local structures. However, unlike a functional measure, the landmark-based measure fails to detect non-plausible deformations of image regions with homogeneous intensity. The contribution of this work is twofold. First, a framework is described for registration validation on a functional level. Second, a method is proposed to automatically choose the elastic modulus based on CT density. This allows the registration scheme to use spatially varying regularization and to achieve a physically meaningful deformation with impact on functional lung analysis.

Acknowledgement

We thank Dr. Udo van Stevendaal for acquiring the phantom dataset, as well as Mrs. Keelin Murphy for providing the software tool for annotating and propagating landmarks.

References

1. West, J., Fitzpatrick, J.M., Wang, M.Y., Dawant, B.M., Maurer Jr., C.R., et al.: Comparison and evaluation of retrospective intermodality brain image registration techniques. J. Comput. Assist. Tomogr. 21(4), 554–566 (1997)
2. Ding, K., Cao, K., Christensen, G.E., Hoffman, E.A., Reinhardt, J.M.: Registration-based regional lung mechanical analysis: retrospectively reconstructed dynamic imaging versus static breath-hold image acquisition. In: SPIE, vol. 7262, pp. 72620D–72620D–9 (2009)
3. Castillo, R., Castillo, E., Guerra, R., Johnson, V.E., McPhail, T., Garg, A.K., Guerrero, T.: A framework for evaluation of deformable image registration spatial accuracy using large landmark point sets. Phys. Med. Biol. 54, 1849–1870 (2009)
4. Murphy, K., van Ginneken, B., Pluim, J.P.W., Klein, S., Staring, M.: Semi-automatic reference standard construction for quantitative evaluation of lung CT registration. In: Metaxas, D., Axel, L., Fichtinger, G., Székely, G. (eds.) MICCAI 2008, Part II. LNCS, vol. 5242, pp. 1006–1013. Springer, Heidelberg (2008)
5. Kabus, S., Klinder, T., Murphy, K., van Ginneken, B., Lorenz, C., Pluim, J.P.W.: Evaluation of 4D-CT lung registration. In: Yang, G.-Z., Hawkes, D., Rueckert, D., Noble, A., Taylor, C. (eds.) MICCAI 2009. LNCS, vol. 5761, pp. 747–754. Springer, Heidelberg (2009)
6. Reinhardt, J.M., Ding, K., Cao, K., Christensen, G.E., Hoffman, E.A., Bodas, S.V.: Registration-based estimates of local lung tissue expansion compared to xenon-CT measures of specific ventilation. Med. Image. Anal. 12(6), 752–763 (2008)
7. Guerrero, T., Sanders, K., Castillo, E., Zhang, Y., Bidaut, L., Pan, T., Komaki, R.: Dynamic ventilation imaging from four-dimensional computed tomography. Phys. Med. Biol. 51(4), 777–791 (2006)
8. Yamamoto, T., Kabus, S., von Berg, J., Lorenz, C., Keall, P.J.: The impact of four-dimensional computed tomography pulmonary ventilation imaging-based functional avoidance for lung cancer radiotherapy. In: IJROBP (accepted 2010)
9. Levitzky, M.G.: Pulmonary Physiology, 7th edn. McGraw-Hill, New York (2007)
10. Modersitzki, J.: Numerical methods for image registration. OUP, Oxford (2004)
11. Kabus, S., Franz, A., Fischer, B.: Variational image registration with local properties. In: Pluim, J.P.W., Likar, B., Gerritsen, F.A. (eds.) WBIR 2006. LNCS, vol. 4057, pp. 92–100. Springer, Heidelberg (2006)
12. Ruan, D., Fessler, J.A., Roberson, M., Balter, J., Kessler, M.: Nonrigid registration using regularization that accomodates local tissue rigidity. In: SPIE, vol. 6144, pp. 614412-1–614412-9 (2006)
13. Kabus, S., Franz, A., Fischer, B.: Spatially varying elasticity in image registration. Methods Inf. Med. 46(3), 287–291 (2007)
14. Yin, Y., Hoffman, E.A., Lin, C.-L.: Mass preserving nonrigid registration of CT lung images using cubic B-spline. Med. Phys. 36(9), 4213–4222 (2009)

Nonlinear Elastic Spline Registration: Evaluation with Longitudinal Huntington's Disease Data

Marc Modat[1], Zeike A. Taylor[1], Gerard R. Ridgway[1], Josephine Barnes[2], Edward J. Wild[2], David J. Hawkes[1], Nick C. Fox[2], and Sébastien Ourselin[1,2]

[1] Centre for Medical Imaging Computing, Department of Medical Physics and Bioengineering, University College London, UK
[2] Dementia Research Centre, Institute of Neurology, University College London, WC1N 3BG, UK

Abstract. Longitudinal brain image studies quantify the changes happening over time. Jacobian maps, which characterize the volume change, are based on non-rigid registration techniques and do not always appear to be *clinically* plausible. In particular, extreme values of volume change are not expected to be seen. The Free-Form Deformation (FFD) algorithm suffers from this drawback. Different penalty terms have been proposed in the past. We present in this paper a regularisation of the B-Spline displacements using nonlinear elasticity. Our work links a finite element method with *pseudo-forces* derived from a similarity measure. The presented method has been evaluated on longitudinal T1-weighted MR images of Huntington's disease subjects and controls. Multiple time point consistency, the Jacobian map homogeneity and statistical power for group separation have been used. Our new method performs better than the *classical* FFD, while keeping similar registration accuracy.

1 Introduction

When studying brain images using non-rigid registration, the determinant of the Jacobian provides a measure of local volume change that is often of interest for quantifying deformations over time or between subjects. However, as each registration method produces a slightly different transformation (and equally importantly, via a different deformation mechanism) the Jacobian determinant maps vary both quantitatively and qualitatively. Moreover, the quality of the map (judged directly by clinicians, or indirectly via results of tensor-based morphometry) is not necessarily correlated with the quantitative accuracy of the registration. For example, using different techniques such as the Free-Form Deformation [1] (FFD), the fluid [2], the diffeomorphic demons algorithm [3] or symmetric normalization (Syn) [4], different Jacobian determinant maps are obtained even though the warped images all match the reference — see Fig. 1.

In order to generate smooth and plausible transformation with the FFD method, efforts have been made to impose constraints on the deformations. Rueckert *et al.* [1] proposed a penalty term based on the bending energy. Rolhfing *et al.* [5] presented another based on the logarithm of the Jacobian determinant. The Jacobian determinant was also embedded in a regularizer by

B. Fischer, B. Dawant, and C. Lorenz (Eds.): WBIR 2010, LNCS 6204, pp. 128–139, 2010.

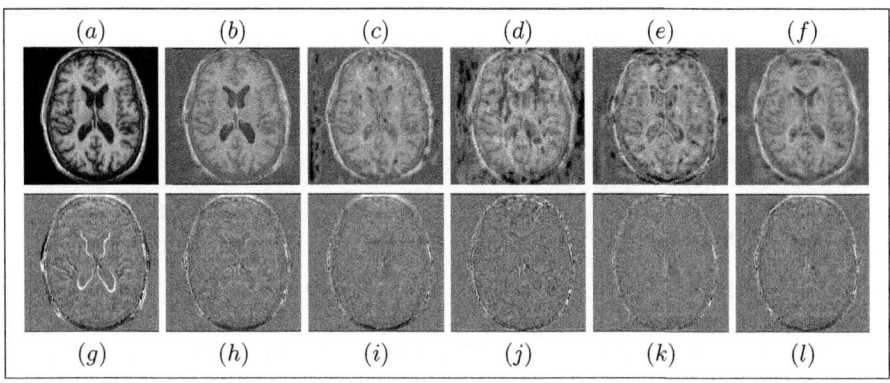

Fig. 1. Variation in volume change distribution with different registration algorithms. A floating image has been registered to a reference image (a) using: fluid (b,h), Syn (c,i), demons (d,j), free-form deformation (e,k) and the proposed method (f,l). It can be appreciated from the difference images (bottom row) that all techniques successfully recovered the initial differences (f). However the Jacobian determinant maps (top row) reveal very different patterns of deformation. $(\log_2(\det(J)))$ is shown with colour range from -0.5 to 0.5).

Sdika [6]. However, simple constraints or penalty terms are either incapable of modelling large deformations or unable to prevent highly variable (or negative) Jacobians. Considering that the general aim of the above penalty terms is to favour physically plausible deformations, a natural alternative is to directly include a biomechanical regulariser, for example based on equations of continuum mechanics. Linear elastic registration has been used since the 1980s [7,8], however, linearity breaks down for large deformations, limiting the flexibility of such methods. Fluid-mechanical regularisation allows large deformation without discontinuities, but also permits unrealistically severe distortions. This paper argues in favour of a nonlinear elastic regulariser coupled with a spline model, that should handle large but realistic deformations while maintaining an anatomically reasonable Jacobian map.

Yanovsky *et al.* [9] also investigated nonlinear elasticity. They developed a variational form which coupled similarity and elasticity functionals, using a linear strain energy function (Saint Venant-Kirchhoff model), and solved the system using finite differences. The development and solution of the coupled system was facilitated by an approximation for the material displacement derivatives.

We present a decoupled regularisation of the FFD algorithm using nonlinear elasticity. Solution of the equations of continuum mechanics is performed using the finite element method, which requires no approximation of the deformation components, and allows for incorporation of elaborate constitutive models. The deformation model is linked to an appropriate similarity metric by so-called *pseudo-forces* derived from the metric's gradient. The scheme is shown to produce both accurate and smooth deformation fields. We emphasise that in employing a continuum mechanics-based model our aim, in this case, is to produce physically consistent smooth transformations, not to model the physiology of the disease process itself; we do not claim, for example, that deformations associated with tissue loss are directly analogous to mechanical compressions.

2   Method

2.1   Deformation Model

We consider the floating image volume to be a continuous (but not necessarily homogeneous) elastic body with initial volume V_0. We assume that loading is entirely in the form of body forces $\mathbf{f}^B$. At any point in the body we define the deformation in terms of the Green-Lagrange strain tensor [10]

$$\mathbf{E} = (\mathbf{F}^T\mathbf{F} - \mathbf{I})/2, \tag{1}$$

where $\mathbf{F} := \mathrm{d}\mathbf{x}/\mathrm{d}\mathbf{X}$ is the deformation gradient, $\mathbf{I}$ is the second order identity tensor, and $\mathbf{x}$ and $\mathbf{X}$ are current and initial material point coordinates, respectively. Standard results from continuum mechanics dictate that deformations within the image volume must satisfy the equation of virtual work [11]:

$$\int_{V_0} \mathbf{S}\,\delta\mathbf{E}\,\mathrm{d}V = \int_{V_0} \mathbf{f}^B\,\delta\mathbf{u}\,\mathrm{d}V, \tag{2}$$

where $\delta\mathbf{E}$ are strain variations corresponding to virtual displacements $\delta\mathbf{u}$, and the left and right hand sides represent internal and external virtual work terms, respectively; Eqn. (2) is an equilibrium equation. $\mathbf{S}$ are second Piola-Kirchhoff stresses, which are related to the strains through the constitutive model [10]: $\mathbf{S} = \partial\Psi/\partial\mathbf{E}$, where Ψ is an appropriate strain energy function. We note that use of kinematically consistent stress and strain measures means this formulation is valid even for large deformations. By seeking deformations of the image volume which satisfy these equilibrium and constitutive constraints we guarantee that a physically plausible transformation is obtained.

Eqn. (2) may be solved for the deformation field throughout the image volume using the finite element method (FEM) [11]. For simulation of large deformations a formulation capable of accommodating geometric nonlinearities must be used. We employ a total Lagrangian explicit dynamic (TLED) algorithm [12], which has been shown to be highly efficient for solving nonlinear soft tissue deformation problems [13,12,14]. The image volume is discretised into a regular hexahedral mesh, similar to the grid used for B-spline-based methods [1], wherein grid points constitute finite element nodes. Each node has three displacement degrees of freedom, and we employ 8-node hexahedral elements with trilinear interpolation and reduced integration [11]. Via standard methods [11] this discretisation renders Eqn. (2) into the following system of differential equations

$$\mathbf{M}\ddot{\mathbf{U}} + \mathbf{C}\dot{\mathbf{U}} + \mathbf{K}\,(\mathbf{U})\,.\mathbf{U} = \mathbf{R}, \tag{3}$$

where $\mathbf{M}$ and $\mathbf{C}$ are mass and structural damping matrices, respectively, $\mathbf{K}(\mathbf{U})$ is the system stiffness matrix, which depends on nodal displacements $\mathbf{U}$, and $\mathbf{R}$ are external loads. The over-dot notation denotes time-derivatives. Appropriate boundary conditions (nodal displacement constraints) are enforced (see Sect. 2.3), and loads in the form of pseudo-forces derived from the gradient of the employed similarity metric (see Sect. 2.2) are applied. Solutions (nodal displacements $\mathbf{U}$) to Eqn. (3) are then computed incrementally in time using the procedure detailed in [12,14].

Once the nodal displacements have been computed for the current loading, interpolation is used to obtain a continuous deformation field. In this final step, rather than the trilinear interpolation functions of the finite elements themselves, we use a cubic B-spline scheme; the C^2 continuity of the deformation $\mathbf{T}$ ensures smoothly varying first derivatives and hence a smooth Jacobian map, $\det_{Jac} = |\nabla\mathbf{T}|$. The elastic model thus constitutes a regulariser for the B-spline model. Note that the Jacobian in this formula is different from $\mathbf{F}$, as it is based on the B-spline interpolation model.

2.2   Metric and Optimisation

To evaluate the quality of the registration and optimise the node positions, we compute the Normalised Mutual Information (NMI) between the reference R and the deformed floating image $F(\mathbf{T})$. NMI is a voxel intensity-based information-theoretic similarity measure [15], which quantifies the shared information of the two images. It is defined as

$$\text{NMI} = \frac{H(R) + H(F(\mathbf{T}))}{H(R, F(\mathbf{T}))} \tag{4}$$

where $H(R)$ and $H(F(\mathbf{T}))$ are the marginal entropies of images R and $F(\mathbf{T})$, and $H(R, F(\mathbf{T}))$ denotes their joint entropy. The computation of each (Shannon) entropy $H = -p(e)\log(p(e))$, is based on the probabilities $p(e)$ of events derived from a joint histogram $\mathbf{H}$. This histogram indicates the probability of each combination of intensities in images R and $F(\mathbf{T})$. In order to fill the histogram we used the Parzen Window technique. This technique has been presented as more accurate than the generalised partial volume method as the joint histogram is less populated near the optimum [16]. Considering r and f as voxel intensities respectively in the reference image and the deformed floating image, the joint histogram $\mathbf{H}$ is filled as

$$\mathbf{H}(r, f) = \sum_{\mathbf{x} \in \Omega} \beta_r^3(R(\mathbf{x}); r)\beta_f^3(F(\mathbf{T}(\mathbf{x})); f) \tag{5}$$

where R is defined over the Ω domain and β_r^3 and β_f^3 are intensity kernels based on cubic splines.

To drive the displacement of the nodes we computed the gradient of the NMI at every node position. It is possible to compute such values for every node using the derivatives of the marginal and joint entropies:

$$\frac{\partial \mathrm{NMI}}{\partial \mu_{i,j,k}^{\xi}} = \frac{\frac{\partial H(R)}{\partial \mu_{i,j,k}^{\xi}} + \frac{\partial H(F(\mathbf{T}))}{\partial \mu_{i,j,k}^{\xi}} - \mathrm{NMI} \times \frac{\partial H(R,F(\mathbf{T}))}{\partial \mu_{i,j,k}^{\xi}}}{H(R,F(\mathbf{T}))} \qquad (6)$$

These entropy derivatives are calculated by taken into account the deformation model $\mathbf{T}$ to fill the derivative of the joint histogram:

$$\frac{\partial \mathbf{H}(r,f)}{\partial \mu_{i,j,k}} = \sum_{\mathbf{x} \in \Omega} \beta_r^3 (R(\mathbf{x}); r) \left. \frac{\partial \beta_f^3(v; f)}{\partial v} \right|_{v=F(\mathbf{T}(\mathbf{x}))} \left. \frac{\partial F(\mathbf{T}(\mathbf{x}))}{\partial p} \right|_{p=\mathbf{T}_x} \frac{\partial \mathbf{T}(\mathbf{x})}{\partial \mu_{ijk}} \qquad (7)$$

This approach provides the mathematical value of the gradient but involves significant computation redundancy, since every voxel is included in the neighborhood of several control points. Moreover it is memory intensive as each node requires one joint histogram per degree of freedom. In order to decrease this redundancy and the memory requirement, we propose a voxel-centric approximation of the node-centric gradient. We first compute the gradient value for every voxel, then gather the information from all voxels to obtain the nodal gradient values.

We computed the voxel-centric gradient values using the formulas in equations 6 and 7 where $\frac{\partial \mathbf{H}(r,f)}{\partial \mathbf{u}_\mathbf{z}^\xi}$ is computed by replacing $\frac{\partial \mathbf{T}(\mathbf{x})}{\partial \mu_{ijk}}$ with $\frac{\partial \mathbf{T}(\mathbf{x})}{\partial \mathbf{u}_\mathbf{z}^\xi}$ where $\frac{\partial \mathbf{T}(\mathbf{x})}{\partial \mathbf{u}_\mathbf{z}^\xi} =$ 1 if $\mathbf{z} = \mathbf{x}$ as $\mathbf{T}(\mathbf{x}) = \mathbf{x} + \mathbf{u}(\mathbf{x})$.

In order to provide one gradient per node we weighted the gradient of each voxel such that voxels close to a node had more impact than voxels further away. However, weighting every voxel in the neighborhood of one node would lead to extra computation because of redundancy, as before. To avoid this, we applied a convolution window to the gradient field and so approximated the gradient for every node. The chosen convolution window was a cubic B-Spline curve which matched the basis functions in the deformation model in terms of node spacing; it was equivalent to $\frac{\partial \mathbf{T}(\mathbf{x})}{\partial \mu_{ijk}}$ in equation 7.

To optimise the tranformation we normalised the NMI gradients of all nodes and applied them as external forces in the TLED solver. Each time the solver was run the floating image was resampled and the metric value re-evaluated. A conjugate gradient ascent was then performed to find the external forces which best transformed the floating image in the direction of the gradient. The gradient was then recomputed and the line ascent re-performed. This loop iterated until no improvement superior to 0.1% of the similarity measure was produced.

2.3   Framework

We implemented our algorithm for graphics processing unit (GPU) execution using the CUDA API from NVidia (http://www.nvidia.com). Our framework can be decomposed into four modules, as presented in figure 2.

Module 1: TLED solver. The first module concerned the TLED solver. As described by Taylor et al. [14], the solver consisted of precomputation and online components. Since we deal with regular meshes in this application (and homogeneous material properties in the first instance), all finite elements have the

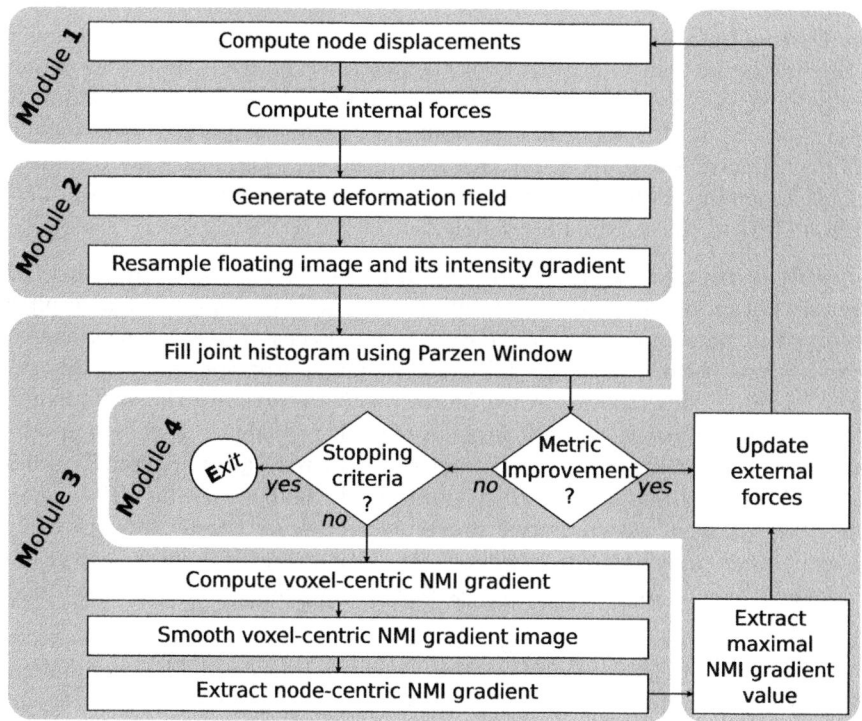

Fig. 2. Framework of the presented algorithm

same properties, which simplifies the computation and considerably decreases memory requirements; variables for only a single element need be precomputed and stored. Node positions and element geometries were computed on-the-fly according to image size and the user-defined node spacing.

The solution time step was estimated from $\Delta t_c = L_e/c$, where L_e is the characteristic element length and c is the dilatational wave speed of the material [11]. This formula provides an estimate of the stable time step in explicit dynamic analyses, assuming linear elasticity. We employed both kinematic and constitutive nonlinearities and consequently used a conservative time step twice smaller than Δt_c.

To avoid any free displacement of the volume, some points must be fixed. For each registration we generated a brain mask using BET [17] and dilated it. All nodes outside of the mask were then fixed.

The GPU computation consisted in two kernels. In the first the internal nodal forces were computed, and in the second the resulting nodal displacements were computed — see [14] for details.

Module 2: resampling of the floating image. The second module dealt with the deformation and resampling of the floating image, and also comprised two kernels. The cubic B-spline interpolation was calculated for every voxel in the reference image in the first kernel. Once the deformation field was generated the floating image was resampled using a second kernel. The latter kernel also returned the intensity derivatives of the deformed image. These were required in the next module for the NMI gradient computation. The deformation field interpolation and the trilinear resampling of the floating image were split into different functions in order to increase the occupancy, and hence performance, of the GPU computation. The occupancy is the ratio of active computation threads on the GPU to the maximum possible.

Module 3: metric and gradient calculation. The third module consisted in the calculation of the NMI and its gradient. The NMI computation result was observed to be sensitive to the floating point precision used. Hence, the computation was performed on the CPU using double precision. As a consequence, after its resampling, the deformed image was transferred to the CPU memory. During this computation the logarithm of each probability was computed. As their computation for the NMI gradient would be redundant we stored each in a second histogram and subsequently transferred this back to the GPU memory. The NMI gradient was computed in a single kernel on the GPU, after which a series of other kernels were invoked for convolution window creation and gradient field smoothing. A last kernel then extracted the gradient value for each node.

Module 4: external force optimisation. The last module was concerned with the update of the pseudo-forces and their optimisation. The maximal norm of the gradient was first extracted using a spread and gather approach, then the pseudo-forces were updated as described in the previous section.

Multi-scale framework. To improve the efficiency of the elastic model we developed a multi-level mesh approach. This allowed the system to recover gross deformations more quickly, and also helped in avoiding local minima. Beginning with a course level mesh (l_n) the deformation field was optimised as described. The next (denser) level mesh (l_{n+1}) was then obtained by subdividing elements in each dimension. Thus, we required the input forces for l_{n+1} which would reproduce the deformation field of l_n. These were computed as follows: (1) the deformed positions of new nodes were obtained by linearly interpolating those of existing nodes; (2) for this configuration the nodal force contributions from each element were computed using kernel 1, module 1 (see [14] for details); (3) these force contributions were summed at each node to give the required l_{n+1} input forces. By construction, these inputs exactly balance the elastic forces in the desired configuration, and were used as the start values in the l_{n+1} optimisation scheme.

3   Evaluation

3.1   Data and Methods

The methods are evaluated on serial MR images of 33 patients with early Huntington's Disease (HD) and 14 healthy age- and gender-matched control subjects, imaged at baseline and 12-month follow-up; 23 and 9 of the respective groups were also scanned after 24 months. Three-dimensional T1-weighted MR images with 1.5 mm coronal slices of in-plane dimension 0.9375×0.9375 mm were acquired with a spoiled GRASS sequence at 1.5 T. Each follow-up image was registered to its baseline using an affine algorithm followed by each non-rigid algorithm. We also registered the 24-month follow-ups to the 12-month scans. The multi-scale approach used 3 levels, with the finest having 2.5 mm isotropic spacing between nodes. The TLED-solver used a Poisson ratio of 0.1. Our FFD implementation [18] used a bending energy penalty term with a 10% weight (the code can be downloaded from http://sourceforge.net/projects/niftyreg).

To derive inter-subject correspondence, we used the group-wise diffeomorphic registration algorithm DARTEL [19]. The resulting transformations were used to spatially-normalise the Jacobian maps, and to inverse-normalise semi-automatic lateral ventricular and intra-cranial segmentations of the DARTEL average back to the original images. DARTEL uses a very different transformation model (exponentiation of velocity fields) to those evaluated here, thus helping to avoid bias.

3.2   Experiments

Validation of non-rigid registration algorithms is a challenging problem [20]. Direct measurement of correspondence errors [21] relies on time-consuming and error-prone manual identification of corresponding landmarks. Furthermore, unambiguous landmarks may only be found in certain locations, away from which errors cannot be reliably determined. Using overlap indices of automatic registration-propagated segmentations and manually performed labellings [20] is also operator-dependent, and provides no information on the behaviour of the transformation inside the labelled objects. These two approaches may also be biased in favour of algorithms driven by landmark-matching or intensity differences respectively, e.g. feature-based methods may appear more successful in terms of matching manually identified landmarks if similar points are considered distinctive by both human and computer vision systems; conversely intensity-based methods could match (MR-visible) boundaries almost perfectly, while misaligning underlying structural homologies that require expert or contextual knowledge to infer.

Attempts have been made to quantify performance via direct comparison of estimated displacement fields [22] or Jacobian maps [23] on images related by simulated and hence known transformations. The key advantages of this are greater objectivity, and the potential for dense voxel-wise measurement of error. However, such a method is clearly only as valid as its simulation model. For physical deformation of breast images [22] a biomechanical FEM model should provide an excellent gold standard. For phenomenological modelling of brain atrophy [23] simulation seems well-suited to evaluating regional or global volume changes, but severely limited for the present application — evaluation of different regularisation approaches at the scale of individual voxels — since the simulation model (which only approximates an unknown biological model) cannot help but bias the evaluation towards similar physical regularisation models. In the hope of overcoming these challenges, we present a sophisticated validation strategy comprising three complementary experiments, described now.

Longitudinal consistency. It is clearly desirable for a registration algorithm to recover equivalent correspondences whether registering follow-up source images to their baseline targets or vice versa — the principle of inverse-consistency [24]. For the specific purpose of comparing regularisation methods, simple (A ← B)∘(B ← A) consistency is flawed, because increasingly strong regularisation will tend towards the 'perfect' but trivial consistency of the identity. We argue here that this limitation can be ameliorated by using three time-point longitudinal imaging to evaluate the discrepancy between the composition of the two 12-month interval transformations (A ← B) ∘ (B ← C) and the direct 24-month interval registration A ← C. The hope being that overly influential regularisation will prevent the 24-month registration from recovering as much deformation as the two combined 12-month interval transformations, thus restoring merit to the consistency measure. The discrepancy in mm for each registration algorithm is summarised by the voxel-wise mean over each subject's intra-cranial mask.

Realism of ventricular changes. To directly address the clinically-motivated question of whether the Jacobian images are biological reasonable, the maps of determinant values are analysed over the segmented lateral ventricle region. We argue that (a) in the homogeneous cerebrospinal fluid (CSF), an ideal registration algorithm should recover homogeneous estimates of volume change, yielding low variance; and (b) in the abscence of gray- or white-matter expansion in either HD or healthy aging in adult subjects, we would expect either stable or expanding ventricles.

Jacobian-based group separation. The first two experiments have been designed to help avoid favouring over-regularised models by including three time-points, and by considering mean ventricular expansion in addition to Jacobian variance. However, to further reduce bias towards constrained transformations, the third experiment is inherently based on quantifying clinically-relevant information, in terms of the registration method's power to discriminate HD from healthy aging. Unlike the commonest form of dementia, (sporadic) Alzheimer's disease, HD status is known from genetic testing, providing a genuine ground truth for classification. We use a linear soft-margin Support Vector Machine (similar to that used in [25]), with a nested cross-validation procedure that leaves out each subject in turn, performs an inner leave-one-out loop to optimise the SVM's C parameter, then classifies the left-out subject, which provides an unbiased estimate of the classification accuracy. The SVM's kernel consists of the image-based inner-products of the subjects' log-transformed determinants, meaning that classification accuracy should closely reflect the clinical information in these maps.

4   Results and Discussion

Registration performance is summarised in table 3. Mean computation times were about 40 minutes per registration for the TLED-based method and

	TLED-based reg		*classical* FFD	
	Follow-up 12 to Baseline	Follow-up 24 to Baseline	Follow-up 12 to Baseline	Follow-up 24 to Baseline
Normalised mutual information	1.2306	1.1908	1.2368	1.1933
Jacobian values range	[0.31 1.92]	[0.43 1.97]	[-1.91 6.93]	[-1.61 6.10]
Consistency mean error	0.29 mm		0.80 mm	
Classification accuracy (%)	74.5	87.5	63.8	71.9

Fig. 3. Summary of quantitative results for registration performance

approximately 40 seconds for our GPU-based implementation of the FFD. The NMI is fractionally higher for the FFD algorithm; the differences being statistically significant when paired over subjects. The FFD algorithm produces widely varying Jacobian values, while the TLED-based method appears to produce more realistically smooth deformation gradients. The nonlinear elastic model has substantially reduced consistency errors compared to the FFD method. Greater consistency at the expense of lower NMI could simply indicate over-regularisation, however, the ventricular measurements indicate that in addition to featuring lower variability (Fig. 4), the TLED-based registration measurements actually show greater mean expansion, and are more biologically plausible in terms of having far fewer subjects with erroneously contracting ventricles.

The TLED algorithm is more powerful at discriminating HD patients from controls than the classical FFD. A 95% confidence interval for the increase in the (paired) accuracies on the 12-month interval is $[-2.23\ 23.1]\%$, and $[-3.59\ 33.9]\%$ for the 24-month interval, indicating that the differences are not statistically significant. However, unlike the changes in NMI, improvements in accuracy of circa 10% and 15% would be *clinically* very significant if shown to generalise.

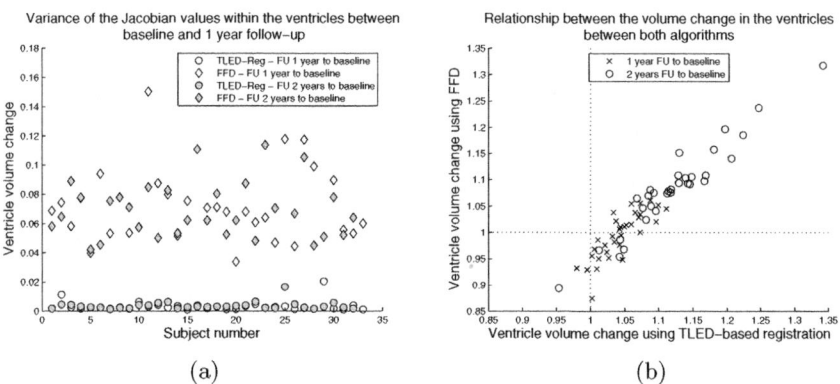

(a)   (b)

Fig. 4. Comparison of ventricular expansion rates

5   Conclusion

We have presented a novel method for efficient GPU-based non-rigid registration, regularised by a nonlinear elastic model. The most closely related work is [9] in which nonlinear elasticity is also used, but with a Jacobian matrix approximation employed to ease computation. The present approach should also be compared with Rueckert *et al.*'s [26] diffeomorphic version of the cubic spline algorithm, which allows large deformations with strictly positive Jacobian by composing a large number of smaller displacement fields.

A thorough evaluation of the method has been performed, showing that the nonlinear elastic regulariser improves the plausibility of the Jacobian maps while increasing the information they contain for automatic classification of neurodegenerative disease. In return for a slight decrease in NMI, the longitudinal consistency is greatly improved. The speed of the GPU-based nonlinear elastic registration will facilitate application to larger cohorts of images in the future, it should also make feasible more sophisticated regularisation models, for example permitting varying material properties in different brain tissues.

Acknowledgment

This work was undertaken at UCLH/UCL who received a proportion of funding from the Department of Healths NIHR Biomedical Research Centres funding scheme. We acknowledge Prof Sarah Tabrizi (UCL Institute of Neurology) for allowing use of data from a longitudinal study of Huntington's disease.

References

1. Rueckert, D., Sonoda, L., Hayes, C., Hill, D., Leach, M., Hawkes, D.: Nonrigid registration using free-form deformations: Application to breast MR images. IEEE Transactions on Medical Imaging 18, 712–721 (1999)
2. Christensen, G., Rabbitt, R., Miller, M.: Deformable Templates Using Large Deformation Kinematics. IEEE Trans. Med. Imag. 5, 1435–1447 (1996)
3. Vercauteren, T., Pennec, X., Perchant, A., Ayache, N.: Diffeomorphic demons: efficient non-parametric image registration. NeuroImage 45, 61–72 (2009)
4. Avants, B.B., Epstein, C., Grossman, M., Gee, J.C.: Symmetric diffeomorphic image registration with cross-correlation: Evaluating automated labeling of elderly and neurodegenerative brain. Medical Image Analysis 12, 26–41 (2008)
5. Rohlfing, T., Maurer Jr., C.R., Bluemke, D.A., Jacobs, M.: Volume-Preserving Nonrigid Registration of MR Breast Images Using Free-Form Deformation with an Incompressibility Constraint. IEEE Trans. Med. Imag. 22, 730–741 (2003)
6. Sdika, M.: A Fast Non Rigid Image Registration with Constraints on the Jacobian using Large Scale Constrained Optimization. IEEE Trans. on Med. Imag. 27, 271–281 (2008)
7. Broit, C.: Optimal registration of deformed images. Ph.D. dissertation, University of Pennsylvania (1981)
8. Bajcsy, R., Kovačič, S.: Multiresolution elastic matching. Comput. Vision Graph. Image Process. 46, 1–21 (1989)

9. Yanovsky, I., Le Guyader, C., Leow, A., Thompson, P., Vese, L.: Nonlinear elastic registration with unbiased regularization in three dimensions. In: Computational Biomechanics for Medicine III, MICCAI 2008 Workshop (2008)
10. Holzapfel, G.: Nonlinear Solid Mechanics: A Continuum Approach for Engineering. John Wiley & Sons, Chichester (2000)
11. Bathe, K.-J.: Finite Element Procedures. Prentice Hall, Englewood Cliffs (1996)
12. Miller, K., Joldes, G., Lance, D., Wittek, A.: Total Lagrangian explicit dynamics finite element algorithm for computing soft tissue deformation. Communications in Numerical Methods in Engineering 23, 121 (2007)
13. Szekely, G., Brechbühler, C., Hutter, R., Rhomberg, A., Ironmonger, N., Schmid, P.: Modelling of soft tissue simulation for laparscopic surgery simulation. Medical Image Analysis 4, 57–66 (2000)
14. Taylor, Z., Cheng, M., Ourselin, S.: High-speed nonlinear finite element analysis for surgical simulation using graphics processing units. IEEE Transactions on Medical Imaging 27, 650–663 (2008)
15. Studholme, C., Hill, D., Hawkes, D.: An Overlap Invariant Entropy Measure of 3D Medical Image Alignment. Pattern Recognit. 32, 71–86 (1999)
16. Loeckx, D.: Automated nonrigid intra-patient image registration using B-splines. Ph.D. dissertation, Katholieke Universiteit Leuven (2006)
17. Smith, S.: Fast robust automated brain extraction. Human Brain Mapping 17, 143–155 (2002)
18. Modat, M., Ridgway, G.R., Taylor, Z.A., Lehmann, M., Barnes, J., Hawkes, D.J., Fox, N.C., Ourselin, S.: Fast free-form deformation using graphics processing units. Comput. Meth. Prog. Bio. 98(3), 278–284 (2010)
19. Ashburner, J.: A fast diffeomorphic image registration algorithm. Neuroimage 38, 95–113 (2007)
20. Crum, W.R., Rueckert, D., Jenkinson, M., Kennedy, D., Smith, S.M.: A framework for detailed objective comparison of non-rigid registration algorithms in neuroimaging. In: Barillot, C., Haynor, D.R., Hellier, P. (eds.) MICCAI 2004. LNCS, vol. 3216, pp. 679–686. Springer, Heidelberg (2004)
21. Hellier, P., Barillot, C., Corouge, I., Gibaud, B., Goualher, G.L., Collins, D.L., Evans, A., Malandain, G., Ayache, N., Christensen, G.E., Johnson, H.J.: Retrospective evaluation of intersubject brain registration. IEEE Trans. Med. Imaging 22, 1120–1130 (2003)
22. Schnabel, J.A., Tanner, C., Castellano-Smith, A.D., Degenhard, A., Leach, M.O., Hose, D.R., Hill, D.L.G., Hawkes, D.J.: Validation of nonrigid image registration using finite-element methods: application to breast MR images. IEEE Trans. Med. Imaging 22, 238–247 (2003)
23. Camara, O., Schnabel, J.A., Ridgway, G.R., Crum, W.R., Douiri, A., Scahill, R.I., Hill, D.L.G., Fox, N.C.: Accuracy assessment of global and local atrophy measurement techniques with realistic simulated longitudinal Alzheimer's disease images. Neuroimage 42, 696–709 (2008)
24. Christensen, G.E., Johnson, H.J.: Consistent image registration. IEEE Trans. Med. Imaging 20, 568–582 (2001)
25. Klöppel, S., Stonnington, C.M., Chu, C., Draganski, B., Scahill, R.I., Rohrer, J.D., Fox, N.C., Jack, C.R., Ashburner, J., Frackowiak, R.S.J.: Automatic classification of MR scans in Alzheimer's disease. Brain 131, 681–689 (2008)
26. Rueckert, D., Aljabar, P., Heckemann, R., Hajnal, J., Hammers, A.: Diffeomorphic Registration Using B-Splines. In: Larsen, R., Nielsen, M., Sporring, J. (eds.) MICCAI 2006. LNCS, vol. 4191, pp. 702–709. Springer, Heidelberg (2006)

Evaluating Image Registration Using NIREP

Joo Hyun Song, Gary E. Christensen, Jeffrey A. Hawley,
Ying Wei, and Jon G. Kuhl

Electrical and Computer Engineering,
and Iowa Institute for Biomedical Imaging The University of Iowa, Iowa City, IA
52246, USA
{joohyun-song,gary-christensen,jeffrey-hawley,
ying-wei,jon-kuhl}@uiowa.edu
http://www.nirep.org/

Abstract. This paper describes the functionality and use of the Non-rigid Image Registration Evaluation Program (NIREP) that was developed to make qualitative and quantitative performance comparisons between one or more image registration algorithms. Registration performance is evaluated using common evaluation databases. An evaluation database consists of groups of registered medical images (e.g., one or more MRI modalities, CT, etc.) and annotations (e.g., segmentations, landmarks, contours, etc.) identified by their common image coordinate system. Prior to analysis with NIREP, each algorithm is used to generate pair-wise correspondence maps/transformations between image coordinate systems. NIREP has a highly customizable graphical user interface for displaying images, transformations, segmentations, overlays, differences between images, and differences between transformations. Evaluation statistics built into NIREP are used to compute quantitative algorithm performance reports that include region of interest overlap, intensity variance of images mapped to a reference coordinate system, inverse consistency error and transitivity error.

Keywords: NIREP, evaluation, non-rigid image registration, transformation, medical imaging.

1   Introduction

Image registration is important for many medical image applications including longitudinal evaluations within the same individual, comparison across individuals, creation of population atlases, computer aided diagnosis, computer aided treatment, evaluation of outcomes and many others. Unfortunately, evaluating non-rigid image registration algorithm performance is difficult since there is rarely if ever ground truth correspondence to judge the performance.

The Non-rigid Image Registration Evaluation Project (NIREP) was established to develop software tools and provide shared image validation databases for rigorous testing of non-rigid image registration algorithms. This paper reports on progress developing the Non-rigid Image Registration Evaluation Pro-

B. Fischer, B. Dawant, and C. Lorenz (Eds.): WBIR 2010, LNCS 6204, pp. 140–150, 2010.

gram (NIREP) for evaluating registration accuracy of nonrigid image registration algorithms.[1]

Under the NIREP model, users process data on their own and evaluate the performance of different nonrigid registration algorithms using evaluation criteria that are built into NIREP. The data can be the user's own data or data downloaded from the central database repository on the NIREP website. This model has the advantage of standardizing the evaluation metrics and distributing the processing load. It provides researchers with a tool to compare the performance of multiple registration algorithms on their own data so they can make an informed decision regarding the best algorithm for their specific application. It also provides researchers with a tool to validate their research results.

NIREP uses a diverse set of evaluation metrics to evaluate registration performance on well documented evaluation image databases. These tests evaluate the performance of image registration algorithms with respect to their transformation properties, agreement with human experts, and other indirect performance tests.

2   Methods

2.1   Evaluation Database

A critical step in making unbiased comparisons of algorithm performance is to evaluate registration algorithms on the same population of images. NIREP assumes that the registration algorithms to be analyzed have been used to register images contained in a common evaluation database. An evaluation database consists of groups of registered images and annotations identified by their common image coordinate system.

An evaluation database consists of a set of images to be registered and associated data for accessing the registration results. An example of an evaluation database would be a set of N 3D MRI images of the brain and N expertly labeled segmentations–i.e., one segmentation per 3D image volume. The registration algorithms are used to register the MRI data and the segmentations are used assess registration performance. The segmentations could be used to assess performance by examining the overlap of a deformed source segmentation with the segmentation of the target. In this example, each MRI image and its associated segmentation image constitutes one entry in the evaluation database.

In general, evaluation database entries consist of multiple image modalities (e.g., one or more MRI modalities collected in register, CT image, etc.) and many different types of data for assessing registration performance (e.g., expertly labeled segmentations, landmarks, contours, surfaces, etc.). All the data associated with one entry in the evaluation database are indexed by their common coordinate system. Indexing database entries by coordinate systems provides a

---

[1] In this paper, the acronym NIREP is used to refer to both the evaluation project and to the evaluation software program. It is our hope that it is clear what NIREP means from the context that it is used. Sometimes, both meanings are appropriate.

vocabulary for describing transformations between coordinate systems. For example, we say that the transformation $h_{i,j}$ is used to transform a segmentation from coordinate system i to coordinate system j.

2.2   Evaluation Statistics

Evaluation statistics are criteria that quantify image registration performance based on particular features of the evaluation data. Examples of evaluation statistics include image intensity difference, landmark distance error, and overlap error. NIREP currently implements four evaluation statistics: 1) relative overlap, 2) inverse consistency error, 3) transitivity error, and 4) intensity variance. The transformations required to compute some of these statistics are performed by NIREP, using the interpolation scheme designated by the user.

Relative Overlap. Relative overlap (RO) assesses how well two equally likely segmentations of the same region of interest (ROI) agree or disagree with each other. For an image pair S and T, relative overlap is defined as

$$RO_i(S_i, T_i) = \frac{|S_i \cap T_i|}{|S_i \cup T_i|} \tag{1}$$

where $|S_i \cap T_i|$ is the volume of voxels that intersect between the ith region of interest of images S and T.

Inverse Consistency Error. Inverse consistency error (ICE) evaluates registration performance based on desired transformation properties [1,2,3,4]. It is a common assumption in image registration that the correspondence mapping between two anatomical images is unique–i.e., each point in the source image S is mapped to its corresponding point in the target image T and vice versa. However, in practice, the forward mapping from S to T and the reverse mapping from T to S are not necessarily inverses of each other for most image registration algorithms. This inconsistency reflects an algorithm's inability to uniquely describe the correspondence between two images [5]. Inverse consistency is defined as the mapping of point x in S to a point in T and subsequently being mapped back to the original point. Then inverse consistency error is defined as the distance between the original point x and its transformed point x', which can be expressed in two different ways as

$$ICE1_j(x) = \left\| h_{ji}(h_{ij}(x)) - x \right\|^2 \tag{2}$$

or

$$ICE2_j(x) = \left\| h_{ij}(x) - h_{ji}^{-1}(x) \right\|^2 \tag{3}$$

where h_{ij} is the forward transformation from image S to T, h_{ji} the reverse transformation from image T to S, and $\|\cdot\|$ the standard Euclidean norm. Note that the transformations are defined in the Eulerian coordinate system–i.e., defined with respect to the target frame of reference. Equation 3 gives another interpretation of inverse consistency which is computed using the inverse of the reverse transformation. Note that $ICE1_j(x)$ and $ICE2_j(x)$ show the inverse consistency error with respect to the coordinate system of image T. While inverse consistency does not measure the accuracy of the transformation, it measures the consistency of the correspondence defined by forward and reverse transformations between two coordinate systems [1]. It is important to note that zero inverse consistency does not imply accuracy of the mapping. For example, an identity mapping between two images have perfect inverse consistency, but the correspondence is inaccurate for non-identical images.

Transitivity Error. Transitivity error (TE) evaluates how well the registration transformation satisfies the transitivity property [2,6]. Similarly to inverse consistency error, transitivity error is a measure of consistency of the correspondence defined by compositions of transformations. More specifically, transitivity error measures the distance of point x in image A to its mapped point in B, which is then subsequently mapped to image C, and finally back to point x' in image A. Another interpretation of transitivity is the difference of the composition of transformation AB with BC to transformation AC. These two definitions are expressed as follows:

$$TE2_k(x) = \|h_{ki}(h_{ij}(h_{jk}(x))) - x\|^2 \tag{4}$$

and

$$TE2_k(x) = \|(h_{ij}(h_{jk}(x)) - h_{ik}(x)\|^2 \tag{5}$$

where h_{ij} is the transformation from image A to B, h_{jk} the transformation from image B to C, h_{ki} the transformation from image C to A, h_{ik} the transformation from image A to C, and $\|\cdot\|$ the standard Euclidean norm. Similar to that of ICE, $TE1_k(x)$ and $TE2_k(x)$ show the transitivity error with respect to the coordinate system of image C.

Intensity Variance. Intensity variance is a measure of similarity between a population of images based on voxel intensity difference. In image registration applications driven by voxel intensity features, the ideal registration should result in zero voxel intensity difference between the registered images. Intensity variance is a population study based on this characteristic, where the voxel-wise intensity variance (IV) of a population of M images registered to image j is computed as:

$$IV_j(x) = \frac{1}{M-1} \sum_{i=1}^{M} (T_i(h_{ij}(x)) - ave_j(x))^2 \tag{6}$$

where

$$ave_j(x) = \frac{1}{M} \sum_{i=1}^{M} T_i(h_{ij}(x)) \tag{7}$$

and T_i is the ith image of the population, and $h_{ij}(x)$ is the transformation from image i to j in a Eulerian coordinate system.

2.3   Non-rigid Image Registration Evaluation Program (NIREP)

The NIREP image registration evaluation software integrates the evaluation statistics defined previously. The built-in evaluation statistics allow users to evaluate registration performance themselves, without having to make submissions to external evaluators. This allows users to have immediate access to registration evaluation results and to use evaluation feedback to tune their algorithms and improve performance.

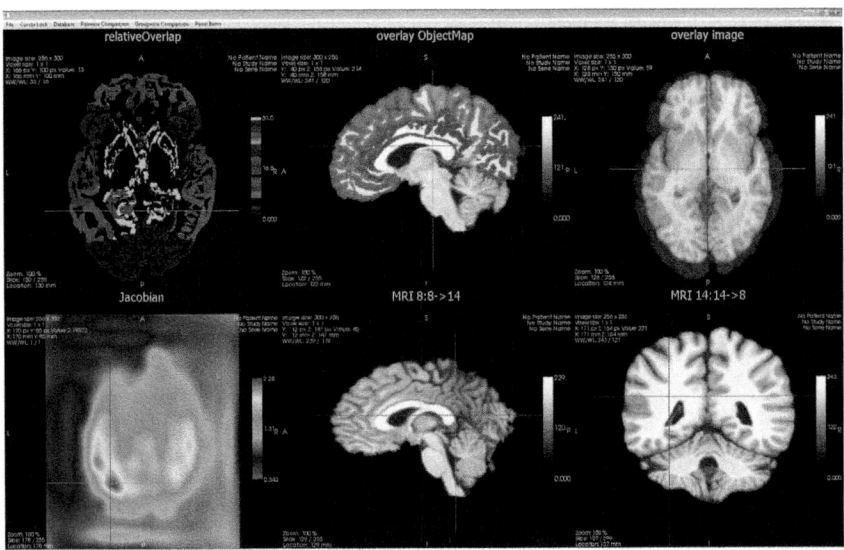

Fig. 1. A typical view of NIREP display showing a 2 × 3 grid of widget panels. The display widgets support various color schemes and transverse, sagittal and coronal planar views. Cursors of each panel can be locked with cursors of other panels, allowing point-to-point comparisons of data in multiple panels. The top-left panel shows the overlay of object maps from the source and the target coordinate systems. The top-center panel shows the object map of the source overlaid on top of the source image. The top-right panel shows the overlay of the source image on top of the target image. The bottom-left panel shows the Jacobian of the forward transformation. The bottom-center and bottom-right panels show the forward and reverse deformed images, respectively.

The primary user interface of NIREP is a display organized as a rectangular grid of panels, as illustrated in Figure 1. The dimensions (number of rows, columns) of the display are user configurable. Each panel can display different visual or textual information (images, evaluation metrics, etc.) and the contents of each can be controlled independently or locked together. The NIREP can display images, difference images, checkerboard and wipe images, several varieties of overlays, and textual information. Examples of evaluation statistics that provide both visual and quantitative textual analysis include the relative overlap, intensity variance, inverse consistency error, and transitivity error statistics.

Characteristics of multiple panels can be locked together so that they all change together. This, for instance, allows a user to set up an evaluation or algorithm comparison scenario, displaying desired evaluation/comparison statistics in visual or textual form. Once such a scenario has been set up, the user can step through different data sets with the contents of all panels automatically updated to reflect each new data set.

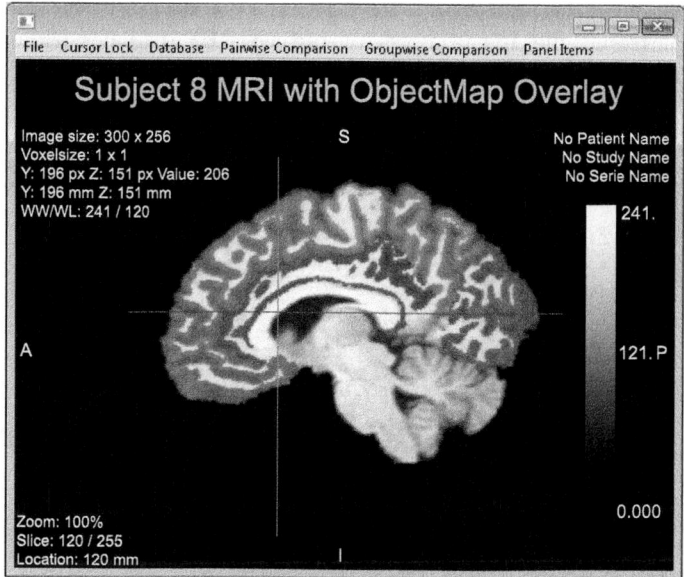

Fig. 2. A NIREP display showing an object map overlay on top of its corresponding MRI data. This display panel widget illustrates the typical information displayed in each panel. The image dimension, voxel size, and voxel intensity at the current cursor location are shown in the top-left corner. The image zoom, slice number, and slice location are shown in the bottom-left corner. The widget popup menu allows users to change widgets, data displayed in the widget, color schemes, the level/window, the zoom factor, and edit titles. The color bar can be positioned anywhere in the panel.

The NIREP software is divided into three main components: the Data Manager, the Evaluator, and the Display Manager. All of these components are managed by their respective configuration files, which will be described below.

Display Manager. The Display Manager is responsible for controlling the content displayed in each panel of the display. Each panel is controlled by a "display widget" which is tailored to the specific type of content to be displayed in that panel. The display panel widgets were adapted from the vtkINRIA3D library developed by INRIA, France (http://www-sop.inria.fr/asclepios/software/vtkINRIA3D/). A human readable "Display Description" specifies the layout and content of the display panels. This description specifies the row/column dimensions of the display and contains a "Widget List" that specifies the type of display widget associated with each panel. The Display Description also contains an "Evaluator List" that describes the specific data that needs to be supplied to the widgets. This may include base and precomputed data (e.g., transformations) from the NIREP image database, as well as results computed on-the-fly by NIREP (e.g., Jacobians). The Display Description is parameterized so that users can switch multiple Evaluator operations and display panels with a single variable change. During start-up, the NIREP software reads the initial Display Description from a file. Fig. 1 shows a typical NIREP display with a 2×3 panel configuration.

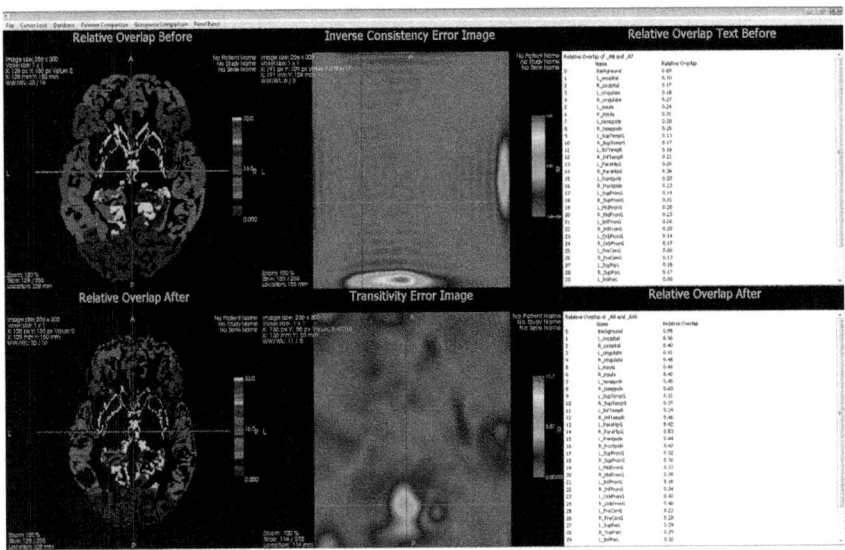

Fig. 3. The display panel can also display text information as shown above. The two right text panels are displaying the relative overlap values for each regions of interest, before and after registration.

Evaluator. The Evaluator is the central processing unit of the NIREP software where all requests and data processing are handled. The display widgets in the Display Manager contact the Evaluator to obtain the necessary data for their respective display functions. The Evaluator is responsible for obtaining data needed by display widgets from the Data Manager and computing new results. The types of data that the Evaluator provides to various display widgets includes images, object maps (annotated segmentation masks), landmarks, contours, surfaces, text tables, and graphs. The Evaluator is designed such that any new data operation or evaluation statistic may be added as a module. The Evaluator uses the Evaluator List, described previously, to determine what data is needed by display widgets. The advantage of a human-readable Evaluator List is that the user can pre-configure desired Evaluator operations by hand before running the NIREP software. This mechanism allows scripting of a large number of operations so that the job can be run in batch mode. An example Display Description is shown in Fig. 4. This description generates the display that visualizes the inverse consistency error for the DEMONS and SICLE registration algorithms.

```
columnSize=2
rowSize=1
Begin WidgetList
   W1,1 = view(iceSicle8-14,ICE 8-14 SICLE)
   W1,2 = view(iceDemons8-14,ICE 8-14 Demons)
End WidgetList
Begin EvaluatorList
   demons8-14    = Transformation(008,014,Demons)
   demons14-8    = Transformation(014,008,Demons)
   iceDemons8-14 = inverseConsistencyErrorImage(demons8-14,
                                         demons14-8,comp)
   sicle8-14     = Transformation(008,014,SICLE_param2)
   sicle14-8     = Transformation(014,008,SICLE_param2)
   iceSicle8-14  = inverseConsistencyErrorImage(sicle8-14,
                                         sicle14-8,comp)
End EvaluatorList
```

Fig. 4. Display Description to generate and visualize the inverse consistency error for the DEMONS and SICLE registration algorithms

Data Manager. The Data Manager manages the loading and storing of data from/to the specified evaluation and algorithm database(s). The Data Manager is responsible for intelligently managing memory by removing data from emery when it is no longer needed by the Evaluator or Display Manager. The Data Manager handles all images supported by ITK (http://www.itk.org) and the Analyze 7.5 (Mayo Clinic, Rochester, MN) format. During start-up, the NIREP software reads an evaluation database resource file, algorithm resource file(s), and optionally, persistent data (pre-computed evaluation data saved to disk) resource file, which contain an exhaustive list of data available for evaluation. The Data Manager provides data to the Evaluator and all data generated by the Evaluator is managed by the Data Manager. This memory management schema stores computed results so they do not need to be recomputed if needed in the future.

3   Results

To demonstrate the NIREP software in evaluating image registration performance, an experiment was performed to compare registration results of Thirion

Demons [7], [8] and SICLE [4], [1], [2], [3] algorithms using the NA0 database. The NA0 database consists of a population of 16 annotated 3D MRI volumes corresponding to eight normal adult males and eight females acquired in the Human Neuroanatomy and Neuroimaging (HNN) Laboratory, The University of Iowa, and each data was segmented into 32 gray matter regions of interests.

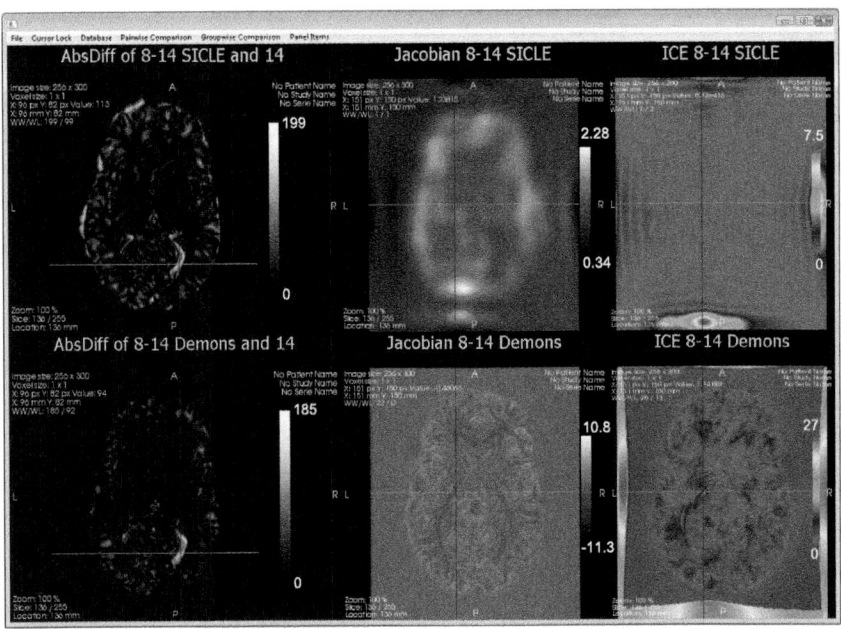

Fig. 5. A display window comparing the registration performances of SICLE and Demons algorithms on subject 8 and 14 of NA0. The left column shows the absolute intensity difference of the deformed source with the target image; the center column shows the Jacobian image of the transformations; and the right column shows the inverse consistency error images of the transformations. Note that the color scales on each of the images are different. The Jacobian for SICLE does not have any zero-crossings (i.e., singularity in transformation), whereas the Jacobian for Demons has many singularities. The cursor location indicates a Jacobian of -0.432701 for Demons and 1.40771 for SICLE. The transformation generated by Demons produced large ICE values, while SICLE produced generally low ICE values inside the brain region. The location pointed by the cursor indicates ICE 8.93467 for Demons, and 0.11022 for SICLE.

Fig. 5 shows a NIREP display window showing the registration results of SICLE and Demons for the registration of subject 8 to subject 14. The left two panels show visually that the absolute intensity difference of the deformed source and the target is smaller for Demons than SICLE. Table 1 shows a portion of the relative overlap values obtained for each region of interest. These results show that the Demons algorithm outperformed the SICLE algorithm based on intensity difference and relative overlap.

Table 1. A subselection of the relative overlap statistics table shown in Fig. 3. The Demons outperformed the SICLE algorithm with respect to relative overlap for this experiment.

Region Name	Relative Overlap (SICLE)	Relative Overlap (Demons)
Background	0.95	0.96
L_occipital	0.36	0.42
R_occipital	0.40	0.48
L_cingulate	0.41	0.48
R_cingulate	0.45	0.53
L_insula	0.44	0.61
R_insula	0.46	0.60
L_temppole	0.45	0.48

However, further evaluation reveals that Demons did not perform as well as SICLE with respect to other evaluation criteria, such as inverse consistency error and distortion measured by the Jacobian of the transformation. Taking advantage of the cursor-lock capability of the NIREP software, it can be seen side-by-side as in the right column of Fig. 5, that the registration made by Demons produced a transformation with high inverse consistency error. In contrast, SICLE, which enforces inverse consistency during registration, had low overall inverse consistency error inside the object boundary as expected.

In addition to inverse consistency error, Demons also performed poorly with the Jacobian of the transformation, with many spots with negative Jacobian values, indicating singularities in the transformation. On the other hand, the SICLE transformation did not contain any singularities.

4   Conclusion

The Non-rigid Image Registration Evaluation Program (NIREP) is a specialized program that makes it easy and intuitive to manipulate data associated with image registration. It differs from other medical image visualization tools in that it can manipulate large amounts of data such as images, deformed images, deformed comparisons specific to image registration. NIREP provides a standard set of evaluation criteria and evaluation databases so that meaningful comparisons between registration algorithms can be made. This standardization ensures that differences in performance are due solely to the algorithms being compared and not other confounding issues. NIREP provides the flexibility for users to create and use their own evaluation databases so that they can investigate how different registration algorithms perform on their own data for their own specific task. Moreover, NIREP provides users the ability make comparisons of their own without being constrained to a predetermined layout. Not only can users compare between any algorithms of choice, the users can make customizations to what kind of comparisons are to be made. The use of a human-readable and user-editable Display Description configuration file for NIREP offers great flexibility to users as to how the display panels are arranged, what types of information are to be displayed, what types of criterion are to be evaluated, what algorithms are to be compared, etc. Another key feature of NIREP is its ability to compute data using transformations of various formats, rather than merely visualizing data. Particularly, NIREP's ability to concatenate multiple transformations and compute inverses of transformations allows users to perform tasks such as computing average shapes based on transformations on the fly.

Acknowledgments

This work is supported in part by NIH grant EB004126.

References

1. Christensen, G.E., Johnson, H.J.: Consistent image registration. IEEE Trans. Med. Imaging 20(7), 568–582 (2001)
2. Christensen, G.E., Johnson, H.J.: Invertibility and transitivity analysis for nonrigid image registration. Journal of Electronic Imaging 12(1), 106–117 (2003)
3. Johnson, H.J., Christensen, G.E.: Consistent landmark and intensity-based image registration. IEEE Trans. Med. Imaging 21(5), 450–461 (2002)
4. Christensen, G.E.: Consistent linear-elastic transformations for image matching. In: Kuba, A., Sámal, M. (eds.) IPMI 1999. LNCS, vol. 1613, pp. 224–237. Springer, Heidelberg (1999)
5. Cao, K.: Local lung tissue expansion analysis based on inverse consistent image registration. Master's thesis, Department of Electrical and Computer Engineering, The University of Iowa, Iowa City, IA 52242 (May 2008)
6. Geng, X., Kumar, D., Christensen, G.E.: Transitive inverse-consistent manifold registration. In: Christensen, G.E., Sonka, M. (eds.) Information Processing in Medical Imaging. LNCS, vol. 3564, pp. 468–479. Springer, Berlin (2005)
7. Thirion, J.P.: Fast non-rigid matching of 3d medical images. Report 2547, Institut National De Recherche en Informatique Et En Automatique (May 1995)
8. Thirion, J.: Image matching as a diffusion process: an analogy with maxwell's demons. Medical Image Analysis 2, 243–260 (1998)

A New Image Database
for 3D/2D Registration
Based on the Visible Human Data Set

Primož Markelj[1], Boštjan Likar[1,2], and Franjo Pernuš[1]

[1] University of Ljubljana, Faculty of Electrical Engineering,
Tržaška 25, 1000 Ljubljana, Slovenia
[2] Sensum, Computer Vision Systems,
Tehnološki park 21, 1000 Ljubljana, Slovenia,
primoz.markelj@fe.uni-lj.si

Abstract. Before an image registration method can be used in the medical theater a rigorous performance assessment of the registration method must be performed. In this paper, a new image database with a reference-based standardized evaluation methodology for objective evaluation and comparison of 3D/2D registration methods has been introduced. CT images of a female from the Visible Human Project® were used and 15 subvolumes each containing one of the vertebrae T3-T12 and L1-L5, and the pelvis were defined. Three pairs of lateral and anterior-posterior 2D fluoroscopic X-ray images were rendered from the CT data. Ray-casting algorithm with an energy conversion function was used to generate realistic fluoroscopic-like DRR images. Furthermore, outliers similar to medical intervention tools were also simulated on the 2D images. The assessment protocol to evaluate four criteria: accuracy, reliability, robustness and algorithm complexity, was defined. The proposed image database with the standardized evaluation methodology comprising ground truth registrations, displacements from the ground truth and target points is available upon request from the authors.

1 Introduction

Assessing the performance of a medical system is a complex and tedious task [1]. When performing assessment studies of an image processing component rather than the whole medical system, the scope and complexity is reduced, although the general framework of assessment remains the same or is slightly adapted for the specific study. In scope of medical image processing, a standardized evaluation (assessment) methodology outlines a reference-based assessment study of an image processing method [2] by defining the image data sets, the corresponding ground truth and its accuracy, the assessment criteria, the assessment metric, the assessment objective and finally the assessment protocol [2]. The guidelines for creating and using such a reference-based evaluation methodology of image processing methods was proposed by Jannin et al. [2]. By using a standardized evaluation methodology the performance and limitations of a proposed method

B. Fischer, B. Dawant, and C. Lorenz (Eds.): WBIR 2010, LNCS 6204, pp. 151–160, 2010.

can be assessed and objectively compared to other methods assessed with the same methodology.

In this paper, we focus on the assessment of 3D/2D registration of CT and X-ray images. To the best of our knowledge, only two publicly available 3D/2D registration evaluation methodologies exist in the literature. Tomaževič et al. [3][1] used a section of cadaveric lumbar spine segment with several millimeters of soft tissue and acquired computed tomography (CT), magnetic resonance (MR) and 18 X-ray images separated by 20° rotation around the axial axis. Similarly, image data in the standardized evaluation methodology proposed by van de Kraats et al. [4][2] consists of 2D fluoroscopic X-ray images and 3D CT, MR and 3D rotational X-ray images of two defrosted segments of a spinal column.

To increase the clinical realism and retain the control over the parameters of the assessment study, we propose a new image database that is based on CT images from The Visible Human Project® [3] [5]. Since this data set does not provide 2D X-ray images, we generated them from the CT data by calculating digitally reconstructed radiographs (DRRs) [6]. Such an approach produces clinically realistic 2D images very similar to the ones acquired during a medical intervention and circumvents the need for calculating the ground truth registration, for instance by fiducial markers, as it is directly available from the projection geometry. In order to further imitate the real clinical scenario, a simulation of medical intervention tools, that can be present in the imaging field-of-view during the interventional image acquisition, was also performed. In addition to the image database with the ground truth, a reference-based evaluation methodology based on the evaluation framework proposed by van de Kraats et al. [4] with the starting positions, target points, metric, and evaluation criteria was also prepared.

2   Methods and Materials

2.1   3D Image Data Set

The Visible Human data set consists of CT, MR and anatomical cryosection images of a representative male and female cadaver [5]. In the scope of the present study, only CT and MR images are of interest. For the present work, the female CT scan was chosen due to the superior image quality of the fresh cadaver, that provides a better contrast between muscle and fat tissues in comparison with the scan of the frozen male cadaver. The chosen CT scan of the thorax, abdomen, and pelvis regions consists of transverse slices with the inter-slice distance of 1 mm, the intra-slice resolution of 0.9375×0.9375 mm^2, and a slice pixel size of 512×512 . The MR images were also considered, however were not used due to the large inter-slice distance of the data (4 mm for both male and female dataset). Further details about the data set can be found in [5].

---

[1] http://lit/tools.php

[2] http://www.isi.uu.nl/Research/Databases/GS/

[3] http://www.nlm.nih.gov/research/visible/visible_human.html

Vertebra T8   Vertebra L3   Pelvis

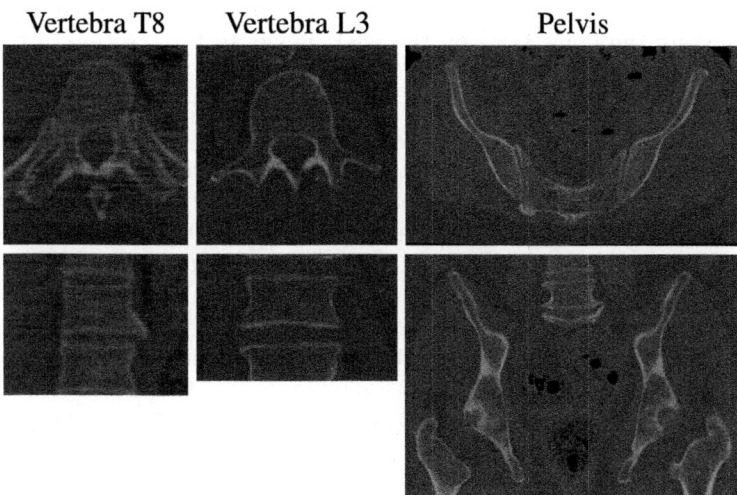

Fig. 1. Transverse (top) and coronal planes (bottom) of sub-volumes containing vertebra T8, vertebra L3 and pelvis (from left to right)

From the CT image of the thorax, abdomen, and pelvis, 15 sub-volumes each depicting one of the thoracic vertebrae T3-T12, lumbar vertebrae L1-L5 and pelvis were determined. The CT resolution of each sub-volume was kept at the $0.9375 \times 0.9375 \times 1$ mm^3 of the original CT image. Furthermore, a world (reference) coordinate system was set as the coordinate system of the chosen 3D CT image defined in the upper left corner of the image. Examples of cross-sections of CT sub-volumes are shown in Fig. 1.

2.2   2D Image Data Set

Since the Visible Human data set does not provide 2D X-ray images and their geometrical setup, 2D images were generated from the CT image. A rendered 2D image - a digitally reconstructed radiograph (DRR) - is most commonly reconstructed from the CT data by ray-casting [6]. Using this approach, the integral of the attenuation function along each ray passing through the volume for a given energy spectrum is computed. However, in order to make this approach practically feasible, several assumption have to be made.

First, the scattered radiation, beam hardening effect and other imaging system characteristics are usually not modeled when generating DRRs. Thereby, only the primary energy attenuation is taken into account yielding the intensity I_{ij} of the DRR image pixel at the point (i,j) as:

$$I_{ij} = \int I_0\left(E\right) \left(e^{-\int_{Q \in l_{ij}} \mu(Q,E)\mathrm{d}l_{ij}}\right) \mathrm{d}E \ , \tag{1}$$

where $I_0(E)$ is the source spectrum, $\mu(Q, E)$ is the attenuation function at point Q for various energies E, and $\mathrm{d}l_{ij}$ is the line integral element corresponding to the point (i, j) in the DRR image I. The direction of the line l_{ij} is determined by connecting the point (i, j) on the DRR image to the position of the X-ray source that is specified by the geometrical setup of the X-ray system. We used a typical geometrical setup with a source-to-center of the volume distance of 1000 mm and source-to-detector distance of 1550 mm.

Second, since the volume is a digital image, a piecewise approximation to the line integral of the linear attenuation coefficient is accumulated along the ray. We use a constant step half the length of the smallest voxel to proceed along the ray from the entrance to the exit point of the volume. At each of the steps, the length of the step is multiplied by the voxel linear attenuation coefficient determined from the CT numbers and accumulated. Trilinear interpolation is used to take into account the contribution of all the neighboring voxels at the current step.

Third, the scanner must be properly calibrated in order for the CT numbers to represent the Hounsfield units (HU) which relate each voxel value to the relative electron density of the tissue. Thereby, the linear attenuation coefficient of each voxel can be calculated as:

$$\mu_x = \mu_w \left(\frac{HU_x}{1000} + 1 \right) , \tag{2}$$

where μ_x is the linear attenuation of the sample, HU_x the CT number of the sample in Hounsfield units, and μ_w is the linear attenuation of water. However, the value of μ_w is only valid for the effective proton energy used to acquire the CT volume, which is not the same as the energy used to obtain a 2D X-ray. To overcome this problem, we assumed that the attenuation function $\mu(Q)$ is obtained at an effective proton energy of E_{CT}, while an X-ray beam effective energy is assumed to be E_{Xray}. If a functional dependency $\mathcal{C}(\cdot)$ is assumed between $\mu(E_{CT})$ and $\mu(E_{Xray})$ (1) can be simplified to:

$$I_{ij} = I_0 \, e^{-\int_{Q \in l_{ij}} \mathcal{C}(\mu(Q, E_{CT})) \mathrm{d}l_{ij}} . \tag{3}$$

The functional dependency $\mathcal{C}(\cdot)$ can be characterized as a linear function within a limited support of $[\mu_l, \mu_h]$, defined by parameters of the width of the support w, the center of the support c and the saturation value o, as shown in Fig. 2 [7,8]. These parameters can be determined by dividing the range of CT numbers into sub-ranges defined by materials of known relative density function and chemical composition. This allows the creation of look-up tables between the HU values and linear attenuation coefficients for all energies of interest [8]. Alternatively, a radiometric calibration can be performed between a sample X-ray image and the corresponding DRR [7] to derive the required parameters. However, as none of these approaches could be applied in our case, a heuristic classification of the background, soft tissues and bone based on the CT number was performed in order to derive suitable parameters for the energy conversion (cf. Fig. 2).

To generate realistic DRRs three sub-volumes of the thorax, abdomen and pelvis CT image were created. The sub-volumes contained the thoracic, lumbar, and pelvis region of the body with all relevant anatomical structures. From each

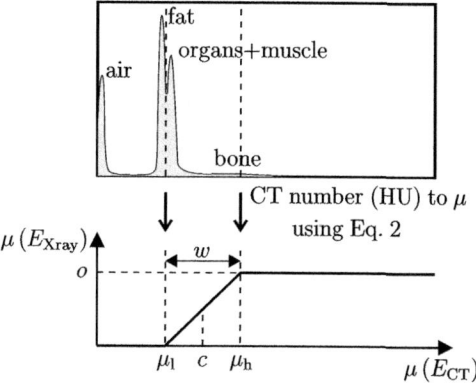

Fig. 2. The conversion function $\mathcal{C}(\cdot)$ and the illustration of the heuristic classification approach to determine its parameters (w, c, and o)

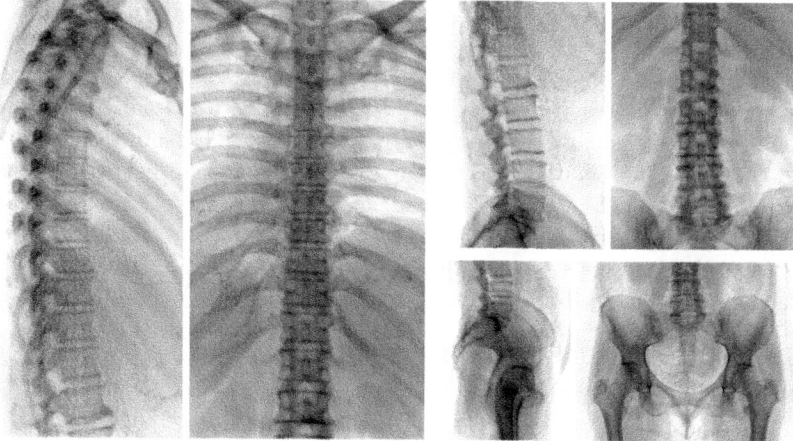

Fig. 3. Rendered lateral and anterior-posterior fluoroscopic DRRs of the thoracic (first and second column), lumbar (third and forth column, top row), and pelvis (third and forth column, bottom row) region

of the three sub-volumes anterior-posterior (AP) and lateral (LAT) DRRs were rendered, yielding six 2D kilo-voltage (kV) X-ray fluoroscopy-like images. In an additional processing step, a suitable region-of-interest without the rendering artifacts on the edges was determined. For all six DRR images the same image resolution of 0.4×0.4 mm^2 was used. Examples of kV fluoroscopic-like images are given in Fig. 3.

2.3 Interventional Tool Simulation

During a real-life intervention different interventional tools might be present in the patients body and therefore in the imaging field-of-view while the fluoroscopic images are being acquired. Furthermore, in some interventions, e.g. percutaneous vertebroplasty [9], 2D imaging is used to guide an interventional tool to the targeted anatomy. In such cases, additional foreign structures are present on projection images which are not present on 3D images acquired before the intervention. Consequently, due to outliers the 3D/2D registration of such images is even more challenging and a decrease in the registration performance can be expected.

To imitate the described clinical scenario and assess the robustness of the registration algorithm to outliers, a simulation of a 13-gauge needle typically used in percutaneous vertebroplasty procedures [9] was performed. The needle was analytically simulated in 3D and projected onto the DRRs by adapting (3) as:

$$
\begin{aligned}
I_{ij}^s &= I_0 \, e^{- \int_{Q \in l_{ij}} C(\mu(Q, E_{CT})) \mathrm{d}l_{ij} - \int_{Q \in l_{ij}} \mu_s \mathrm{d}l_{ij}} \\
&= I_{ij} \, e^{- \int_{Q \in l_{ij}} \mu_s \mathrm{d}l_{ij}} ,
\end{aligned}
\tag{4}
$$

where I_{ij}^s is the simulated intensity at point (i, j) and μ_s is the linear attenuation coefficient of the simulated interventional tool.

A single stainless steel 13-gauge cannula was simulated for each vertebra of interest and positioned typical of the intervention in question. The attenuation coefficient of the needle μ_s was set to 7.64 cm^{-1}, taken from Foster and Evans [10] for Type 304 Stainless Steel at effective proton energy of 60 keV. The obtained AP and LAT DRR images with the simulated needles are shown in Figure 4.

To determine how our DRR images with the superimposed needles compare to real fluoroscopic images obtained during a vertebroplasty procedure a visual comparison to published image data was performed [9,11]. First of all, we found that the real fluoroscopic images themselves taken at various institutions can be quite different due to different imaging equipment, image acquisition settings, needle materials, preferences of the interventionalist etc. Considering all the examined real images and our simulated images we believe that the generated image data compares reasonable well to real data and is suitable for conducting pre-clinical evaluation studies of 3D/2D registration methods.

2.4   Evaluation Criteria, Metric and Protocol

To enable the objective evaluation of the 3D/2D registration methods the evaluation framework proposed by van de Kraats et al. [4] was utilized, according to which a 3D/2D registration method is assessed by four evaluation criteria: accuracy, reliability, robustness and algorithm complexity. Accuracy is measured by the mean target registration error (mTRE) metric [4,12], which is the mean of distances between target points transformed by the ground truth and by the registration obtained with the evaluated method. The target points determine the region for which the accuracy is evaluated and are therefore directly associated with the reason for the registration. Since we focus on the registration of the vertebrae and the pelvis, positions of 12 anatomical target points on the vertebrae of interest and 18 anatomical target points on the pelvis were manually defined on each of the 15 sub-volume CT images. The positions of selected target points are illustrated in Fig. 5. To assess the accuracy, 400 starting positions defined by rigidly displacing each sub-volume from the ground truth were

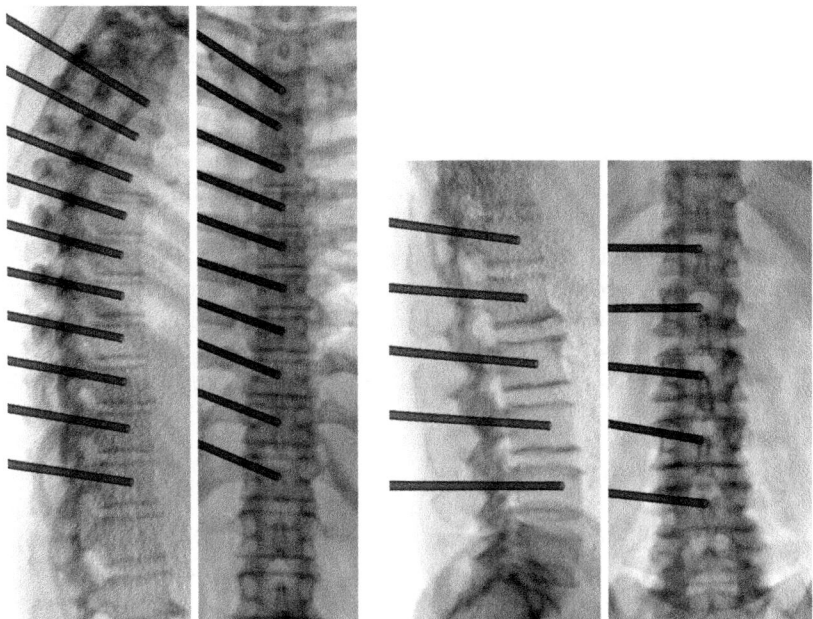

Fig. 4. Rendered lateral and anterior-posterior fluoroscopic DRRs of the thoracic (first and second image from the left) and lumbar (third and forth image from the left) vertebrae with the simulated needles.

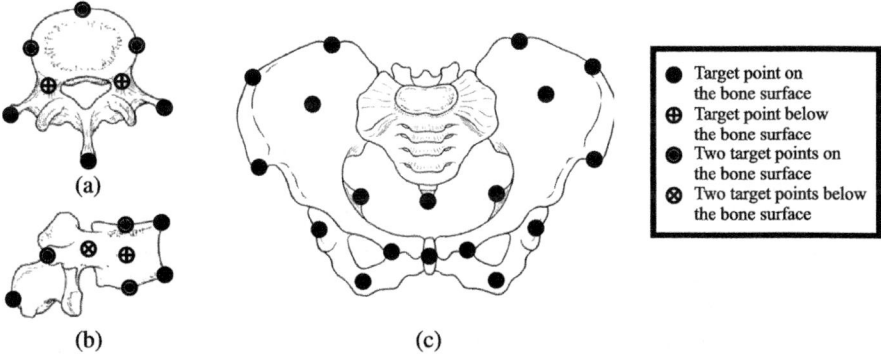

Fig. 5. The positions of 12 anatomical target points on lateral (a) and axial (b) illustrations of the vertebra, respectively, and the positions of 18 anatomical target points on an illustration of the pelvis (c). (Source: [13])

generated. The displacements were thus defined by three translations and three rotations. The translations and rotations were chosen to yield mTRE values of the starting positions uniformly distributed in an interval from 0 to 20 mm, with 20 starting positions in each of the 1 mm wide subintervals [4]. A registration is classified as successful if the mTRE after the registration is smaller than a pre-specified threshold of 2 mm. The overall registration accuracy is computed as the root-mean-square mTRE value of all successful registrations.

To assess the reliability of the registration algorithm, the success rate and capture range are calculated. The success rate is defined as the number of successful registrations against the number of all registrations, while the capture range is defined as the distance from the reference position to the first 1 mm subinterval for which the registration is successful in less than 95 % of all cases [4]. Furthermore, robustness is determined by performing registrations using the DRRs with the simulated needles and comparing the registration results to the results obtained using DRRs without the outliers. Besides the accuracy, success rate and capture range of registrations using 2D images with and without outliers, the registration times should also be reported to indicate the algorithm complexity.

3   Discussion and Conclusion

A new image database with a standardized evaluation methodology for objective comparison of 3D/2D registration methods has been introduced. CT image of a female thorax, abdomen and pelvis from the Visible Human Project® was used and sub-volumes with vertebrae T3-T12 and L1-L5, and the pelvis were defined, while AP and LAT 2D images were rendered from the complete anatomical CT data of the chosen regions of the body. Ray-casting with an energy conversion function was used to compensate for the difference between the CT and X-ray effective proton energies resulting in realistic 2D X-ray fluoroscopy-like images. Furthermore, outliers similar to medical intervention tools were also simulated on the 2D images to enable the evaluation of robustness of the registration method.

In comparison to the two existing publicly available standardized evaluation methodologies [3,4] where cadaver phantoms with little soft tissue were used, the proposed methodology increases the clinical realism of the data by providing images with soft tissues and clinical scenario outliers in the 2D images. Furthermore, the rendering and simulation approach enables a better control over the parameters of the assessment study and the ground truth. Obviously, the rendered 2D images cannot fully mimic the real fluoroscopic images and as the 2D images are generated directly from the 3D images, the deformations of predominantly soft tissue anatomical structures between 3D image acquisition and intervention are not present. Nevertheless, we believe that such a methodology offers an optimal trade-off between the clinical realism on the one hand and control of parameters to be studied on the other.

In this paper, we focused on CT and kV fluoroscopic images, and on the spine and pelvis anatomy. However, the proposed image database could also be extended to other anatomical structures and imaging modalities like 3D MR images and/or rendered 2D portal-like images. Unfortunately, due to the poor quality of the visible human CT and, especially, MRI data in respect to todays imaging standards, the extension to other modalities would probably require an a 3D image data set of superior quality. Other extensions to the proposed methodology include the application of realistic deformation models to the 3D images before rendering to account for the anatomical changes that may occur between 3D image acquisition and intervention. Furthermore, medical tools typical of other medical interventions could be simulated onto the fluoroscopic images making the methodology applicable to a broader field of interventions. Therefore, the proposed image data set can serve as a prototype for building a database of gold standard data sets for evaluating 3D/2D registration methods for image guided interventions.

The aim of this paper is to provide objective comparison and unbiased evaluation of new and existing 3D/2D registration methods. Therefore, the proposed standardized evaluation methodology with the image data sets, registration ground truths, displacements from the ground truth, and target points as described in this paper is available upon request from the authors.

Acknowledgements

This work was supported by the Ministry of Higher Education, Science and Technology, Republic of Slovenia under the grants P2-0232, L2-7381, L2-9758, Z2-9366, J2-0716, L2-2023, and J7-2246.

References

1. Jannin, P., Korb, W.: Assessment of image-guided interventions. In Peters, T.M., Cleary, K., eds.: Image Guided Interventions Technology and Applications. Springer (2008) 531–549
2. Jannin, P., Grova, C., Maurer, C.: Model for defining and reporting reference-based validation protocols in medical image processing. Int. J. CARS 1(2), 63 (2006)
3. Tomaževič, D., Likar, B., Pernuš, F.: Gold standard" data for evaluation and comparison of 3D/2D registration methods. Comput. Aided Surg. 9(4), 137–144 (2004)
4. van de Kraats, E.B., Penney, G.P., Tomaževič, D., van Walsum, T., Niessen, W.J.: Standardized evaluation methodology for 2-D-3-D registration. IEEE Trans. Med. Imaging 24(9), 1177–1189 (2005)
5. Spitzer, V., Ackerman, M.J., Scherzinger, A.L., Whitlock, D.: The visible human male: a technical report. J. Am. Med. Informat. Assoc. 3(2), 118–130 (1996)
6. Sherouse, G.W., Novins, K., Chaney, E.L.: Computation of digitally reconstructed radiographs for use in radiotherapy treatment design. Int. J. Radiat. Oncol. Biol. Phys. 18(3), 651–658 (1990)
7. Khamene, A., Bloch, P., Wein, W., Svatos, M., Sauer, F.: Automatic registration of portal images and volumetric CT for patient positioning in radiation therapy. Med. Image Anal. 10(1), 96–112 (2006)
8. Milickovic, N., Baltas, D., Giannouli, S., Lahanas, M., Zamboglou, N.: CT imaging based digitally reconstructed radiographs and their application in brachytherapy. Phys. Med. Biol. 45(10), 2787–2800 (2000)
9. Mathis, J.M.: Percutaneous vertebroplasty. In: Mauro, M.A., Murphy, K.P.J., Thomson, K.R., Venbrux, A.C., Zollikofer, C.L. (eds.) Image Guided Interventions, Saunders. Expert Radiology, vol. II, pp. 1675–1682 (2008)

10. Foster, B.E., Evans, J.W.: X-ray mass attenuation coefficients in the range of 50 to 150 kVp with data for several reactor material. ORNL 3552, Oak Ridge National Laboratory (1964)
11. Kallmes, D.F., Schweickert, P.A., Marx, W.F., Jensen, M.E.: Vertebroplasty in the mid- and upper thoracic spine. Am. J. Neuroradiol. 23(7), 1117–1120 (2002)
12. Fitzpatrick, J.M., West, J.B., Maurer, C.R.: Predicting error in rigid-body point-based registration. IEEE Trans. Med. Imaging 17(5), 694–702 (1998)
13. Cull, P. (ed.): The Sourcebook of Medical Illustration. Parthenon Publishing Group (1989)

Unifying Characterization of Deformable Registration Methods Based on the Inherent Parametrization
An Attempt at an Alternative Analysis Approach

Darko Zikic[1], Ali Kamen[2], and Nassir Navab[1]

[1] Computer Aided Medical Procedures (CAMP), TU München, Germany
[2] Siemens Corporate Research (SCR), Princeton, NJ, USA

Abstract. We propose to characterize deformable registration methods in a unified way, based on their parametrization. In contrast to traditional classifications, we do not apply this characterization only to standard "parametric" methods such as B-Spline Free-form deformations, but we explicitly include elastic and fluid-type "non-parametric" methods, such as the classic variational approach, and the fluid demons method. To this end, we consider parametrizations by linear combinations of arbitrary basis functions. While for the variational approach we simply utilize piecewise linear bases, for the fluid demons method we provide a new interpretation by showing that it can be seen as inherently parametrized by densely located Gaussian basis functions. Furthermore, we show that the semi-implicit discretization of the variational approach can be seen as steepest descent, with a displacement parametrized by densely located bases, based on Green's functions corresponding to the regularization. This provides a further connection to the demons approaches. The proposed characterization is widely applicable and provides a simple and intuitive way of relating some of the arguably most commonly used methods to each other.

1 Introduction

Dense, intensity-based estimation of nonlinear motion from images has gained tremendous popularity in the last 30 years [1,2], resulting in a plethora of methods. Early reviews of registration methods [3,4], as well as more recent ones [5,6,7,8,9] include overviews of the work on deformable registration at the respective times of publication. These reviews have a focus on linear methods and do not treat deformable registration exclusively. An early survey of nonlinear techniques is given in [10], with focus on hierarchical aspects. More recent overviews and classifications of deformable techniques [11,12,13,14] have in common that they in general distinguish - among other properties - between "parametric" methods, such as B-Spline Free-form deformations (FFD), and the so called "non-parametric" methods.[1] Here, "parametric" methods are classified

---

[1] In some of these publications, different terms are used for generally same groups: [9] distinguishes *Spline models* and *Elastic registration* (defined as "not to use any

B. Fischer, B. Dawant, and C. Lorenz (Eds.): WBIR 2010, LNCS 6204, pp. 161–172, 2010.
© Springer-Verlag Berlin Heidelberg 2010

by a parametrization which leads to a reduction of the number of the degrees of freedom, compared to "dense" parametrizations featuring a displacement vector at every voxel. For the "non-parametric" methods, no explicit parametrization is performed during the modeling of the energy. Hence, during the derivation of the optimization criterion, the unknown is a continuous function, so that the "non-parametric" approach is referred to as *variational*. The term "non-parametric" is used for (at least) two different groups of methods. For the first group, a regularization energy term is defined in the model, and then an optimization of the model is performed [12]. The second "non-parametric" group are the so called demons approaches, for which (in the original formulation) no explicit regularization term is defined in the model, and the regularization is performed by applying a low-pass filter to the displacement. In order to concisely distinguish between the two "non-parametric" groups, we will refer to the first group as *variational*, and the second one as *demons* methods.

Our work in this paper is guided by the fact that for any method, a parametrization must be performed in order to compute an actual solution. However, in most "non-parametric" cases, this inherent parametrization is not explicitly stated. For example, for the "non-parametric" cases, the parameters are usually the displacement vectors located at all sampling points (voxels) of the volume. In this work, we focus on such inherent parametrizations for the variational and the fluid demons approach. These two methods can be seen as prototypal examples for the wider classes of elastic-type and fluid-type methods. While for the variational approach many different basis functions can be used for parametrization, we identify tensor products of piecewise linear functions as the natural choice, which is effectively used in many implementations. For the demons approach, we propose a novel interpretation by showing that the fluid demons method can be seen as optimization of a given similarity measure, with the displacement parametrized by a linear combination of densely located Gaussian bases.

We see the contribution of this paper in the focus on the inherent parametrization as a characterization criterion. This enables the treatment of some of the arguably most commonly used deformable registration methods in a unified framework, and allows for an intuitive way of relating the different methods to each other. In Sec. 2 we present a derivation for the standard parametric approach which is used as the general framework in the paper, and we introduce the elastic and fluid method groups. Following this, we give a brief overview of the parametric (Sec. 3), variational (Sec. 4) and the demons methods (Sec. 5), and show how they can be cast in the parametrization-based framework. In Sec. 6, we discuss the use of parametrization as a criterion for characterization.

2   General Framework Based on Parametrization

Common to all intensity-based registration methods is the goal to estimate the transformation φ between the domains of the target image I_T and the

---

parametric mapping functions"); [11] uses *parametric models* and *competitive regularization* ; [13] differentiates *physically based models* and *basis function expansions*.

source image I_S by optimizing an appropriate similarity measure E_D. This results in

$$\varphi = \arg \min_{\varphi'} E_D(I_T, I_S \circ \varphi') \; , \tag{1}$$

with d-dimensional $I_{\langle S|T \rangle} : \Omega \rightarrow \mathbb{R}$ with $\Omega \subseteq \mathbb{R}^d$, and the transformation $\varphi : \Omega \rightarrow \Omega$, where mostly $\varphi \in L^2$ is assumed. The discretization of the images in Ω is supposed to result in N samples. The deformation φ is usually expressed in terms of the displacement u, as $\varphi = \mathrm{Id} + u$, with the identity operator Id.

Without modification and with $\varphi \in L^2$, Eq. (1) does not offer enough constraints to solve for φ.[2] With the similarity measure being modular in most modern methods, these differ primarily in the strategy to deal with the underconstraintment of (1). There are basically two approaches to this problem.

The first strategy is by defining an explicit regularization term in the energy model. This path is taken for variational methods (Sec. 4).

The second way of dealing with the above problem is by restriction of the deformations to a lower-dimensional function space. The "parametric" approaches (Sec. 3) are the classical example for this solution. In practice, an explicit energy is mostly defined additionally to the restriction of the deformation. This way, many "parametric" approaches combine the two discussed strategies.

Another way of restricting deformations to lower-dimensional manifolds is by treating them in Sobolev spaces, which contain only functions with a certain degree of regularity by construction [15,16,17,18]. In [15,17], it is pointed out that the fluid demons approach can be seen as minimization of (1) in a Sobolev space, which corresponds to a manifold containing only diffeomorphisms. The parametrization of the fluid demons as discussed in this paper can be seen as a discrete analogon to the use of Sobolev spaces in [15,17].

In our framework, we use the general model, which includes the explicit regularization energy term E_R, that is

$$E(u) = E_D(I_T, I_S \circ (\mathrm{Id} + u)) + \alpha E_R(u) \; . \tag{2}$$

Here, approaches with no regularization energy are included by setting $\alpha = 0$. Depending on the problem at hand, different regularization terms such as diffusion, curvature, or linear elasticity can be employed [12]. Since the problem in (2) is non-linear, it is solved in an iterative manner by computing an update du to an initial displacement estimate u. In the following we drop the argument u in the notation for simplicity where it is not necessarily required.

The minimization problem in each iteration is solved by computing the update du. Most commonly, du is based on the gradient of the energy E with respect to the displacement, resulting in a gradient descent scheme

$$du \equiv \frac{\partial u}{\partial t} \quad \text{with} \quad \frac{\partial u}{\partial t} \equiv -\frac{\partial E}{\partial u} \; , \tag{3}$$

cf. e.g. [19,12]. For shorter notation, we set $\partial E / \partial u = \nabla E$.

---

[2] Note that (1) can be well posed in other spaces such as Sobolev spaces [15].

In order to solve the non-linear partial differential equation (PDE) in (3), discretization has to be performed. For time discretization, two common choices are: 1) the *explicit discretization*, leading to the update rule

$$du = -\tau(\nabla E_D + \alpha \nabla E_R) \,, \tag{4}$$

which results in the standard steepest gradient descent, and 2) the *semi-implicit discretization* (cf. e.g. [12,20]), resulting in a linear system

$$(\mathrm{Id} + \tau\alpha\nabla E_R)du = -\tau(\nabla E_D(u) - \alpha\nabla E_R(u)) \,. \tag{5}$$

The spatial discretization is performed by representing the deformation by parameters p. As parametrizations, we consider linear combinations of arbitrary basis functions $B_k : \Omega \to \Omega$, resulting in

$$u_p(x) = \sum_k p_k B_k(x) \,. \tag{6}$$

The parameters $p_k \in \mathbb{R}^d$ can be seen as representative displacement vectors. The set of all p_k constitutes the parameter vector p. With the parametrization from (6), the derivative of (2) with respect to the parameters reads

$$\nabla_p E = \frac{\partial E}{\partial u}\frac{\partial u}{\partial p} \,. \tag{7}$$

Please note that due to the linearity of (6), Eq. (7) can be written for each parameter as a scalar product of ∇E with the corresponding basis function as

$$(\nabla_p E)_k = \left\langle B_k \,, \nabla E \right\rangle \,, \tag{8}$$

which can be seen as the projection of the continuous updates onto the space of parameters. We can use the gradient (7) in (4) or (5) to obtain the evolution rules for the parameters. For example, for the explicit discretization (4) we get

$$dp = -\tau\nabla_p E \,. \tag{9}$$

2.1   Elastic and Fluid Registration Modes

In this work, we treat the variational and the fluid demons methods as representatives of two groups of approaches: the elastic-type, and the fluid-type methods. In this context, the terms *elastic* and *fluid* present generalizations of the original linear elasticity [2] and viscous fluid [21] approaches to more general regularization terms, compare e.g. [22,23]. This generalization classifies methods as *elastic* if the regularization is performed on the displacement field, which is the case for standard minimization of (2). On the other hand, a methods is *fluid*, if the regularization is performed only on the displacement updates (i.e. velocities) in every iteration. A characteristic of fluid approaches is that the regularization energy is not conserved in the iteration process, in contrast to elastic methods.

Variational and parametric methods as described in Sec. 3 and 4 of this paper implement the elastic approach. The original form of the demons method [24] proposes the smoothing of the complete displacement field in every iteration, which was shown to constitute an elastic-type method [23]. This provides a connection between the approaches with explicit regularization energy, and the original demons method. For the demons methods, also combinations of elastic and fluid approaches have also been discussed [23,25].

Fluid-type approaches comprise the viscous fluid methods [21,22], approaches employing Sobolev spaces [16,17,15,18], and the fluid-type demons method [22,23]. Equivalence between these methods is established [22,15,17], with different regularization resulting in different flow models. In Sec. 5 we discuss the fluid demons method from [16] as a representative of this group.

Finally, one can note that elastic-type methods can in general be rendered fluid by applying the resulting evolution rules to displacement updates du instead of the displacement u. In this case, the original energy is no longer optimized.

3   Classic Parametric Methods

Classic "parametric" methods can be derived as shown in Sec. 2. In the following we consider two general groups of parametrizations, and discuss briefly one popular example of each class. The first group employs local basis functions B_k, each of which is centered at the position $c_k \in \Omega$. This is exemplified by B-Spline based Free-form Deformations (Sec. 3.1). This group further includes the parametrization by radial basis functions (RBF) such as Thin-Plate Splines (TPS), Wavelets, or parametrizations used by the Finite Element (FE) method.[3] The second class features global basis functions, which cannot be assigned a geometrical center of influence. This group is represented by the parametrization based on trigonometric functions (Sec. 3.2).

3.1   B-Spline Free-form Deformations (FFD)

The parametrization of deformations by FFDs based on cubic B-Splines is a common technique for registration of medical images. Early uses are reported in [27,28,29], and the methods has become very widely used since [30,31,32,33].

The B-Spline basis B is the tensor product of the one-dimensional basis functions b, defined as

$$b(x) = \begin{cases} 2/3 - (1 - |\tilde{x}|/2)\tilde{x}^2 & \text{for } 0 < |\tilde{x}| < 1 \\ (2 - |\tilde{x}|)^3/6 & \text{for } 0 < |\tilde{x}| < 1 \\ 0 & \text{otherwise} \end{cases}, \qquad (10)$$

---

[3] In [26], a link between FE-based methods, which are commonly used for parametrization of variational methods, and B-Spline FFDs is discussed, providing further motivation to discuss variational methods in the context of parametrization.

with $\tilde{x} = x/H$, where H is the spacing between two control points along the respective dimension on a regular grid. The actual bases B_k, located at points c_k, are defined as

$$B_k(x) = B(x - c_k) . \tag{11}$$

A visualization of the one dimensional B-Spline representation is given in Fig. 1a. More details on B-Splines can be found in [34,35] while [13] gives an overview of the historical development.

3.2   Trigonometric Functions

Parametrization by trigonometric functions is also a popular choice in many applications. The general approach is to parametrize the displacement field by Discrete Fourier Transformation (DFT) [36,37], or Discrete Cosine Transformation (DCT) [38] basis functions. For space reasons, at this point we only note that the corresponding basis functions B_k are global and represent a signal of frequency k, and refer the reader to the respective papers for the definitions. Mostly, only a certain number of low-frequency basis functions is used for parametrization. This provides an inherent regularization since only smooth functions can be generated by construction. For an exemplary visualization, please see Fig. 1b. A further motivation for the use of trigonometric functions is that in some cases, the trigonometric bases form the eigenfunctions to the linear operator in (5), which facilitates the solution of the linear system.

4   Variational Methods

The variational approach for deformable registration is very common, cf. e.g. [39,12]. The actual derivation of the methods is mostly performed in the spirit of the first part of the derivation in Sec. 2, resulting in evolution rules (4) and (5).

4.1   Variational Methods Parametrized

For numerical realization of variational methods, parametrization of the resulting PDE in (3) (i.e. discretization of the displacement) is inevitable. There are different parametrization approaches in the context of image registration, most notably the Finite Difference (FD), and the Finite Element (FE) methods. The discretization of the displacement by FE as a linear combination of a set of chosen basis functions is obviously parametric in the classical sense according to Sec. 3. On the other hand, classical "non-parametric" approaches mostly employ the FD discretization on a regular grid. In this approach, the differential operators are discretized by evaluating the underlying data (images and displacement) at all given sampling points in the image domain, and the parameters are the values of the displacement field vectors at the sampling points. This discretization approach can be seen as a parametrization of the displacement by a linear combination of basis functions covering only one sampling point by their support, and having the value 1 at the corresponding sampling point position. A natural choice for such a basis is the tensor product of piecewise linear "hat" basis functions, as these bases are often used for interpolation of the displacement field at inter-voxel positions in practice. Other possible choices include constant unity box function (nearest neighbor interpolation), or simply a function equal to one at the respective control point and zero everywhere.

So, corresponding to (6), we again perform the parametrization with bases $B_k(x) = B(x - c_k)$. Here, the basis B is a tensor product of d one-dimensional functions b, defined as $b(x) = 1 + h^{-1}$ for $x \in [-h, 0]$, $b(x) = 1 - h^{-1}$ for $x \in (0, h]$, and $b(x) = 0$ elsewhere, with h being the distance between sampling points.

The resulting update rules are equivalent to those in Sec. 2. After discretization of (7), the derivative of the displacement with respect to the parameter p_k vanishes everywhere except at the corresponding sampling point c_k. This can be also directly seen from (8), as we have $(\nabla_p E)_k = \langle B_k, \nabla E \rangle = (\nabla E)_k$. This is the case since after discretization it holds that $B_k(c_k) = 1$ and $B_k = 0$ everywhere else. Thus, the equation (7) effectively boils down to (3) in this case.

Please note that such a parametrization is always performed for variational approaches, but often not explicitly stated. Our goal is not to propose a new parametrization, but rather to point out its inherent usage, and employ it for characterization in the hope that it facilitates comparison to other approaches.

Semi-Implicit Version of Variational Methods. An alternative interpretation for the semi-implicit version of the variational approach from (5), is gained by observing that (5) can be solved by

$$du = -\tau \, F * \big(\nabla E_D(u) - \alpha \nabla E_R(u)\big) = -\tau \, F * \nabla E(u) \, . \tag{12}$$

Here, F is the Green's function depending on the choice of regularization and defined as $\big(\mathrm{Id} + \tau \alpha \nabla E_R\big) F(x, s) = \delta(x - s)$, with the Dirac delta δ [22]. For regularization settings, the Green's function is F is a low-pass filter. For certain choices of E_R, it equals a Gaussian, while for others, the Gaussian is a good approximation [22,16]. With $B_k(x) = \widetilde{F}(x - c_k)$, with $F = \widetilde{F} * \widetilde{F}$, the semi-implicit approach can be seen as a standard steepest gradient descent, with the displacement parametrized densely based on the appropriate Green's functions, cf. Fig. 1d. The detailed derivation of the above follows closely the argument for fluid demons in Sec. 5.1, as (12) has the same form as (13). This interpretation provides a further connection between the variational and the demons methods.

5   Fluid Demons

The original demons algorithm was proposed by Thirion [40,24]. This seminal work contains a number of different heuristic variants, motivated by an analogy to Maxwell's Demons. The variant 1, which entailed most interest, consists of defining forces at all sampling points in the image domain, iteratively adding them to the already computed deformation, and smoothing the new resulting deformation field at the end of each iteration. In contrast to methods in Sec. 3 and 4, no explicit energy model was assumed.

Since the initial publication, a lot of work was dedicated to the interpretation and extension of the method, and a solid theoretical context has been developed. A connection between a fluid version of the demons method and the so called viscous fluid method [21] is discussed in [22]. An interpretation of the forces as approximation to second order optimization of the SSD similarity was given in [23]. Furthermore [23] discusses fluid and elastic variants of the demons algorithm, depending on whether the smoothing is applied to the accumulated displacement or the displacement updates only. In [16,17], the fluid demons approach is interpreted as gradient descent on the similarity measure in a Sobolev space representing diffeomorphisms. Also, in this work, derivatives of different similarity measures as forces are employed, as discussed in [39]. In [11], a connection is provided between the minimization of an explicit regularization energy term, and the elastic version of demons. Recent developments include efficient diffeomorphic versions of the demons approach [41]. Furthermore, in the recent years, the compositional update rule has gained popularity as the natural composition operator in the space of transformations [16,25,41].

In summary, a fluid version of the demons approach can be stated as minimization of (1), in which the regularity of the deformation is ensured by convolution with a Gaussian G^σ with variance σ. In every iteration, the following update rule is performed

$$du = -\tau\ G^\sigma * \nabla E_D(u) \tag{13}$$
$$\varphi = \varphi \circ (\mathrm{Id} + du) \ . \tag{14}$$

It was shown in [22] that the application of the Gaussian in (13) corresponds to fluid approach for the diffusion regularization term. Different smoothing kernels, corresponding to certain regularization terms such as linear elasticity or curvature have also been discussed [22,42].

5.1   Parametrized Fluid Demons

Here, we show that the fluid demons approach in (13) can be seen simply as the optimization of a similarity criterion (1), with a displacement function parametrized by Gaussians G^β with a standard deviation of $\beta = \sigma/2$, that is

$$u_p(x) = \sum_{k=1}^{N} p_k G^\beta(x - c_k) \ . \tag{15}$$

Following the derivation in (7), the Eq. (8) now corresponds to

$$(\nabla_p E)_k = \left\langle G_k^\beta\ , \nabla E \right\rangle , \tag{16}$$

where we use $B_k = G_k^\beta$ with $G_k^\beta(x) = G^\beta(x - c_k)$. Since in this case, the bases functions are located at every sampling point c_k, the resulting gradient can be written in terms of discrete convolution as

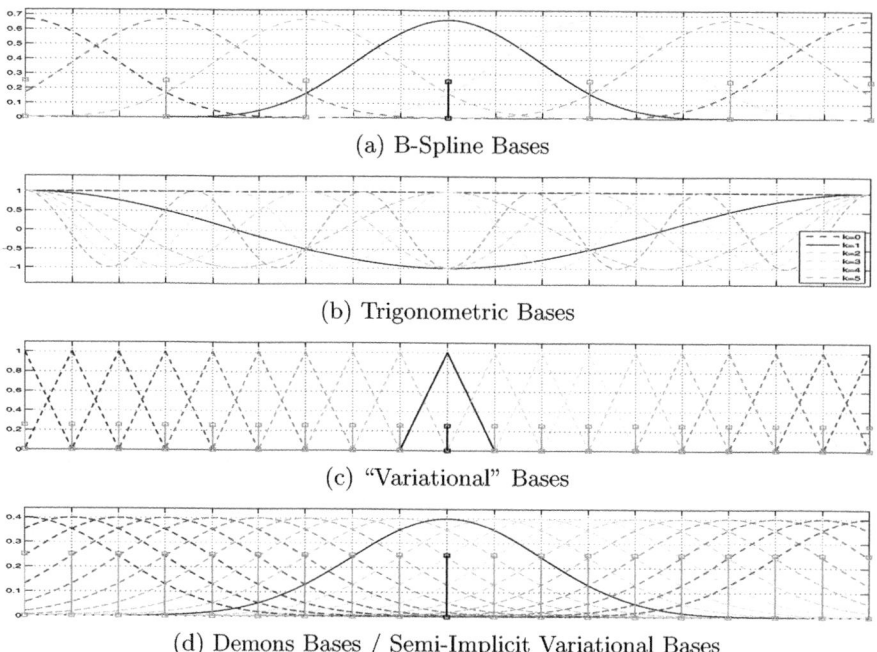

(a) B-Spline Bases

(b) Trigonometric Bases

(c) "Variational" Bases

(d) Demons Bases / Semi-Implicit Variational Bases

Fig. 1. 1D illustrations of discussed parameterizations. Parameters (vertical lines) and corresponding basis functions are given. Please note that for the trigonometric bases (b), the influence of parameters is not localized in space.

$$\nabla_p E = G^\beta * \nabla E \ , \tag{17}$$

According to (9), this gives us the evolution $dp = -\tau \, G^\beta * \nabla E_D$ for the parameters, and the corresponding displacement is then, according to (15),

$$u_{dp}(x) = \sum_{k=1}^{N} dp_k G^\beta (x - c_k) = -\tau \, G^\sigma * \nabla E_D \ . \tag{18}$$

This corresponds to the fluid demons evolution rule (13), and shows that fluid demons can be interpreted as a gradient descent on (2), with $\alpha = 0$ and the displacement parametrized as in (15). For a visualization please see Fig. 1d.

6   Discussion of Parametrization-Based Characterization

With the results from the previous sections, we can provide a characterization of the discussed methods based on their parametrizations. More specifically, the characterization criteria are: type of the basis function, location of the basis function, and support of the basis function. An example of such a characterization is given in Tab. 1. It can be seen as a description of the parametrizations

Table 1. Exemplary characterization of some common deformable registration methods, based on parameterization

Method	Basis Function	Basis Location	Basis Support
FFD	tensor product B-Splines	sparse (regular)	extended
Trigonometric	DFT, DCT, DST	global	global
Variational	"hat functions"	dense	local
Variational (semi-impl.)	low-pass filter	dense	extended
Demons	Gaussian	dense	extended
FE-based	different options	sparse, irregular	extended
TPS-based	TPS	sparse, irregular	global

illustrated in Fig. 1. The proposed characterization can be used to gain insight into the relations between the single methods. We give two examples.

For instance, there is a striking similarity between the parametrizations of the B-Spline FFD approach (1a) and the demons approach (1d) in Fig. 1. With the respective choice of standard deviation, the B-Spline and Gaussian bases have very similar shapes. This observation extends to higher dimensions. So the major difference between the two approaches seems to be the sparsity of the basis locations in the FFD parametrization. With dense setting of the control points for the FFD approach, and the standard deviations for demons adjusted accordingly, the two methods can be expected to behave in a very similar way.

A further possible relation which can be established by inspecting the parametrizations is that the demons method can be seen as an approximation to the Fourier-based methods employing only a certain number of low-frequency functions. Since the demons method is parametrized by dense Gaussian bases, the resulting displacement does not contain high-frequency signals by construction. This corresponds to a Fourier-based parametrization, from which the corresponding high-frequency bases have been excluded.

7   Summary and Conclusion

In this paper, we propose to use the parametrization of deformable registration methods for their characterization. To this end, we demonstrate that also methods often described as "non-parametric" feature an inherent parametrization. For the variational methods, we employ simple "hat functions", and for the semi-implicit version, we demonstrate equivalence to steepest descent with a certain dense parametrization. For the demons approach, the inherent parametrization yields an interesting new interpretation. The proposed parametrization-based characterization provides a compact and precise way for comparing and distinguishing some of the most popular groups of deformable methods. Thus, it can be used for a classification of deformable registration methods, and could prove a useful tool to gain further insight into the single approaches.

Acknowledgments. We would like to thank Maximilian Baust of CAMP for his extremely helpful feedback on the organization of this manuscript.

References

1. Horn, B., Schunck, B.: Determining optical flow. Artificial Intelligence (1981)
2. Broit, C.: Optimal Registration of Deformed Images. PhD thesis (1981)
3. Brown, L.: A survey of image registration techniques. ACM Computing Surveys (1992)
4. Van den Elsen, P., Pol, E., Viergever, M.: Medical image matching - a review with classification. IEEE Engin. in Medicine and Biology Magazine (1993)
5. Maintz, J., Viergever, M.: A survey of medical image registration. Medical Image Analysis (1998)
6. Fitzpatrick, J., Hill, D., Maurer Jr., C.: Image registration. In: Handbook of medical imaging - Medical Image Processing and Analysis (2000)
7. Hill, D., Batchelor, P., Holden, M., Hawkes, D.: Medical image registration. Physics in Medicine and Biology (2001)
8. Hajnal, J., Hill, D., Hawkes, D. (eds.): Medical Image Registration. CRC Press, Boca Raton (2001)
9. Zitova, B., Flusser, J.: Image registration methods: a survey. Image and Vision Computing (2003)
10. Lester, H., Arridge, S.: A survey of hierarchical non-linear medical image registration. Pattern Recognition (1999)
11. Cachier, P., Bardinet, E., Dormont, D., Pennec, X., Ayache, N.: Iconic feature based nonrigid registration: the pasha algorithm. Computer Vision and Image Understanding (2003)
12. Modersitzki, J.: Numerical methods for image registration. Oxford University Press, Oxford (2004)
13. Holden, M.: A review of geometric transformations for nonrigid body registration. IEEE Trans. Medical Imaging (2008)
14. Modersitzki, J.: FAIR: Flexible Algorithms for Image Registration. SIAM, Philadelphia (2009)
15. Trouvé, A.: Diffeomorphisms groups and pattern matching in image analysis. Int. Journal of Computer Vision (1998)
16. Chefd'hotel, C., Hermosillo, G., Faugeras, O.: Flows of diffeomorphisms for multimodal image registration. In: Int. Symp. on Biomedical Imaging (2002)
17. Chefd'hotel, C.: Geometric Methods in Computer Vision and Image Processing: Contributions and Applications. PhD thesis, L'Ecole Normale Superieure de Cachan (2005)
18. Beg, M., Miller, M., Trouvé, A., Younes, L.: Computing large deformation metric mappings via geodesic flows of diffeomorphisms. Int. Journal of Computer Vision 61 (2005)
19. Alvarez, L., Weickert, J., Sánchez, J.: Reliable estimation of dense optical flow fields with large displacements. Int. Journal of Computer Vision (2000)
20. Khamene, A., Schwarz, L., Zikic, D., Azar, F., Rietzel, E., Navab, N.: A unified and efficient approach for free-form deformable registration. In: Int. Conf. on Computer Vision (2007)
21. Christensen, G.: Deformable Shape Models for Anatomy. PhD thesis, Washington Uuniversity, Sever Institute of Technology (1994)

22. Bro-Nielsen, M., Gramkow, C.: Fast fluid registration of medical images. In: Höhne, K.H., Kikinis, R. (eds.) VBC 1996. LNCS, vol. 1131. Springer, Heidelberg (1996)

23. Pennec, X., Cachier, P., Ayache, N.: Understanding the demon's algorithm: 3d non-rigid registration by gradient descent. In: Medical Image Computing and Computer Assisted Intervention (1999)

24. Thirion, J.: Image matching as a diffusion process: an analogy with maxwell's demons. Medical Image Analysis (1998)

25. Stefanescu, R., Pennec, X., Ayache, N.: Grid powered nonlinear image registration with locally adaptive regularization. Medical Image Analysis (2004)

26. Tustison, N., Avants, B., Sundaram, T., Duda, J., Gee, J.: A generalization of free-form deformation image registration within the itk finite element framework. In: Workshop on Biomedical Image Registration (2006)

27. Feldmar, J., Declerck, J., Malandain, G., Ayache, N.: Extension of the icp algorithm to non-rigid intensity-based registration of 3d volumes. Computer Vision and Image Understanding (1997)

28. Declerck, J., Feldmar, J., Goris, M., Fabienne, B.: Automatic registration and alignment on a template of cardiac stress rest reoriented spect images. IEEE Trans. Medical Imaging (1997)

29. Rueckert, D., Sonoda, L., Hayes, C., Hill, D., Leach, M., Hawkes, D.: Nonrigid registration using free-form deformations: application to breast mr images. IEEE Trans. Medical Imaging (1999)

30. Kybic, J., Unser, M.: Fast parametric elastic image registration. IEEE Trans. Image Processing (2003)

31. Rohlfing, T., Maurer, C.R., Bluemke, D.J., Jacobs, M.: Volume-preserving nonrigid registration of mr breast images using free-form deformation with an incompressibility constraint. IEEE Trans. Medical Imaging (2003)

32. Glocker, B., Komodakis, N., Tziritas, G., Navab, N., Paragios, N.: Dense image registration through mrfs and efficient linear programming. Medical Image Analysis (2008)

33. Klein, S., Staring, M., Murphy, K., Viergever, M., Pluim, J.: Elastix: A toolbox for intensity-based medical image registration. IEEE Trans. Medical Imaging (2010)

34. Unser, M., Aldroubi, A., Eden, M.: B-spline signal processing. part i. theory. IEEE Trans. Signal Processing (1993)

35. Unser, M., Aldroubi, A., Eden, M.: B-spline signal processing. part ii. efficient design and applications. IEEE Trans. Signal Processing (1993)

36. Amit, Y.: A nonlinear variational problem for image matching. SIAM Journal on Scientific Computing (1994)

37. Christensen, G., Johnson, H.: Consistent image registration. IEEE Trans. Medical Imaging (2001)

38. Ashburner, J., Friston, K.: Nonlinear spatial normalization using basis functions. Human Brain Mapping (1999)

39. Hermosillo, G., Chefd'Hotel, C., Faugeras, O.: Variational methods for multimodal image matching. Int. Journal of Computer Vision (2002)

40. Thirion, J.: Non-rigid matching using demons. Computer Vision and Pattern Recognition (1996)

41. Vercauteren, T., Pennec, X., Perchant, A., Nicholas, A.: Diffeomorphic demons: Efficient non-parametric image registration. NeuroImage (2009)

42. Cahill, N., Noble, J., Hawkes, D.: Demons algorithms for fluid and curvature registration. Int. Symp. on Biomedical Imaging (2009)

Reliability-Driven, Spatially-Adaptive Regularization for Deformable Registration

Lisa Tang[1], Ghassan Hamarneh[1], and Rafeef Abugharbieh[2]

[1] Medical Image Analysis Lab., School Computing Science, Simon Fraser University
{hamarneh,lisat}@cs.sfu.ca
[2] Biomedical Signal and Image Computing Lab.,
Department of Electrical and Computer Engineering, University of British Columbia
rafeef@ece.ubc.ca

Abstract. We propose a reliability measure that identifies informative image cues useful for registration, and present a novel, data-driven approach to spatially adapt regularization to the local image content via use of the proposed measure. We illustrate the generality of this adaptive regularization approach within a powerful discrete optimization framework and present various ways to construct a spatially varying regularization weight based on the proposed measure. We evaluate our approach within the registration process using synthetic experiments and demonstrate its utility in real applications. As our results demonstrate, our approach yielded higher registration accuracy than non-adaptive approaches and the proposed reliability measure performed robustly even in the presences of noise and intensity inhomogenity.

1   Introduction

The goal of deformable image registration is to recover a local transformation, T, that best aligns two images. Generally, the problem involves minimizing a weighted sum of two penalty terms [1,2,3,4], e.g.:

$$\hat{T} = \arg \min_{T} \mathcal{D}(F, T \circ M) + \alpha \mathcal{R}(T) \tag{1}$$

where $\mathcal{D}$ denotes a data term, which measures how well T aligns two images, F and M, $\mathcal{R}$ denotes a regularization term that ensures T maintains certain smoothness properties (e.g. being continuous or homeomorhpic), and α is a weight that balances these two terms.

Literature in medical image registration has generally focused on the development of either image metrics [5], regularization models [6,7], or optimization algorithms [1,3], the three main ingredients of a registration method. In this paper, we attempt to address all three aspects of the problem, with a particular focus on adapting the regularization of deformations to local image content.

Commonly known as *inhomogeneous deformability* [6], deformable registration incorporating adaptive regularization allows one to obtain smooth deformations in some parts of an anatomy and highly varying ones in other regions. Inhomogeneous deformability is particularly useful when we wish to model the various

B. Fischer, B. Dawant, and C. Lorenz (Eds.): WBIR 2010, LNCS 6204, pp. 173–185, 2010.

types of motions different tissues undergo, so that, for example, soft tissues can deform elastically while hard bones are restricted to move only rigidly. Most researchers to date achieve adaptive regularization by incorporating anatomical models. An example is the variable-elasticity registration algorithm of Davatzikos [7], where anatomical segmentations were used in an elastic registration algorithm to adjust the amount of regularization according to tissue types. Regions that were labeled as soft tissues (e.g. skin and fat) were regularized less than regions that were identified as hard tissues or rigid structures (e.g. bone). Similar works include [8], where Rexilius et al. derived the inhomogeneous elasticity parameters probabilistically using a statistical atlas, and [9], where Kabus et al. performed elastic registrations and suppressed smoothness constraints at the interfaces between identified structures via a spatially-dependent weight. In [10], Pitiot and Guimoid developed a geometrically-driven regularization for a block-matching algorithm where the regularization of displacement vectors were localized to regions that were fitted to the geometry of the anatomy.

Several adaptive regularization methods have also been incorporated into registration frameworks that formulate image matching and regularization as separate processes, as opposed to minimizing the combined data and regularization energies directly. In [11], Stefanescu et al. incorporated an adaptive regularization approach into a compositive demons algorithm, which iteratively composed a correction field and a tentative displacement field. They proposed to regularize the deformation field by smoothing it with a variable Gaussian kernel whose size depended on a scalar field, which encoded the expected amount of deformation and was estimated from a region-based segmentation of the anatomy. The authors also proposed to filter the correction field using a measure called *local confidence* to estimate local intensity variance. In the template-matching framework of [12], after each iteration of deformation estimation, Suarez et al. smoothed the estimated field with a variable Gaussian kernel whose size was determined by a scalar measure of local structure.

In summary, adaptive regularization as formulated in all of the methods highlighted above have some inherent problems. The methods of [6,7,8,9,10] all required prior information (e.g. manual segmentation), making them impractical, especially when anatomical models are laborious to prepare, and difficult to define in cases containing pathologies. On the other hand, the data-driven regularization approaches of [11,12], where regularization depended on image gradients or local structures, suffered from sensitivity to noise. Unfortunately, the reliability and effectiveness of regularization become questionable when regularization depended on such noise-sensitive functions.

To address these issues, we propose a data-driven, spatially-adaptive regularization approach that is robust to noise and does not require prior information (e.g. segmentation or knowledge of material properties). As image forces computed in uncertain regions (e.g. suffering from high noise level, or bounded by weak or missing boundaries) should play a smaller role in estimating the transformation solution, we propose a robust *reliability* measure that analyzes local noise levels and image structures from which we derive data-driven, adaptive regularization. In our reliability-based regularization, the amount of regularization is increased in regions that have high noise level, or decreased otherwise. Similarly, data-derived forces computed in highly structured and uncorrupted regions should have low regularization because they are derived from reliable and discriminative information. Fig. 1a provides an illustration of these concepts. By accounting for local noise levels when measuring image cues, our proposed reliability measure can better distinguish reliable regions from unreliable, noise-corrupted regions more robustly than previously proposed measures (Fig. 1b-c).

To the best of our knowledge, this is the first work in the context of registration that examines reliability of image data as a means to balance the data and regularization terms in an image-dependent manner. We are also the first to incorporate spatially varying regularization into two Markov Random Field (MRF)-based registration frameworks. Formulating deformable registration as MRF-energy minimization has become a growing trend due to the recent developments of efficient solvers [13,14,15,16]. With these solvers, volumetric, multi-resolution registration can be achieved in minutes, a significant speedup over previous methods [17]. While efficient, the regularization adopted in these frameworks had always been controlled globally (across the whole image) by a scalar weight [3,2,1]. Determination of this weight also required empirical experiments, which were often done through a rather ad-hoc and tedious process. For that reason, as another part of our major contribution, we will illustrate how our

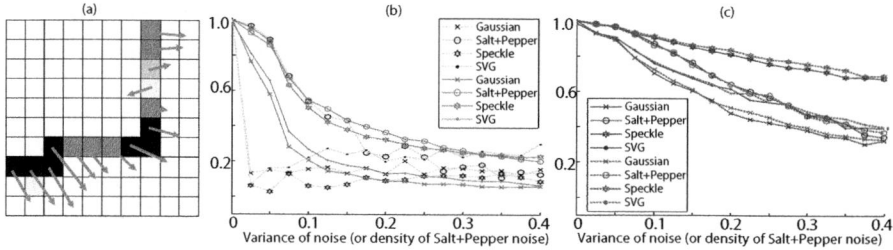

Fig. 1. (a) An illustrative example of a deformation field obtained from a non-parametric registration. Displacement vectors computed at the boundary of an object are shown as arrows. Gray values at each pixel along this boundary indicate the measured reliability (dark gray indicates high reliability). With our proposed reliability measure, the outlier vector (one pointing to left) will be regularized more than the rest, while those that are reliable and located along salient structures (e.g. corners) will be regularized relatively less, subject to the influence of the data term. (b) and (c) a measure's sensitivity to noise, which was defined as the correlation between the measure computed before and after noise corruption. Each curve shows the effect of one noise type: Gaussian, speckle, Salt+Pepper, and spatially varying Gaussian (SVG). Sensitivity of (b) local confidence [11] (magenta) and local structure [12] (black), and (c) our reliability measure. In (c), two different parameter settings (discussed in Sec. 2.2) were used to evaluate the performance of our measure. Under all noise types, local confidence and local structure were more sensitive to noise than our proposed measure.

reliability-based regularization can be easily incorporated into these frameworks to improve their accuracies.

In the past, few researchers have proposed the use of measures of certainty or saliency of image data to improve registration, e.g. [5]. However, these measures were solely used to improve the fidelity of the data term and not for regularization, as we propose in this work. In dealing with noisy images, Paquin et al. [18] proposed multi-scale decomposition of images to iteratively register the obtained decomposed components. Their method, however, did not employ adaptive regularization either. Accordingly, our contributions are: 1) adapting image regularization according to local image information using an image-derived measure, as opposed to use of prior information; 2) improving registration robustness by enhancing the fidelity of the data term using this measure; 3) introducing the novel use of a spatially varying weight to a discrete optimization-based registration framework; 4) proposing and examining various techniques to encode the proposed reliability-based regularization; and 5) validating the overall method with synthetic and real data.

2   Methods

2.1   Deformable Registration via MRF-Minimization

Let F and M be discrete representations of a fixed and moving image, respectively, in a domain $\Omega \subset \mathbb{R}^d$, where d is the image dimension, i.e. $F : \Omega \to \mathbb{R}$, $M : \Omega \to \mathbb{R}$. Our goal is to recover a displacement field T, $T : \Omega \to \mathbb{R}^d$, that maps each pixel location $\mathbf{x} = (x^1, x^2, \cdots, x^d)$ in M to F by minimizing the energy in Eq. 1. To formulate deformable registration as an MRF optimization, the pixel coordinates of M are usually converted to a graph $\mathcal{G} = (\mathcal{V}, \mathcal{E})$, where vertex $p \in \mathcal{V}$ represents a spatial coordinate $\mathbf{x}_p$ and the set of edges $(p, q) \in \mathcal{E}$ describe a 4-neighbourhood system of the image grid of M. Next, the deformation space (e.g. $\mathbb{R}^2$ in 2D) is discretized into a finite set of translations $\mathcal{L}$ of size L, where each element represents a translation vector t_i, i.e. $\mathcal{L} = \{t_1, \cdots, t_L\}$. We then seek to label each p with a label in $\mathcal{L}$ to obtain T that minimizes:

$$E(T) = \sum_{p \in \mathcal{V}} \psi_i(p, t_i) + \alpha \sum_{(p,q) \in \mathcal{E}; i, j \leq L} \psi_{ij}(p, q, t_i, t_j) \qquad (2)$$

where ψ_i denotes the cost of assigning t_i to p, ψ_{ij} denotes the cost of assigning t_i to p and t_j to its neighbour q, and α denotes a global weight between the two terms. Essentially, ψ_i and ψ_{ij} correspond to the data term $\mathcal{D}$ and regularization term $\mathcal{R}$ in Eq. 1, respectively. This energy can then be minimized via combinatorial optimization algorithms of [13,14,16].

In this work, we propose the use of spatially adaptive regularization by replacing α with a function that is spatially dependent on pairwise neighbours, i.e. $\lambda(p, q)$. Thus, if the data term is, for example, based on the absolute difference (AD) between image intensities and ψ_{ij} is a distance-based metric, the energy minimization becomes:

$$\hat{T} = \arg\min_{T} \sum_{p \in \mathcal{V}} \frac{1}{I_{max}} |F(p + t_i(p)) - M(p)| + \sum_{(p,q) \in \mathcal{E}} \frac{\lambda(p, q)}{4 \times 2\, d_{max}} ||t_i(p) - t_j(q)||$$

$$(3)$$

where I_{max} denotes the maximum intensity difference between F and M, $t_i(p)$ denotes translating $\mathbf{x}_p$ with the i-th label in $\mathcal{L}$ and d_{max} denotes the maximum displacement allowed (as set by the user)[1].

2.2 Adaptive Regularization via Measure of Image Reliability

As motivated earlier, regularization of T should be adapted according to the local image content of M. Here, we advocate adaptive regularization based on local noise levels and image structures. When images are corrupted with spatially varying noise levels, the amount of regularization should be increased in noise-corrupted regions so that the local registration of these regions can be better driven by their more reliable neighbours. Regularization should also be decreased in regions with high signal-to-noise ratio and meaningful local structures because their local content have sufficient discriminatory information to provide reliable motion estimates.

To adaptively regularize T, we propose a *reliability measure*, $R(\mathbf{x})$, that analyzes two types of cues of an image I: data fidelity and local image structure. Here, we define the fidelity of a pixel as a function of noise levels and edge evidence. The local noise levels, $N(\mathbf{x})$, is estimated using the spectral flatness measure defined in [19]. To estimate local edge strength, $G(\mathbf{x})$, we compute the image gradient and employ the noise-gating strategy of [19] to dampen strong responses that might have been provoked by noise, yielding:

$$G_{gated}(\mathbf{x}) = |\nabla I(\mathbf{x})|(1 - N(\mathbf{x}))^{\alpha_G} \qquad (4)$$

where the scalar α_G controls the level of noise-gating on the image gradient.

In estimating the local image structures, $\kappa(\mathbf{x})$, we first smooth I using a Gaussian kernel of size σ. The local curvature of the smoothed image, denoted as I_σ, is then computed in scale space as shown in [20]:

$$\kappa(\mathbf{x}; \sigma) = (I_{y,\sigma}^2 I_{xx,\sigma} - 2I_{x,\sigma} I_{y,\sigma} I_{xy,\sigma} + I_{x,\sigma}^2 I_{yy,\sigma})(\sqrt{I_{x,\sigma}^2 + I_{y,\sigma}^2})^{-1} \qquad (5)$$

where $I_{x,\sigma}$ and $I_{y,\sigma}$ denote the image derivatives of I_σ along x and y, respectively, and $I_{yy,\sigma}$ denote the second-order image derivatives of I_σ along y, etc. We then use the normalized scale coordinates of [21] to address the scale-selection problem. Specifically, to compare curvature values across different scales, we scale-normalize $\kappa(\mathbf{x}; \sigma)$, yielding $\kappa_n(\mathbf{x}) = \max_\sigma \sigma^3 \kappa(\mathbf{x}; \sigma)$. Finally, to weaken the strong responses at non-structural and noisy regions, we also apply noise-gating, yielding:

---

[1] Since each node of a 4-neighbourhood grid system contributes to ψ_{ij} four times and contributes to ψ_i once, the constant 4 is used to equalize the contribution of ψ_{ij} and ψ_i in the total energy cost. $2d_{max}$ is the maximum difference between two assigned displacement vectors.

(a)   (b)   (c)

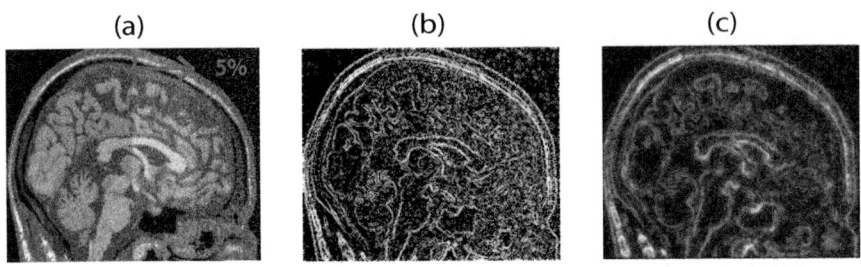

Fig. 2. (a) An image from BrainWeb [23] corrupted with spatially varying Gaussian white noise, 2% and 5% noise level on left and right side of image, respectively. (b) Its local confidence measure [11], and (c) our proposed reliability measure, which has successfully identified important image cues (e.g. local curvatures) despite of noise-corruption. Conversely, (b) assigned higher emphasis to the local image gradients located on the more noise-corrupted, right side of the image.

$$\kappa_{gated}(\mathbf{x}) = \kappa_n(\mathbf{x})(1 - N(\mathbf{x}))^{\alpha_C} \tag{6}$$

where the scalar α_C controls the level of noise-gating on the local curvatures.

With $N(\mathbf{x})$, $G_{gated}(\mathbf{x})$, and $\kappa_{gated}(\mathbf{x})$ estimated, the reliability measure R at $\mathbf{x}$ is then computed as:

$$R(\mathbf{x}) = G_{gated}(\mathbf{x})^{(1-\kappa_{gated}(\mathbf{x}))} \tag{7}$$

where the exponential term is adopted as a cue-gating strategy as proposed in [22] to suppress gradient information in highly textured regions. R is subsequently normalized to a range of [0,1]. Fig. 2c shows the reliability map computed from an image corrupted with spatially varying noise. Observing Fig. 2c, we note that despite of data corruption, the change in R is small, indicating that it is relatively insensitivity to noise. In general, as presented in Fig. 2b-c, R is much more robust to noise than some of the measures proposed in the literature, e.g. [11]. Details of how parameters of R were chosen will be discussed in Sec. 2.6.

We next present how the proposed reliability measure is used in MRF-based registration, augmented with adaptive regularization. For this task, we compute R over F and M to create reliability maps R_F and R_M, respectively.

2.3   Reliability Encoded as Edge-Weights for Regularization

In the context of MRF-based registration, $\lambda(p, q)$ is the regularization weight assigned to two neighbouring pixels p and q. The higher the value of $\lambda(p, q)$, the higher the required coherence between the deformations at p and q. To incorporate adaptive regularization into such a framework, we propose to determine $\lambda(p, q)$ based on $R_M(\mathbf{x}_p)$ and $R_M(\mathbf{x}_q)$. To this end, three encoding schemes have been conceived for determining $\lambda(p, q)$ from R_M.

1. Continuous scheme (CONT). This scheme enforces minimal regularization if both $\mathbf{x}_p$ and $\mathbf{x}_q$ have the highest reliability scores, or enforces maximal regularization otherwise. It does so by defining the weight function as: $\lambda(p,q) = exp(-R_M(\mathbf{x}_p)R_M(\mathbf{x}_q))$.

2. Clustered scheme (CLUST). This scheme follows the ideas presented in [24] (for matching of stereo images) where regularization weights are quantized. It computes $\lambda(p,q)$ as in CONT but further clusters the set of weights into K values using K-means. As shown in our experiments, the smaller the size of the set of all possible edge weights, the faster the convergence of MRF-optimization due to fewer number of 'graph reparameterizations' [16] needed to minimize the MRF energy.

3. Discrete scheme (DISCR). Based on CLUST, DISC incorporates the use of intensity cues for adapting λ (referred to as 'contextual information' in the segmentation work of [16]) and assumes that a change in intensity values indicates presence of boundary between different tissues types. It examines the noise-gated edge strength $G(\mathbf{x})$ given in Sec. 2.2 and assigns $\lambda(p,q)$ to one of four discrete values $w = \{w_1, w_2, w_3, w_4\}$, where $w_1 < w_2 < w_3 < w_4$, as similarly done in [16]. Specifically, if both p and q are identified as reliable pixels, as determined by a threshold τ_{rely}, and they both have high edge strengths, i.e. $G(\mathbf{x}_p)$ and $G(\mathbf{x}_q)$ are both greater than a threshold τ_{edge}, then we assume that p and q belong to different tissue types and assign the lowest regularization weight possible, i.e. $\lambda(p,q) = w_1$. If both pixels are reliable, but their edge strengths are lower than τ_{edge}, then we set $\lambda(p,q) = w_4$, hence assuming that they belong to same tissue type. However, if one of the two pixels or both pixels are unreliable, we assign intermediate weights, depending on their noise-gated local edge strengths: we set $\lambda(p,q) = w_3$ if their edge strengths are greater than τ_{edge}, or $\lambda(p,q) = w_2$ otherwise. Finally, to minimize the number of free variables introduced in this scheme, we parameterize w with the variable μ and set $w = \{w_1 = \mu, w_2 = 2\mu, w_3 = 3\mu, w_4 = 4\mu\}$.

2.4   Truncation of the Unary Term Based on Reliability (DTrunc)

Since the reliability measure readily reflects the quality of local image content, we can improve the fidelity of the data term by lowering the influence of the unary costs of all unreliable pixels via truncation [16]. If the pixel values $M(\mathbf{x}_p)$ and $F(\mathbf{x}_p + t_i(\mathbf{x}_p))$ are reliable, then the unary cost computed at the corresponding locations are also reliable. If either of the pixel values is considered unreliable, then we can enforce higher regularization at p by modifying the corresponding unary costs of p. In other words, if $R_M(\mathbf{x}_p)$ and $R_F(t_i(\mathbf{x}_p) + \mathbf{x}_p)$ are both above τ_{rely}, then we leave $\psi_i(t_i, p)$ unmodified; otherwise, we assign $\psi_i(t_i, p) = \eta$. We shall denote this truncation strategy as DTrunc.

2.5   Implementation Details

To illustrate the generality of our adaptive regularization approach, we implemented two versions of MRF-based deformable registration with spatially adaptive regularization to compute $\hat{T}$. The first, denoted as DENSE, follows the construction of Tang and Chung in [2] and computes $\hat{T}$ explicitly as described in Sec. 2.1. The second, denoted as BSPLINE, employs a B-Spline transform model to compute $\hat{T}$ as done in [1,3]. BSPLINE registration minimizes a similar energy function[2] as DENSE, but $\hat{T}$ is produced from a B-Spline transform grid. Thus, in 2D, each p represents a control point in a grid of size $C_x \times C_y$, with grid spacing δ, and we seek to label the set of control points with a label in $\mathcal{L}$ (Sec. 2.1). Displacement at $\mathbf{x}$ is then computed using a cubic B-Spline model as similarly done in [1,3].

Both DENSE and BSPLINE were implemented in MATLAB R2009b (Mathworks Natwick, MA) and employed the FastPD software [14]. We used DENSE if a registration trial involved $d_{max} \leq 8$ pixels or BSPLINE otherwise, although the two algorithms may be used sequentially (employ BSPLINE to pre-align images and refine the alignment using DENSE). To illustrate the robustness of our proposed regularization method to noise and to intensity inhomogenity, we derive the data term from the absolute difference image similarity metric (Sec. 3), which normally fails under noise and intensity inhomogenity corruptions.

2.6   Summary of Parameters

The parameters involved in our algorithm are τ_{edge}, τ_{rely}, μ, K, η, α_G, α_C, d_{max}, d_{res}, and δ. We emphasize that most of these parameters are only related to the efficiency of MRF optimization and does not relate to our proposed regularization approach. For DISCR, based on emperical evaluation, we chose $\mu = \{0.8, 1.5\}$ and computed τ_{rely} as the 25th percentile of R, τ_{edge} as the 75th percentile of G, and η to be the mean of all reliable unary costs. Preliminary results did not indicate sensitivity to these values, thanks to the robustness of R. This is demonstrated in 1c which shows that the sensitivity of R to different noise corruptions is minimal (the blue curves in the figure represent results using parameters $\alpha_G = .8$ and $\alpha_C = .4$ and those in red represent results using $\alpha_G = .4$ and $\alpha_C = .1$). For CLUST, we set $K = 10$ or if the clustering algorithm that we employed did not converge, we rerun the clustering algorithm with K increased by one. The value of d_{res} was restricted by d_{max} so that at most 250 labels were used ($L \leq 250$ best balances between optimization time and the optimal accuracy of $\hat{T}$) and d_{max} was set to half the diagonal length of the image.

3   Results

We performed validation of our method with both synthetic deformations and real clinical data. Our test data comprised of a pair of magnetic resonance imaging (MRI) brain slices from BrainWeb [23], and a set of 18 sagittal brain slices from the Internet Brain Segmentation Repository (IBSR)[3].

---

[2] The data term is modified slightly, rather than computing a similarity metric at each point, we compute the metric over a 3×3 neighbourhood of each control point. $R(\mathbf{x}_p)$ is computed as a distance-weighted sum of R over the neighborhood of $\mathbf{x}_p$.

[3] http://www.cma.mgh.harvard.edu/ibsr/

Table 1. Synthetic experiments involving random TPS-warped BrainWeb images. Shown are registration accuracies obtained by different schemes, under various types of noise corruption and intensity inhomogenity (IIH). Accuracy is computed as the average MED obtained over all trials. U denotes best uniform regularization. Bolded numbers indicate better performance. Note how the proposed data term truncation strategy improved registration results in 8 out of 12 cases, irrespective of noise type and level of intensity inhomogeneity. In general, results obtained with adaptive regularization had higher accuracies than those obtained with uniform regularization.

IIH	Under random speckle noise				Under random Gaussian noise			
	U	U+DTrunc	DISCR	DISCR+DTrunc	U	U+DTrunc	DISCR	DISCR+DTrunc
6%	4.69	**3.93**	2.85	**2.76**	4.23	**3.81**	2.85	**2.39**
18%	3.49	**3.43**	2.70	2.96	3.61	**3.20**	2.55	**2.49**
30%	**4.89**	4.99	**2.75**	2.96	**4.64**	4.78	3.37	**2.60**

We first studied the effects of employing DTrunc, the procedure described in Sec. 2.4. Following the approach of [25], we simulated groundtruth data by applying random thin-plate-spline (TPS) warps, denoted as T_{GT}, to an image from BrainWeb, with T_{GT} containing maximum displacement of 5 pixels in each dimension, yielding 20 sets of F, M and T_{GT} (10 such trials generated for each BrainWeb image). We then corrupted the images by adding intensity inhomogenity at different levels and added Gaussian or speckle noise (at 5%), as similarly done in [15,18]. We subsequently performed DENSE registration with and without DTrunc. We discretized the deformation space with $d_{max} = 6$, $d_{res} \geq 0.5$ in the x and y dimensions.

Registration accuracy of each registration trial was computed as the mean Euclidean distance (MED) of every pixel between T_{GT} and $\hat{T}$, the one recovered from registration. For all tests on uniform regularization, we repeated trials with different values of α in $\{0.05, 0.1, \cdots, 0.95\}$ and the trial with the lowest MED was selected as the final result. The obtained results are summarized in Table 1, which indicates that the registration errors obtained with DTrunc are generally lower than those obtained without DTrunc.

We next compared the registration performance of our proposed reliability-based regularization using the encoding schemes outlined in Sec. 2.3. We generated a set of groundtruth data as described before, but the maximum displacement introduced by the TPS-warps was set to 8 pixels and the generated images were corrupted with spatially varying Gaussian noise (additive Gaussian noise patterns of different variances at random locations). We then performed DENSE registration to register the images with $d_{max} = 10$ and $d_{res} = 1.2$.

Fig. 3a presents a quantitative comparison between our proposed schemes against uniform regularization. Results demonstrate that the use of the proposed reliability measure for adaptive regularization using DISCR can reduce MED by as much as 2.45 pixels. We also examined the accuracy of $\hat{T}$ by examining the Euclidean distance between T_{GT} and $\hat{T}$ on a per-pixel basis as shown in Fig. 4. Clearly, adaptive regularization (Fig. 4) allowed for much more accurate deformations than those generated with uniform regularization. As the proposed reliability measure was able to identify unreliable regions and the amount of regularization

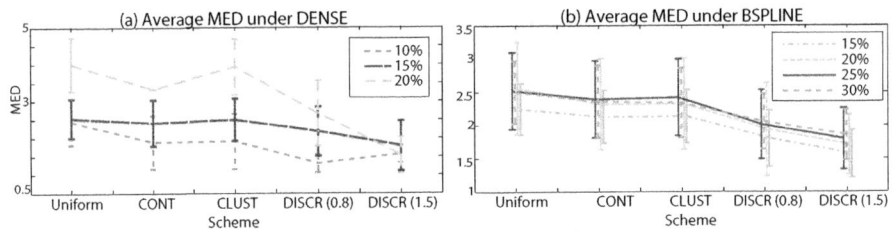

Fig. 3. Results of registration under different levels of spatially varying noise applied to BrainWeb images. Plots show the average MED obtained when registration was incorporated with adaptive regularization. Uniform denotes registration without reliability-based adaptive regularization; CONT, DISCR, CLUST each denotes one of our proposed schemes as presented in Sec. 2.3. For DISRC, the number in brackets are the values of parameter μ. Results involving (a) DENSE to recover TPS warps ($d_{max} = 8$) and (b) BSPLINE to recover B-Spline warps ($d_{max} = 12$). The differences in trend were due to differences in registration schemes, types of warp used, and discretization levels. Reliability-based regularization encoded with DISCR generally yielded low MED.

was increased in these regions accordingly, errors at these unreliable regions were relatively lower than those obtained with uniform regularization.

We next tested BSPLINE registration incorporated with adaptive regularization. We applied synthetic B-Spline warps containing maximum displacement of 12 pixels and evaluated results by comparing the known warps with the recovered ones. Results from this experiment are summarized in Fig. 3b, which shows that reliability-based regularization using DISCR had reduced MED by as much as 0.90 pixels.

Finally, we performed pairwise registrations on the clinical brain MR images from the IBSR dataset. Segmentations of these images are also available (each slice was segmented into 3 structures) so registration validation could be done with segmentation-based measures (as performed in [26]), which allows us to examine registration accuracy in relation to the anatomical structures of interest. In absence of pathologies, more accurate registration will result in better overlap of corresponding regions.

A total of 153 DENSE registrations (all 18 images with repetitions) were done per registration scheme, e.g. uniform regularization and reliability-based regularization encoded with CONT, CLUST, and DISCR (we selected $\mu = 1.5$ based on evaluaton in Fig. 3). For each registration, we applied $\hat{T}$ to the label field of M, using nearest-neighbour interpolation and compared the warped segmentation to the label field of F. After registration, we computed target overlap (TO) and distance error (DE) as defined in [26]. The obtained results were as follows, which are reported in (TO,DE) pairs, with TO expressed in fraction and DE expressed in pixels: uniform regularization obtained (0.712,7.82), while reliability-based regularization with CONT obtained (0.758,6.46), CLUST obtained (0.766,6.89); and DISCR obtained (0.768,7.12).

Overall, results from synthetic experiments have demonstrated that the use of reliability-based, adaptive regularization can recover TPS and B-Spline warps more accurately than those recovered with non-adaptive approaches: up to 2.45 and 0.90 improvement in MED for BSPLINE and DENSE registration, respectively. This is true regardless of the severity of intensity inhomogenity and noise types, e.g. (spatially varying) Gaussian and speckle. The reliability-based data term truncation strategy was also shown to improve registration results in general (adaptive and uniform regularization). Results from our segmentation-based evaluation also showed that our proposed method increased TO by 0.056 ($> 5\%$).

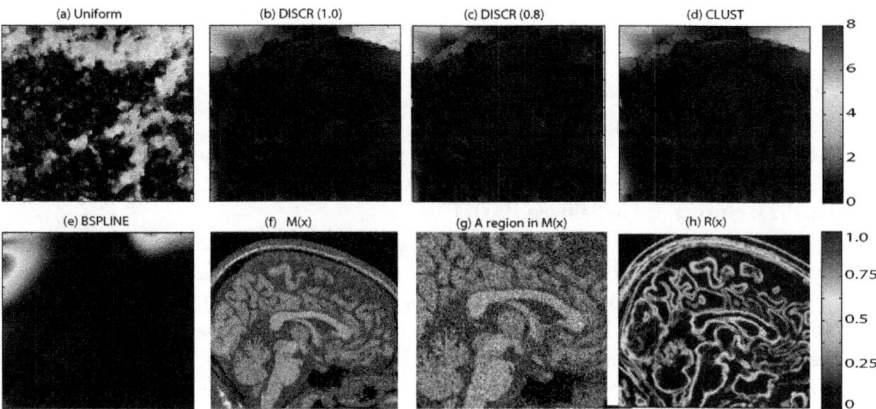

Fig. 4. Results obtained from a DENSE registration trial. Sub-figures (a)-(e) show the Euclidean distance between $T_{GT}(\mathbf{x})$ and $\hat{T}(\mathbf{x})$, which was obtained using one of the following registration schemes: (a) uniform regularization; reliability-based regularization encoded with (b) DISCR ($\mu = 1.0$), (c) DISCR ($\mu = 0.8$), and (d) CLUST ($K = 10$). Although the input image (f) was corrupted with 5% Gaussian noise, R was capable of capturing important image cues as shown in (h). An enlarged view of a region in (f) is shown in (g). Our propsed approach (b-d) gave more accurate results than (a) uniform regularization. Incorrect deformation estimation occurred mostly in background regions where discriminative information was lacking (note the upper left and right corners of (b-e)). Obtained displacement fields were also smoother than the one obtained in (a) as reflected by the abrupt changes in colour. (e) A result of BSPLINE registration (R encoded with CONT).

4 Conclusions

We have proposed a data-driven, spatially-adaptive regularization approach for deformable registration. The amount of regularization enforced on the spatial transformation was dependent on an image reliability measure that we developed. As shown in our experiments, the reliability measure can also be used to improve the fidelity of the data term via reliability-based truncation. Different encoding schemes have been proposed to transform our measure to a weight function for use in an MRF-based registration framework. Use of the DISCR encoding scheme achieved better and more consistant performance over other schemes. Evaluations of our method based on synthetic and real data have demonstrated that our regularization approach can greatly improve registration accuracy of existing MRF-based registration algorithms. Preliminary results on 3D test data already suggest improvement our approach brings, and thus we intend to conduct a thorough evaluation of our approach on full 3D clinical datasets. Future work will include multi-resoluton implementation of the proposed method and incorporation of the reliability measure into region-based image similarity metrics to be applied to a wider class of registration problems.

References

1. Glocker, et al.: Dense image registration through MRFs and efficient linear programming. Med. Image Anal. 12(6), 731–741 (2008)
2. Tang, T., Chung, A.: Non-rigid image registration using graph-cuts. In: Ayache, N., Ourselin, S., Maeder, A. (eds.) MICCAI 2007, Part I. LNCS, vol. 4791, pp. 916–924. Springer, Heidelberg (2007)
3. Kwon, D., et al.: Nonrigid image registration using dynamic higher-order MRF model. In: Forsyth, D., Torr, P., Zisserman, A. (eds.) ECCV 2008, Part I. LNCS, vol. 5302, pp. 373–386. Springer, Heidelberg (2008)
4. Hellier, et al.: Hierarchical estimation of a dense deformation field for 3-d robust registration. IEEE Trans. Med. Imaging 20(5), 388–402 (2001)
5. Luan, et al.: Multimodality image registration by maximization of quantitative-qualitative measure of mutual information. Pattern Recognit. 41, 285–298 (2008)
6. Lester, et al.: Non-linear registration with the variable viscosity fluid algorithm. In: IEEE IPMI, pp. 238–251 (1999)
7. Davatzikos, C.: Spatial transformation and registration of brain images using elastically deformable models. Comput. Vision Image Understand. 66, 207–222 (1997)
8. Rexilius, J., Warfield, S., Guttmann, C.: A novel nonrigid registration algorithm and applications. In: Niessen, W.J., Viergever, M.A. (eds.) MICCAI 2001. LNCS, vol. 2208, pp. 923–931. Springer, Heidelberg (2001)
9. Kabus, S.: Multiple-Material Variational Image Registration. PhD thesis, der Universitat zu Lubeck (October 2006)
10. Pitiot, A., Guimond, A.: Geometrical regularization of displacement fields for histological image registration. Med. Image Anal. 12(1), 16–25 (2008)
11. Stefanescu, et al.: Grid powered nonlinear image registration with locally adaptive regularization. Med. Image Anal. 8(3), 325–342 (2004)
12. Suarez, et al.: Nonrigid registration using regularized matching weighted by local structure. In: MICCAI, pp. 581–589 (2003)
13. Ishikawa, H.: Exact optimization for markov random fields with convex priors. IEEE Trans. Pattern Anal. Mach. Intell. 25(10), 1333–1336 (2003)
14. Komodakis, et al.: Performance vs computational efficiency for optimizing single and dynamic MRFs. Comput. Vision Image Understand. 112(1), 14–29 (2008)
15. Shekhovtsov, A., Kovtun, I., Hlavac, V.: Efficient MRF deformation model for non-rigid image matching. Comput. Vision Image Understand 112, 91–99 (2008)
16. Boykov, Y., Veksler, O., Zabih, R.: Fast approximate energy minimization via graph cuts. IEEE Trans. Pattern Anal. Mach. Intell. 23, 1222–1239 (2001)

17. Glocker, et al.: Dense image registration through MRFs and efficient linear programming. Med. Image Anal. 12(6), 731–741 (2008)
18. Paquin, D., Levy, D., Xing, L.: Multiscale deformable registration of noisy medical images. Math. Biosc. Engin. 5(1), 125–144 (2008)
19. Rao, J., et al.: Adaptive contextual energy parameterization for automated image segmentation. In: Bebis, G. (ed.) ISVC 2009. LNCS, vol. 5875, pp. 1089–1100. Springer, Heidelberg (2009)
20. Donias, M., Baylou, P., Keskes, N.: Curvature of oriented patterns: 2-d and 3-d estimation from differential geomery. In: ICIP, vol. 70, pp. 236–240 (1998)
21. Lindeberg, T.: On scale selection for differential operators. In: Proc. 8th Scandinavian Conf. on Image Analysis, pp. 857–866 (1993)
22. Leung, et al.: Contour and texture analysis for image segmentation. Int. J. Comput. Vision 43(1), 7–27 (2001)
23. Kwan, D., et al.: MRI simulation-based evaluation of image-processing and classification methods. IEEE Trans. Med. Imaging 18(11), 1085–1097 (1999)
24. Zhang, L., Seitz, S.: Estimating optimal parameters for MRF stereo from a single image pair. IEEE Trans. Pattern Anal. Mach. Intell. 29(1), 331–342 (2007)
25. Hamarneh, G., et al.: Simulation of ground-truth validation data via physically- and statistically-based warps. In: Metaxas, D., Axel, L., Fichtinger, G., Székely, G. (eds.) MICCAI 2008, Part I. LNCS, vol. 5241, pp. 459–467. Springer, Heidelberg (2008)
26. Klein, et al.: Evaluation of 14 nonlinear deformation algorithms applied to human brain MRI registration. NeuroImage 46(3), 786–802 (2009)

Large Deformation Diffeomorphic Registration Using Fine and Coarse Strategies

Laurent Risser[1,2], François-Xavier Vialard[1], Maria Murgasova[2],
Darryl Holm[1], and Daniel Rueckert[2]

[1] Institute for Mathematical Science, Imperial College London, 53 Prince's Gate,
SW7 2PG, London, UK*
[2] Visual Information Processing, Imperial College London, Huxley Building,
Department of Computing, SW7 2BZ, London, UK

Abstract. In this paper we present two fine and coarse approaches for the efficient registration of 3D medical images using the framework of Large Deformation Diffeomorphic Metric Mapping (LDDMM). This formalism has several important advantages since it allows large, smooth and invertible deformations and has interesting statistical properties. We first highlight the influence of the smoothing kernel in the LDDMM framework. We then show why approaches taking into account several scales simultaneously should be used for the registration of complex shapes, such as those treated in medical imaging. We then present our fine and coarse approaches and apply them to the registration of binary images as well as the longitudinal estimation of the early brain growth in preterm MR images.

1 Introduction

Non-rigid image registration has various applications such as motion tracking, shape comparison, atlas creation or image segmentation. Recent years have seen the development of new non-rigid registration techniques allowing large diffeomorphic deformations. Diffeomorphic deformations are by definition smooth and invertible, properties that are highly desirable in image registration and that most of the classical registration techniques have. Importantly, since the pioneering work of [12], an increasing number of registration techniques transform the images using the concept of deformation flow characterized by a velocity vector field. This makes possible large deformations while preserving diffeomorphic properties. Note that the velocity fields can be either steady or time-dependent. Such approaches have led to new problems: First, how to find the optimal deformation flow between two shapes and secondly how to regularize spatially the deformations. Similarly, the issues of the computational complexity and memory requirements are also important, especially in the context of 3D medical image registration.

* We thank the Imperial College Strategic Initiative Fund for partial support. The work of DDH was also partially supported by the Royal Society of London Wolfson Research Merit Award.

B. Fischer, B. Dawant, and C. Lorenz (Eds.): WBIR 2010, LNCS 6204, pp. 186–197, 2010.
© Springer-Verlag Berlin Heidelberg 2010

In the work of [12], the registration was formulated in a Bayesian setting. Statistical prior distributions of the deformations were modelled using stochastic PDEs controlling the displacement field according to driving forces. Later, the framework of Large Deformation Diffeomorphic Metric Mapping (LDDMM) [21, 23, 4, 27, 18], in which the optimal velocity fields are time-dependent and geodesic, was developed. Finding geodesic flows between two registered shapes is fundamental in the framework of LDDMM since it ensures that the optimal flow is the shortest path between the shapes according to a metric regularizing the deformation. We will discuss later the influence of this metric. The LDDMM has therefore convenient properties for the statistical comparison of images and shapes as well as the creation of atlases. A practical implementation of the LDDMM for image registration, considered as the reference, has been proposed in [4]. It solves the registration between two images in an Euler-Lagrange framework using a gradient descent to minimize the registration energy as a function of the velocity vector field of the deformation flow. Algorithms based on [4] have been applied to inter-subject local shape comparison or atlas creation. In [6, 16], the approach has been used to measure shape variations between segmented hearts, in order to highlight the structural remodelling of dyssynchronous failing heart. In [9, 8] the LDDMM has been extended to vector- and tensor-valued images. Finally a symmetric extension of [4] has been proposed in [5]. However, despite its interesting statistical properties, the LDDMM approach is particularly time and memory consuming. Similarly, although it were designed to allow very large deformations, its practical use remains limited to relatively small deformations in the literature.

Interestingly, alternatives to the LDDMMs, faster, requiring less memory or adapted to multi-modal images have been proposed: A symmetric interpretation of [4] using cross correlation to measure the image similarity between the source and target images was proposed in [3]. This interpretation was used in [11] to measure the cortical grey matter thickness in segmented brain images. Another interpretation [19] allowing multimodal registration for atlas creation estimates the transformations in a Bayesian framework. Correspondences between the underlying tissue classes are found by using Kullback-Leibler divergence on the space of posteriors probabilities. More recently, [4] has been formulated as an optimal control problem in [15] leading to an improvement of the convergence speed and robustness. Note finally that interesting approaches making use of the Navier-Stokes equation of fluid dynamics, have been proposed [10]. Such approaches allow large diffeomorphic deformations but are not designed to provide geodesic transformations.

Another class of large diffeomorphic registration techniques, using stationary velocity fields, emerged with [1]. Such parameterizations, have been applied as an evolution of the LDDMM framework [2, 17] and an extension of the demons algorithm [25]. Stationary parameterizations are efficient in terms of memory required and computational time while providing registrations similar to those obtained using time-dependent velocity fields in most cases. However, the optimal flows found using these techniques are usually not geodesic at convergence except for very simple deformations. Statistical comparisons may therefore be less valid using these techniques than what can be provided by the LDDMM framework and the estimation of mean shapes out of an atlas is not as straightforward as using geodesic deformations. Moreover, the range of possible deformations is theoretically limited compared to time-varying velocity fields.

In an attempt to extend the utility of the LDDMM framework in the context of 3D medical image registration, we discuss in this paper one of its fundamental aspects: the choice of the smoothing kernel. Indeed, the kernel is directly related to the metric of the deformations and therefore controls its spatial regularization. In practice, small kernels favour deformations that match local details and large kernels favour deformations that match global structures. Since 3D medical images often contain complex shapes, such as the cortical surface of the brain, small kernels may provide unsatisfactory deformations. Similarly, commonly used coarse-to-fine strategies, are inappropriate to register complex shapes in the LDDMM framework. In addition, statistics on the deformations depend on the kernel used at the finest scale. Moreover, due to the use of gradient descent during the search for the optimal path, first at large scales and then at small scales, the algorithm can converge to local minima that would be unreachable by using only small kernels. Deformation statistics are biased in that case. In this paper we present two different multiscale extensions of [4]: The first one consists of the use of kernels that are the sum of Gaussian kernels of different scales while the second one consists in using a series of such kernels. Note, that the second extension can be related to the work of J. Glaunes where time-dependent kernels were used in the context of surface registration [13]. Similarly, the idea underlying these extensions is close to the coarse to fine strategy developed in [14]. Though these natural ideas might not be new in the literature they deserve a detailed comparison as provided in this paper.

In section 2, we present the method of [4] and discuss the influence of the kernel. Two multiscale extensions are then presented in section 3 and tested on synthetic and real images in section 4. Finally, the methodology and tests are discussed in section 5.

2   3D Image Registration Using LDDMM

2.1   Registration Technique

We give here an overview of the LDDMM approach and the classical algorithm to find optimal registrations described in [4]. This framework enables the registration of a source image I_S on a target image I_T defined on a spatial domain Ω through a time dependent diffeomorphic transformation of Ω, ϕ_t, $t \in [0, 1]$. Such a transformation is generated by a time dependent velocity field v as follows:

$$\partial_t \phi_t = v_t(\phi_t), \quad t \in [0, 1], \tag{1}$$

where $\phi_0 = Id$. The velocity field v_t deforms the image coordinates at time t and ϕ_t is the induced deformation. For notational convenience we introduce

$\phi_{t,s} \doteq \phi_s \circ \phi_t^{-1}$. The LDDMM framework assumes the velocity field at each time to be smooth enough so that the flow ϕ_t is well defined, as described in [26]. The registration problem then consists in finding the velocity field v_t that minimizes the energy $E(v)$, defined by:

$$E(v) = \int_0^1 \frac{1}{2} \|v_t\|_V^2 dt + \frac{1}{2} \|I_S \circ \phi_1^{-1} - I_T\|_{L^2}^2. \tag{2}$$

The similarity measure here is the sum of the squared differences between the intensities in the target and the deformed image. The time dependent velocity field v is assumed to lie in $L^2([0,1], V)$, where V is a Hilbert space of vector fields, and the norm on V can be any norm which satisfies for any $u \in V$: $\|u\|_{1,\infty} \leq m\|u\|_V$, for a positive constant m (we denote by $\|.\|_{1,\infty}$ the sup norm on the vector field and its first derivative). Importantly, underlying the space of velocity fields V, there exists a smooth matrix-valued kernel $k(.,.)$ which describes the velocity fields that can be used for the registration. Conveniently, the space V can be defined from this kernel as the completion of the linear space spanned by $v(x) = \sum_{i=1}^n k(x, y_i)p_i$, where $y_i \in \Omega$ and $p_i \in \mathbb{R}^d$ (d the spatial dimension of Ω) with respect to the norm defined as $\|v\|_V^2 = \sum_{i,j=1}^n p_j^T k(y_j, y_i)p_i$. Therefore any vector field in V is efficiently approximated by using a finite sum of elementary vector fields $k(., y)p$. Interestingly, there exists a wide family of available kernels. Among various properties, the space of admissible kernels must be stable under addition and under multiplication by a positive constant. For critical computational issues, we consider here Gaussian kernels that are translation invariant ($k(x, y) = K(x - y)$) and separable:

$$K(x) = (2\pi)^{-d/2} |\Sigma|^{-1/2} \exp\left(-\frac{1}{2} x^T \Sigma^{-1} x\right), \tag{3}$$

where Σ is the covariance matrix. We restrict our study to isotropic covariances, i.e. such that $\Sigma = \sigma Id_{\mathbb{R}^d}$. The key parameter σ then controls the spatial correlation of the deformations. We discuss this point in Subsection 2.2.

The minimization algorithm is described hereafter. We denote $J_t^S = I_S \circ \phi_{t,0}$, $J_t^T = I_T \circ \phi_{1,t}$ and $|D\phi_{t,1}|$ the Jacobian of $\phi_{t,1}$ at time t. We consider an homogeneous discretization of the time $t_i = i\Delta t$, $i \in \{1, \cdots, I\}$. The minimization of the variational problem of Eq. 2 is performed by using a steepest gradient descent approach. Practical resolution then involves the iterative use of the gradient of the functional E, denoted by $\nabla_v E_t$, in the space $L^2([0,1], V)$ at time t:

$$K \star \nabla_v E_t = v_t - K \star \left(|D\phi_{t,1}^v| \nabla J_t^S (J_t^S - J_t^T)\right), \tag{4}$$

where $\star$ denotes the convolution operator. The velocity field is then updated by computing:

$$v^{k+1} = v^k - \epsilon K \star \nabla_{v_{t_j}^k} E, \tag{5}$$

where ϵ is the step size during the gradient descent step. The optimal time dependent diffeomorphism should be a geodesic path in the group of diffeomorphisms for which the associated velocity field satisfies the Euler-Lagrange equation:

$$\hat{v}_t - K \star \left(|D\phi_{t,1}^{\hat{v}}| \nabla J_t^S (J_t^S - J_t^T) \right) = 0, \quad \forall t \in [0,1]. \tag{6}$$

In such a case, the optimal path has shooting properties [20] from the velocity field at time $t = 0$ that can be used to statistically compare shapes [24]. We emphasize that these statistics depend critically on the choice of the metric on V as shown in the next subsection.

2.2 Influence of the Kernels

As discussed briefly in the Introduction, the kernel controls the spatial behaviour of the deformations. For isotropic Gaussian kernels of standard deviation σ, the parameter σ is the characteristic length defining the scale at which the registration is performed. To give a practical interpretation of the influence of σ, let us focus on the right hand side of Eq. 4, which provides the energy gradient that is used to update the velocity field at each iteration (Eq. 5). Its second term $|D\phi_{t,1}^v| \nabla J_t^S (J_t^S - J_t^T)$ pushes locally the source image I_S onto the target image I_T since the direction is defined by the gradient ∇J_t^S. This term is then smoothed by using the filter K so the deformations are more or less correlated according to the choice of σ. Figures 2 and 3 illustrate the influence of the kernel on the 2D binary images $I_S^1, I_T^1, I_S^2, I_T^2$ of Fig. 1. In Fig. 2, we register the

Fig. 1. 2D binary images to illustrate the influence of the kernel. **From left to right:** Source image I_S^1, target image I_T^1, source image I_S^2, target image I_T^2

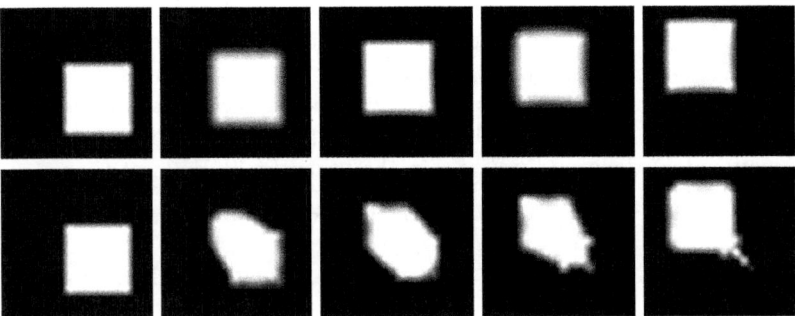

Fig. 2. Deformation of I_S^1 to I_T^1 for (from left to right) $t = 0$, $t = 0.25$, $t = 0.5$, $t = 0.75$, $t = 1.0$. **Row 1:** I_S^1 to I_T^1 using a large kernel ($\sigma = 8$ pixels). **Row 2:** I_S^1 to I_T^1 using a small kernel ($\sigma = 2$ pixels).

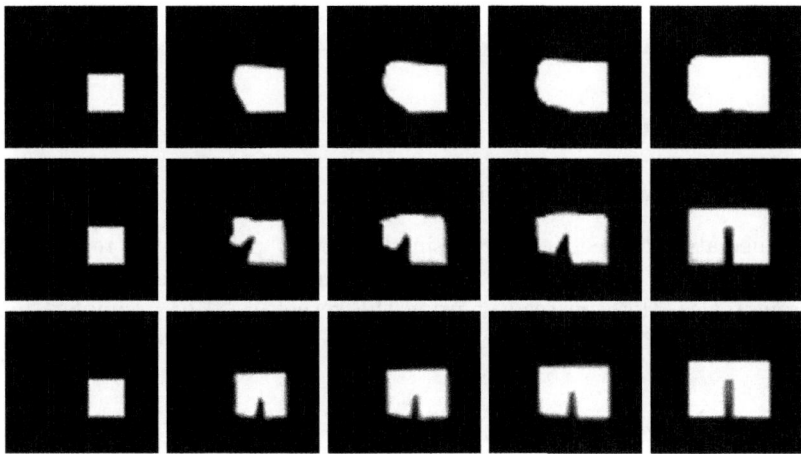

Fig. 3. Deformation of I_S^2 to I_T^2 for (from left to right) $t = 0$, $t = 0.25$, $t = 0.5$, $t = 0.75$, $t = 1.0$. **Row 1:** I_S^2 to I_T^2 using a large kernel ($\sigma = 5$ pixels). **Row 2:** I_S^2 to I_T^2 using a small kernel ($\sigma = 1.5$ pixels). **Row 3:** I_S^2 to I_T^2 registration with a small kernel ($\sigma = 1.5$ pixels) and initialized by the output of Row 1.

square I_S^1 on its translated I_T^1. In order to obtain a translation-like deformation using LDDMMs, the standard deviation σ of the gaussian kernel must be of a size at least similar to the size of the square ($\sigma = 8$ pixels here). Using a smaller kernel ($\sigma = 2$ pixel), the square is not considered as a whole object but as a set of details. Therefore some parts of I_S^1 are compressed and other are expanded during the registration. In Fig. 3, the square I_S^2 is now registered on a rectangle containing a slot I_T^2. As expected, at a large scale ($\sigma = 5$ pixels) the square is registered on the rectangle with a small perturbation while at a small scale ($\sigma = 1.5$ pixels) the registration fully takes into account the slot. Note that, in the latter case, the registration makes use of invertible large deformations. We show the corresponding deformation grid at $t = 1$ in Fig. 5. Even though the transformation appears non-invertible, a closer inspection shows that the deformation is actually invertible but with very high values of the Jacobian. Such behaviour is not desirable. We have registered I_S^2 on I_T^2 using the same small kernel as in row 1 by taking as initial guess the flow of row 2, computed with a large kernel, instead of a null flow. Theoretically, the initial guess should have no influence on the final result, so the estimated flows should be the same in rows 2 and 3. However, even though the final deformations look similar, the estimated flows are completely different, the one obtained with the coarse to fine technique obviously not enjoying shooting properties at $t = 0$. This deformation is therefore not the global optimum. The convergence to a local minimum is due here to the use of a gradient descent. Hence, in the context of LDDMM, the size of the kernels has a strong influence on the scale of the registration. Moreover, the use of inappropriate kernels or coarse to fine strategies can lead to unrealistic deformations. To tackle the presented issues in the context of medical image registration, where the registered shapes may contain several scales of interest, we propose two fine and coarse extensions of [4] in the next section.

3   Multi-kernel LDDMM

3.1   Sum of Gaussian Kernels

An immediate extension of [4] to simultaneously perform the registration at several scales is to define the kernel K as the sum of several kernels having different scales. Here, instead of using the kernel of [4] or a simple Gaussian function, we build K as the sum of N Gaussian kernels as follows:

$$K(x) = \sum_{n=1}^{N} a_n K_{\sigma_n}(x) = \sum_{n=1}^{N} a_n (2\pi)^{-3/2} |\Sigma_n|^{-1/2} \exp\left(-\frac{1}{2} x^T \Sigma_n^{-1} x\right), \quad (7)$$

where Σ_n and a_n are respectively the covariance matrix and the weight of the nth Gaussian function. An important property of reproducing kernel Hilbert spaces is:

$$|w|^2_{K_1+K_2} = \inf\left\{ |u|^2_{K_1} + |v|^2_{K_2} \mid w = u + v \text{ with } u \in H_{K_1} \text{ and } v \in H_{K_2} \right\}. \quad (8)$$

The optimization is then performed simultaneously at the fine and coarse scales. Note that an extension of this idea to the space of diffeomorphisms can be argued according to [7]. Equation (7) then allows one to construct a wide range of kernels with several scales of interest while preserving all the promising statistical properties of the LDDMM. Note that the choice of the weights $(a_n)_{n\in[1,N]}$ is a key issue here since it controls the influence of the structures at different scales for the deformation. For instance, one would want an equivalent influence of the large and small structures in the registration. This point is discussed in Subsection 3.3.

3.2   Chain of Gaussian Kernels

Our second extension of [4] consists of using a chain of N deformations between I_S and I_T, each having its own kernel. The idea of a time dependent kernel already appeared in [13] for surface registration where the width of the kernel was chosen C^1 and decreasing in time. We still register I_S on I_T through a time dependent diffeomorphic transformation ϕ_t, where $t \in [0,1]$, related to the velocity vector field v_t by equation (1). Here, however, we minimize the following energy as a function of v_t, $t \in [0,1]$:

$$\operatorname*{argmin}_{v=v_t, t\in[0,1]} \frac{1}{2} \|I_S \circ \phi_1^{-1} - I_T\|^2_{L^2} + \sum_{n=1}^{N} \int_{(n-1)/N}^{n/N} \frac{1}{2} \|v_t\|^2_{V_{\sigma_n}} \, dt \quad (9)$$

where $\|.\|_{V_{\sigma_n}}$, $n \in \{1, \cdots, N\}$ represents the norm related to Gaussian kernels $K_{\sigma_n}(x)$ of width σ_n and weighted by a_n. As in a coarse-to-fine approach,

$(\sigma_n)_{n \in [1,N]}$ decreases as n increases, which implies that the sequence of Hilbert spaces is increasing for the inclusion. Therefore the group of diffeomorphisms is the same as the one generated by V_{σ_N}. However, the cost of the transformation in (9) does not give a Riemannian metric on this group contrary to the classical framework and it does not even give in general a distance due to this non-symmetric cost. Despite these drawbacks, the shooting property of the initial setting is still conserved. Implementation of this scheme differs slightly from that of [4], as described below. Table 1 presents the resolution algorithm where, for readability, we recall that the symbol $\forall$ means "for all". Note that, in this algorithm, the gradient descent parameter ϵ must be small enough to ensure the invertibility of the deformation.

Table 1. Gradient descent for multi-kernel LDDMM

(1) Initialize the velocity field $v(x, t_i) = 0$, $\forall x$, $\forall i$.
(2) While not convergence
(3)   Estimate $\phi(x, t_i)$ and $\phi^{-1}(x, t_i)$ by forward/backward integration of v, $\forall x$, $\forall i$.
(4)   For $i = 1 : I$
(5)   Estimate $J_{t_i}^S(x)$ and $J_{t_i}^T(x)$ by using ϕ and ϕ^{-1}, $\forall x$.
(6)   Compute $M(x) = |D\phi(x, t_i)| \nabla J_{t_i}^S(x)(J_{t_i}^S(x) - J_{t_i}^T(x))$, $\forall x$.
(7)   Smoothing: $M_s(x, t_i) = K_{\sigma_n}(M(.))$, $\forall x$ and where $\frac{n-1}{N} \leq i\Delta t < \frac{n}{N}$.
(8)   Update: $v(x, t_i) = v(x, t_i) - \epsilon(v(x, t_i) - M_s(x, t_i))$, $\forall x$, $\forall i$.

3.3   Weight of the Kernels

The fine and coarse registration techniques presented in Subsections 3.1 and 3.2 depend on a set of parameters a_n, $n \in [1, N]$ each of them controlling the weight of the deformations at scale n. The deformations are strongly related to the velocity field updates iteration after iteration. These updates do not only depend on the values of a_n but also on the kernels as well as the registered images. To set the weights, we then introduce the apparent weights a_n', $n \in [1, N]$ such that $a_n = a_n'/g(K_{\sigma_n}, I_S, I_T)$ where g represents the typical amplitude of the velocity field updates for a given smoothing kernel and two registered images. We then set g as the norm of the maximum gradient computed (Eq. 4) at the first iteration of the algorithm, when registering I_S on I_T using K_{σ_n}:

$$g(K_{\sigma_n}, I_S, I_T) = K_{\sigma_n} \star (\nabla I_S(I_S - I_T)). \tag{10}$$

In the context of fine and coarse registration, all a_n' should then be similar in order to have equivalent deformations at each scale considered. If the value of a_n' is significantly higher than the other apparent weights, the registration will be almost the same as the registration at the scale n only. This technique has the advantage of being simple to use and was shown to be efficient both on 2D synthetic images and 3D CT and MR images. Importantly, for images of the same type (*e.g.* MR brain images with the same acquisition protocol) and the same kernels K_{σ_n}, the values of g were observed to be stable. The method can then be used for an atlas creation by systematically using the same kernels with same weights.

4 Results

4.1 Evaluation on Synthetic Images

We evaluate here the behaviour of the two techniques presented in Section 3 in the registration of I_S^2 on I_T^2 (cf. Fig. 4). Note that the interpretation of the deformations of I_S^1 on I_T^1 is similar. We use the characteristic scales to $\sigma_1 = 5$ and $\sigma_2 = 1.5$ pixels, the values at which the registration were performed using simple Gaussian kernels in Subsection 2.2, and equal apparent weights at both scales. One can observe that the flow obtained using the sum of kernels (Fig. 4, 1st row) looks similar to the one obtained using small kernels (Fig. 3, 2nd row) for an almost equivalent overlap between the deformed and target images. The flow obtained using the chain of kernels (Fig. 4, 2nd row) matches the shape at a large scale between $t = 0$ and $t = 0.5$ and then matches the details between $t = 0.5$ and $t = 1$ and the final matching is good even if slightly less accurate than using a small kernel or the sum of kernels. The comparison of grid deformations at $t = 1$ in Fig. 5 is particularly interesting. It shows that the deformations obtained using the multi-kernel approaches are smoother and visually more natural than using small kernels. This key property and the good final matching are due to the simultaneous consideration of two scales that are pertinent to the registered shape.

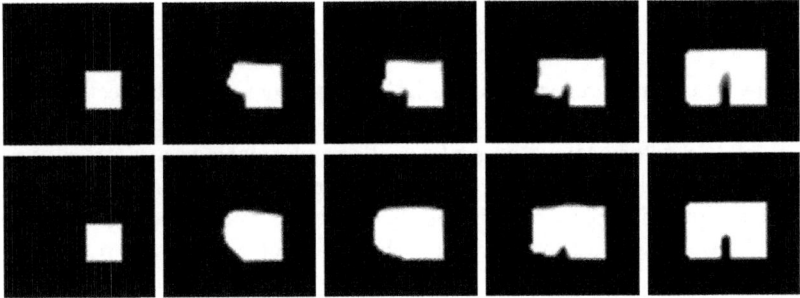

Fig. 4. Deformation of I_S^2 to I_T^2 for (from left to right) $t = 0$, $t = 0.25$, $t = 0.5$, $t = 0.75$, $t = 1.0$ by using sum (Row 1) and chain (Row 2) of kernels, each having $\sigma_1 = 5$ and $\sigma_2 = 1.5$ pixels

4.2 Evaluation on Brain MR Images

We apply now our techniques to the longitudinal estimation of the early brain development out of MR brain images. Here we limit our study to the comparison of two brains of 29.86 and 33.86 weeks of gestational age for the same preterm infant. The images have a spatial resolution of 0.85mm and bias field correction has been performed using N3 [22]. Two characteristic lengths are considered here, a large one ($\sigma_1 = 5$mm) and a small one ($\sigma_2 = 1.5$mm) and equal apparent weights are used for the fine and coarse deformations. As shown in Fig. 6, using a

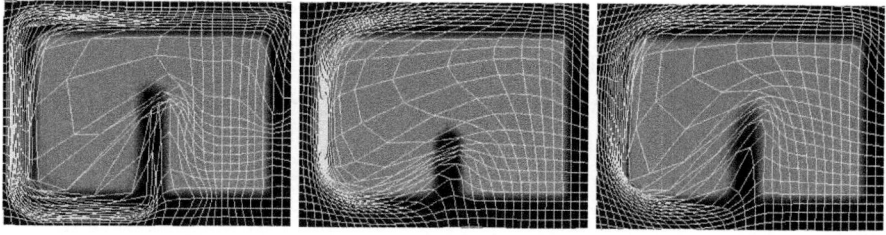

Fig. 5. Deformation grids at time $t = 1$ of the registration of I_S^2 to I_T^2 using a small kernel (left) the chain (center) and the sum (right) of kernels. Each square of the grid represents a deformed pixel.

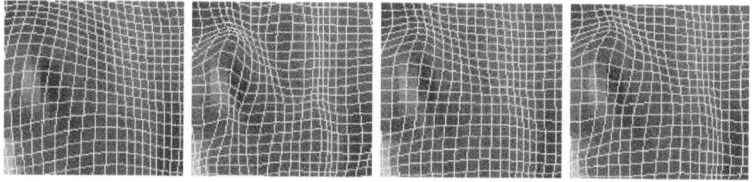

Fig. 6. Effect of the kernel on the deformation of a MR brain image. Grid size is one voxel. **From left to right:** large kernel ($\sigma_1 = 5$mm), small kernel $\sigma_2 = 1.5$mm), chain of the two kernels, sum of the two kernels.

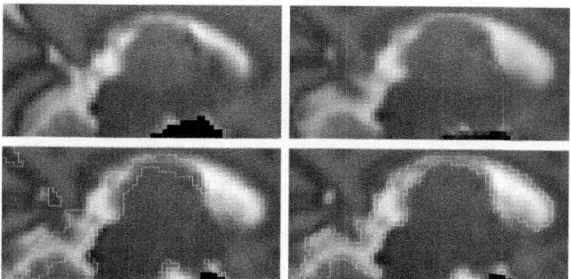

Fig. 7. Registration using the sum of kernels ($\sigma_1 = 5$mm, $\sigma_2 = 1.5$mm). **Top-left:** Source image. **Top-right:** Deformed source image at $t = 1$. **Bottom-left:** Target image and isovalues of the source image showing the surface of a lateral ventricle. **Bottom-right:** Target image and isovalues of the deformed source image at $t = 1$ showing the surface of a lateral ventricle.

small kernel leads to unnatural looking deformations while the deformations look more plausible when using a large kernel. The matching is however much better using small kernels instead of large ones. The multi-kernel approaches provide visually more natural deformations that also match the details. We can observe that they deform the grid at fine and coarse scales simultaneously. In Fig. 7, we can first observe that the deformations obtained using the sum of kernels look natural and are accurate. In comparison, when using the chain of kernels with the same number of iterations the matching seems slightly less accurate both at large and small scales. It appears therefore that the sum of kernels produces more accurate deformations and higher statistical power.

5   Conclusion

We have presented examples of the use of fine and coarse approaches in the context of LDDMM for the registration of 3D medical images. The approaches we developed make use of either a time dependent kernel, or a constant kernel defined by the sum of several Gaussians. Our tests have shown that these methods estimate natural deformations on complex images with diffeomorphic properties. In particular, using the sum of Gaussian kernels leads to natural-looking, accurate registrations that have a strong statistical power, even on complex images. Future work will pursue the development of extensions with other similarity measures and use of a multi-resolution approach. More experiments and applications will also be carried out on MR cerebral images, as well as on CT cardiac images.

References

1. Arsigny, V., Commowick, O., Pennec, X., Ayache, N.: A log-Euclidean framework for statistics on diffeomorphisms. In: MICCAI 2006, Part I. LNCS, vol. 4190, pp. 924–931. Springer, Heidelberg (2006)
2. Ashburner, J.: A fast diffeomorphic image registration algorithm. NeuroImage 38, 95–113 (2007)
3. Avants, B.B., Epstein, C.L., Grossman, M., Gee, J.C.: Symmetric diffeomorphic image registration with cross-correlation: Evaluating automated labeling of elderly and neurodegenerative brain. Medical Image Analysis 12, 26–41 (2008)
4. Beg, F.M., Miller, M.I., Trouvé, A., Younes, L.: Computing large deformation metric mappings via geodesic flows of diffeomorphisms. International Journal of Computer Vision 61(2), 139–157 (2005)
5. Beg, M., Khan, A.: Symmetric data attachment terms for large deformation image registration. IEEE Transactions on Medical Imaging 26(9), 1179–1189 (2007)
6. Beg, M.F., Helm, P.A., McVeigh, E., Miller, M.I., Winslow, R.L.: Computational cardiac anatomy using MRI. Magnetic Resonance in Medecine 52(5), 1167–1174 (2004)
7. Bruveris, M., Gay-Balmaz, F., Holm, D., Ratiu, T.: The momentum map representation of images. J. Nonlin. Sci. (February 20, 2010) (submitted), JNLS-D-10-00024
8. Cao, Y., Miller, M.I., Mori, S., Winslow, R.L., Younes, L.: Diffeomorphic matching of diffusion tensor images. In: CVPRW 2006: Proceedings of the 2006 Conference on Computer Vision and Pattern Recognition Workshop, p. 67 (2006)
9. Cao, Y., Miller, M.I., Winslow, R.L., Younes, L.: Large deformation diffeomorphic metric mapping of vector fields. IEEE Trans. Med. Imaging 24(9), 1216–1230 (2005)
10. Crum, W., Tanner, C., Hawkes, D.: Anisotropic multi-scale fluid registration: evaluation in magnetic resonance breast imaging. Physics in Medicine and Biology 50(21), 5153–5174 (2005)

11. Das, S.R., Avants, B.B., Grossman, M., Gee, J.C.: Registration based cortical thickness measurement. NeuroImage 45, 867–879 (2009)
12. Dupuis, P., Grenander, U., Miller, M.I.: Variational problems on flows of diffeomorphisms for image matching. Q. Appl. Math. LVI(3), 587–600 (1998)
13. Glaunes, J.: Transport par difféomorphismes de points, de mesures et de courants pour la comparaison de formes et l'anatomie numérique. Ph.D. thesis, Université Paris 13 (2005)
14. Haber, E., Modersitzki, J.: Cofir: coarse and fine image registration. In: SIAM Real-Time PDE-Constrained Optimization, pp. 37–49 (2007)
15. Hart, G., Zach, C., Niethammer, M.: An optimal control approach for deformable registration. In: Computer Vision and Pattern Recognition Workshop, pp. 9–16 (2009)
16. Helm, P., Younes, L., Beg, M., Ennis, D., Leclercq, C., Faris, O., McVeigh, E., Kass, D., Miller, M., Winslow, R.: Evidence of structural remodeling in the dyssynchronous failing heart. Circulation Research 98, 125–132 (2006)
17. Hernandez, M., Bossa, M.N., Olmos, S.: Registration of anatomical images using paths of diffeomorphisms parameterized with stationary vector field flows. Int. J. Comput. Vision 85(3), 291–306 (2009)
18. Younes, L., Arrate, F., Miller, M.I.: Evolutions equations in computational anatomy. Neuroimage (November 2008)
19. Lorenzen, P., Prastawa, M., Davis, B., Gerig, G., Bullitt, E., Joshi, S.: Multi-modal image set registration and atlas formation. Med. Image. Anal. 10(3), 440–451 (2006)
20. Miller, M., Trouvé, A., Younes, L.: Geodesic shooting for computational anatomy. J. Math. Imaging Vis. 24(2), 209–228 (2006)
21. Miller, M., Younes, L.: Group actions, homeomorphisms, and matching: A general framework. International Journal of Computer Vision 41(1-2), 61–84 (2001)
22. Sled, J., Zijdenbos, A., Evans, A.: A nonparametric method for automatic correction of intensity nonuniformity in MRI data. IEEE Transactions on Medical Imaging 17(1), 87–97 (1998)
23. Trouvé, A., Younes, L.: Metamorphoses through lie group action. Foundations of Computational Mathematics 5(2), 173–198 (2005)
24. Vaillant, M., Miller, M., Trouvé, A., Younes, L.: Statistics on diffeomorphisms via tangent space representations. Neuroimage 23(S1), S161–S169 (2004)
25. Vercauteren, T., Pennec, X., Perchant, A., Ayache, N.: Diffeomorphic demons: Efficient non-parametric image registration. NeuroImage 45(1), S61–S72 (2009)
26. Younes, L.: Shapes and Diffeomorphisms. Springer, Heidelberg (2008)
27. Younes, L., Qiu, A., Winslow, R.L., Miller, M.I.: Transport of relational structures in groups of diffeomorphisms. Journal of Mathematical Imaging and Vision 32, 41–56 (2008)

Log-Domain Diffeomorphic Registration of Diffusion Tensor Images

Andrew Sweet and Xavier Pennec

Asclepios, INRIA Sophia-Antipolis, France
andrew.sweet@sophia.inria.fr

Abstract. Diffusion tensor imaging provides information about deep white matter anatomy that structural magnetic resonance images typically fail to resolve. Non-linear registration of diffusion tensor images, for which a few methods already exist, allows us to capture the deformations of these structures that would otherwise go unobserved. Here, we build on an existing method for diffeomorphic registration of diffusion tensor images, so that it fully incorporates the useful log-domain parameterization of diffeomorphisms. Initially, this allows us to easily include a registration symmetry constraint that is highly desirable for pair-wise registration. More importantly, the parameterization allows simple and proper calculation of statistics on the transformations obtained. We show that the symmetric log-domain method exhibits the most preferable trade-off between image correspondence and deformation smoothness on real data and also achieves the best recovery of synthetic warps.

Keywords: Diffusion tensor imaging, computational anatomy, diffeomorphic registration, exponential map.

1 Introduction and Motivation

Although linear registration allows proper visual comparison of images and can also account for subject movement during image acquisition, its major limitation is that it only accounts for features of global transformations between images, such as position, orientation and scale. Capturing local anatomical differences, such as the size or shape of particular brain regions, requires non-linear registration, which overcomes these limitations by allowing images to transform differently at each point.

The discipline of computational anatomy aims to use these non-linear transformations to compute deformation statistics of anatomical structures that can potentially account for biological variability within a population [1]. Therefore, any method of registration used in this discipline must be able to provide deformations that can easily be used for statistical analysis. One such method makes use of the diffeomorphic demons registration framework [2], described in Sect. 2, and can be adapted to directly estimate a vector space parameterization of the transformation [3], allowing simple statistical calculation.

B. Fischer, B. Dawant, and C. Lorenz (Eds.): WBIR 2010, LNCS 6204, pp. 198–209, 2010.

In this work, we specifically consider non-linear registration of diffusion tensor images (DTIs), which represent the diffusion of water in the brain using a second-order symmetric tensor at each voxel [4]. DTI registration is of particular interest because it provides unique information about deep white matter structures, the deformations of which we propose may be more significant than changes observed from scalar image registration. In a purely mathematical sense, it is also the case that DTI registration can be considered better determined to estimate a transformation from one image to another simply because each voxel of a DTI contains a tensor defined by six unique values, as opposed to the single value of a scalar image. It is for both these reasons that we propose DTI to be a suitable choice for the study of computational anatomy.

Although the diffeomorphic demons framework has already been suitably developed for DTI registration [5], we contribute further developments in Sect. 3 by describing how the previously referenced parameterization, which has already been used for scalar image registration, is also feasible for DTI registration. This section continues by explaining how our method can easily incorporate a registration symmetry constraint, which ensures that the registration process is independent of the order of input images. This constraint has previously been shown as a desirable feature in non-linear pair-wise registration [6] and we also show, in Sect. 5, that it specifically improves the performance of our method as well. The experiments and results in this section also show that the parameterization alone does not significantly affect the registration process.

2   The Diffeomorphic Demons Framework

Throughout this work, it is assumed that there is a non-parametric spatial transformation s from a moving image, M, to a fixed image, F. The 'demons' framework, initially described in [7], provides one approach to find this transformation and has seen many developments. Its most recent general form [2] works by attempting to iteratively minimize an energy

$$E(F, M, s, c) = \sigma_i^{-2}\mathrm{Sim}(F, M \circ c) + \sigma_x^{-2}\mathrm{Dist}(s, c) + \sigma_T^{-2}\mathrm{Reg}(s) \qquad (1)$$

where c is a non-parametric transformation that should achieve point correspondences between the images, σ_i weights the uncertainty of the images, σ_x weights the spatial uncertainty between c and s and σ_T weights the spatial uncertainty of s alone. This means that solving (1) is equivalent to finding a small update transformation u to compose with the current one such that $c = s \circ u$. The introduction of the hidden variable, c, allows the energy to be split into two forms, each of which can be optimized alternately in the following scheme [8].

1. **Correspondence:** given the current s, find the c that minimizes

$$E_c(F, M, s, c) = \sigma_i^{-2}\mathrm{Sim}(F, M \circ c) + \sigma_x^{-2}\mathrm{Dist}(s, c). \qquad (2)$$

2. **Regularization:** given the c found from step 1, find the s that minimizes

$$E_s(s, c) = \sigma_x^{-2}\mathrm{Dist}(s, c) + \sigma_T^{-2}\mathrm{Reg}(s). \qquad (3)$$

The regularization step in the demons framework constrains the smoothness of s, but it does not guarantee the smoothness, or even existence, of its inverse transformation. However, for s to be a meaningful transformation in biomedical image registration it is desirable that finding an s from M to F implies the existence of a smooth s^{-1} from F to M. Formally, we require s to be a *diffeomorphism*. Such a constraint can be imposed by exploiting the log-Euclidean framework for diffeomorphisms [9]. This uses the log map to parameterize the update transformation as a stationary velocity field $\mathbf{u} = \log(u)$, which when put through the exponential map gives a diffeomorphic update $u = \exp(\mathbf{u})$.

Although we are free to choose the similarity, distance and regularization criteria in (1), it is typically the case that $\text{Sim}(F, M \circ c) = ||F - M \circ c||^2$, $\text{Dist}(s, c) = ||s - c||^2 = ||u||^2$ and $\text{Reg}(s) = ||\nabla s||_K^2$, where it should be noted that the regularization criterion makes use of a norm defined in a space K. These choices have the advantage that (2) has an approximate closed form solution that can be found independently at each point of a scalar image [2] and that (3) can be approximately solved by convolution with a Gaussian related to K [8]. Additionally, the number of free parameters in the model is typically reduced by defining $\sigma_i = ||F - M \circ c||$.

With all these assumptions, a single iteration of the diffeomorphic demons algorithm consists of the two following steps

1. $\mathbf{u}^* = \underset{\mathbf{u}}{\arg\min} \left[E_c^{\text{diffeo}}(F, M, s, \mathbf{u}) \right]$

   $= \underset{\mathbf{u}}{\arg\min} \left[\sigma_i^{-2} ||F - M \circ (s \circ \exp(\mathbf{u}))||^2 + \sigma_x^{-2} ||\exp(\mathbf{u})||^2 \right]$

2. $s \leftarrow K_{\text{diff}} \star \exp(K_{\text{fluid}} \star \mathbf{u}^*)$

where $\star$ represents convolution, $K_{\text{fluid}} = \mathcal{G}[\mathbf{0}, \sigma_{\text{fluid}}^2 \mathbf{I}]$ is used to performed fluid-like regularization of the update to the transformation and $K_{\text{diff}} = \mathcal{G}[\mathbf{0}, \sigma_{\text{diff}}^2 \mathbf{I}]$ is used to perform diffusion-like regularization of the updated transformation. We use $\mathcal{G}[\mu, \Sigma]$ to denote a Gaussian distribution with mean μ and covariance Σ.

3   Diffeomorphic Demons Registration of DTIs

3.1   General DTI Registration

While the regularization step in the diffeomorphic demons framework only operates on vector fields, and is therefore independent of the image type, the correspondence step includes a few operations that must be explicitly defined for tensor images.

First of all, there should be a way to perform arithmetic on tensor images, so that the sum of squares similarity criterion can continue to be used. This is achieved by exploiting the log-Euclidean framework for tensors [10], which allows a tensor $T(n)$ at voxel n in image T to be parameterized by a log-tensor $\log(T(n))$. As log-tensors belong to a vector space, tensor arithmetic is accomplished by performing vector arithmetic on the log-tensors and exponentiating the result. Secondly, we must also define how to correctly warp the DTIs. As we work with discrete images, there must be a way to interpolate tensors so that images can always be compared at the same points. Continuing to use the log-tensor representation means that interpolation is simply achieved by linear component-wise vector interpolation, an approach which has exhibits reasonable performance [10].

However, non-rigid transformations of tensor images also causes the local orientation of the tensors to be lost. The orientation of diffusion tensors is vital, as it is groups of locally aligned tensors that represent anatomical white matter structures in the brain. There are two possible reorientation schemes that attempt to correct for this [11]. The preservation of principal direction (PPD) approach finds the rotation matrix, $R(n)$, which ensures that the principal axis of $T(n)$ is the same as it was before the warp was applied. By contrast, the finite strain (FS) approach finds the $R(n)$ that minimizes the Frobenius distance to the local transformation Jacobian matrix $J(n)$. In practice, this minimization is computed from the polar decomposition of the Jacobian, so that $R(n) = (J(n)J(n)^T)^{-\frac{1}{2}}J(n)$. In both cases, the corrected tensor is given by $T'(n) = R(n)^T T(n)R(n)$ and the log-tensor is corrected in the same way to give $\log(T'(n)) = R(n)^T \log(T(n))R(n)$.

Given the advantages of using log-tensors in all these aspects of DTI registration, we compute these beforehand, use them in the registration, then take their exponential to produce the final warped image. Therefore, all references to the fixed and moving images, F and M, hereby refer to the log-tensor images.

3.2   DT-REFinD

The DT-REFinD method [5], hereby denoted as DTR, provides a way of performing diffeomorphic demons registration of tensor images and importantly incorporates FS reorientation directly into the energy to be minimized

$$E_c^{\text{DTR}}(F, M, s, \mathbf{u}) = \sigma_i^{-2}||F - R^T(M \circ (s \circ \exp(\mathbf{u})))R||^2 + \sigma_x^{-2}||\exp(\mathbf{u})||^2 \quad (4)$$

where R can be thought of as an image of rotation matrices, which specifies the tensor reorientation at each voxel. The direct incorporation of the reorientation into the optimization has been shown to improve performance compared to a scheme where orientation is simply corrected after each standard update. Following the notation of [5], we can express the correspondence energy as

$$E_c^{\text{DTR}}(F, M, s, \mathbf{u}) = \left|\left|\begin{matrix}\varphi_1(F, M, s \circ \exp(\mathbf{u})) \\ \varphi_2(\mathbf{u})\end{matrix}\right|\right|^2 = ||\varphi_c(F, M, s, \mathbf{u})||^2 \quad (5)$$

where $\varphi_1(F, M, s\circ\exp(\mathbf{u})) = \sigma_i^{-1}[F - R^T(M\circ(s\circ\exp(\mathbf{u})))R]$, $\varphi_2(\mathbf{u}) = \sigma_x^{-1}\exp(\mathbf{u})$ and $\varphi_c(F, M, s, \mathbf{u}) = [\varphi_1(F, M, s \circ \exp(\mathbf{u})), \varphi_2(\mathbf{u})]^T$.

In general, the demons algorithm approximates this energy by the 0th and 1st order terms of its Taylor expansion with respect to $\mathbf{u}$

$$E_c^{\text{DTR}}(F, M, s, \mathbf{u}) \approx \left|\left|\begin{bmatrix}\varphi_1(F, M, s \circ \exp(\mathbf{0})) \\ \varphi_2(\mathbf{0})\end{bmatrix} + \begin{bmatrix}D^{\varphi_1}(F, M, s \circ \exp(\mathbf{0})) \\ D^{\varphi_2}(\mathbf{0})\end{bmatrix}\mathbf{u}\right|\right|^2$$

$$(6)$$

which means that finding $\mathbf{u}^*$ by minimizing (6) is equivalent to solving the least squares problem $||\mathbf{b} - \mathbf{Au}||^2$ where $\mathbf{b} = [\varphi_1; \varphi_2]$ and $\mathbf{A} = -[D^{\varphi_1}; D^{\varphi_2}]$. For scalar image registration, the matrix $\mathbf{A}$ has a block diagonal structure which means that each vector component of $\mathbf{u}^*$ can be individually solved. However, DTR's incorporation of FS reorientation into the energy means that $\mathbf{A}$ is sparse, but no longer has a simple block diagonal structure because the optimal displacement of a tensor at one point affects the reorientation, and therefore optimal displacement, of a tensor at a neighboring point. Accordingly, the current implementation of DTR finds a solution using a least squares conjugate gradients solver in Gmm++ [12], but is memory and processor intensive due to the large size of the sparse matrix $\mathbf{A}$.

4 Log-Domain Diffeomorphic Registration of DTIs

4.1 Log-Domain DT-REFinD

On first appearances, the basic diffeomorphic demons framework satisfies the need for statistical computation because the log map of the final transformation should be its stationary velocity field representation. However, in practice the log map acts as a high-pass filter, and exhibits a lack of stability between the transformation and its stationary velocity field representation [13]. To overcome this problem an alternative approach [3] extends the demons framework by not only parameterizing the update field in the 'log-domain', but the current transformation as well, so that the update is directly applied to a stationary velocity field $\mathbf{v}$ whose exponential is s. This direct update on the velocity field is achieved using the Baker-Campbell-Hausdorff function, denoted as $Z(.)$, to approximate the composition for small updates such that $\exp(Z(\mathbf{v}, \epsilon\mathbf{u})) \approx \exp(\mathbf{v}) \circ \exp(\epsilon\mathbf{u})$ [14]. As a result, the two iterative steps of log-domain DTR (LDDTR) are

1. $\mathbf{u}^* = \underset{\mathbf{u}}{\operatorname{argmin}} \left[E_c^{\text{DTR}}(F, M, \exp(\mathbf{v}), \mathbf{u}) \right]$
2. $\mathbf{v} \leftarrow K_{\text{diff}} \star Z(\mathbf{v}, K_{\text{fluid}} \star \mathbf{u}^*)$

where it should be noted that E_c^{DTR} is the same as in the original algorithm. In other words, exactly the same method can be used to find $\mathbf{u}^*$ because the log-domain approach only affects the representation of the transformation. However, the consequence of using this representation directly is that the regularization is defined for the stationary velocity field $\mathbf{v}$ which parameterizes the transformation, rather than the transformation itself. More specifically, the regularization energy is modified to become $Reg(s) = ||\nabla \log(s)||_K^2 = ||\nabla \mathbf{v}||_K^2$.

4.2 Symmetric Log-Domain DT-REFinD

The diffeomorphic parameterization in the general framework ensures s^{-1} exists and is smooth, but the classic demons algorithm only ever finds the forwards transformation $s : M \to F$. Running the algorithm with the images exchanged will certainly produce a diffeomorphism $t : F \to M$, but there is no guarantee that $t = s^{-1}$. This registration symmetry, or inverse consistency, can be easily achieved in the log-domain by performing two unconstrained optimisations of the current transformation and projecting these onto a new symmetric transformation [3]. The first is the same as usual and finds an update $\mathbf{u}_{\text{forw}}^*$ for s, while the second finds an update $\mathbf{u}_{\text{back}}^*$ for s^{-1} with the fixed and moving images exchanged. As DTR can be performed in the log-domain, the same approach can be exploited to define the two steps of symmetric LDDTR (SLDDTR)

1. (a) $\mathbf{u}_{\text{forw}}^* = \underset{\mathbf{u}}{\text{argmin}} \left[E_c^{\text{DTR}}(F, M, s \circ \exp(\mathbf{v}), \mathbf{u}) \right]$

   (b) $\mathbf{u}_{\text{back}}^* = \underset{\mathbf{u}}{\text{argmin}} \left[E_c^{\text{DTR}}(M, F, s \circ \exp(-\mathbf{v}), \mathbf{u}) \right]$

2. $\mathbf{v} \leftarrow \frac{1}{2} K_{\text{diff}} \star \left(Z(\mathbf{v}, K_{\text{fluid}} \star \mathbf{u}_{\text{forw}}^*) - Z(-\mathbf{v}, K_{\text{fluid}} \star \mathbf{u}_{\text{back}}^*) \right)$

where it should be noted that R will be different for the steps 1a and 1b and the second term in step 2 is negated in order to invert the updated inverse transformation, so that the average of both updated transformations is found in the forwards direction. Note that projection of the two updated transformations onto the space of symmetric transformations is simply performed by averaging because the representative stationary velocity fields belong to a vector space.

5   A Comparison of DTI Registration in and Out of the Log-Domain

In order to implement the LDDTR and SLDDTR methods described in Sect. 4.1 and Sect. 4.2 respectively, we have adapted the implementation of symmetric and non-symmetric log-domain diffeomorphic demons registration of scalar images [15], so that it uses the implementation of the energy function from [5].

5.1   Validation on Real Data

Diffusion weighted imaging data are provided by the Neuradapt study group and the authors would like to acknowledge M. Vassallo, C. Lebrun and S. Chanalet for making these available. Here we consider a sub-group of 7 subjects from this study. For each subject, a single unweighted ($b = 0$) was acquired along with 23 gradient weighted ($b = 700\text{s}/\text{mm}^2$) images with data dimensions of $256 \times 256 \times \tilde{2}6$ and spatial dimensions of $0.9375\text{mm} \times 0.9375\text{mm} \times 5.5\text{mm}$. While the anisotropy of the spatial dimensions is particularly high, we still believe that the data can highlight any differences between the registration methods considered.

DTI reconstructions are performed assuming the usual log-Gaussian noise model and any non-positive tensors, which are physically meaningless, are replaced with a local tensor mean [16]. Each subject's $b = 0$ image is linearly registered to that of the 2mm ICBM-DTI-81 template [17] using the affine version of the robust method described in [18], which is available in [19]. The resultant affine transformations are applied to their corresponding DTIs, using FS reorientation. Finally, the brain extraction toolkit [20] is used to generate a brain foreground mask from each $b = 0$ image, which is applied to the affinely registered DTI to remove any tensors outside of the brain. Although this tool is primarily designed for use on T1 images, we find that the masks generated using the T2 weighted $b = 0$ images are reasonable after a small erosion.

Every possible unique pair-wise registration is performed between the subjects' DTIs, giving 42 registrations for the non-symmetric methods and 21 for SLDDTR. All algorithms are allowed to iterate ten times using $\sigma_x = 1$, which is enough to ensure reasonable convergence of the solutions. A multi-resolution scheme is not used because it does not significantly improve the convergence or performance, possibly due to the initial affine registration. As LDDTR and SLD-DTR optimize a different regularization energy compared to DTR, we register over a range of regularizaton parameter values $\sigma_T = \{0.6, 0.8, \ldots, 2.0\}$ so that the final transformations produced by each of the methods can be compared at a range of harmonic energies (HEs). The HE is defined as the mean square Frobenius norm of the transformation Jacobian and therefore corresponds to the irregularity of the transformation.

Figure 1 demonstrates that at low HEs, the mean square error between the log-tensor images, referred to from here as the log mean square error (LMSE), is relatively similar for all of the methods. One difference is that LDDTR produces a higher LMSE than DTR at the same HE. This difference is accentuated at higher HEs. By contrast, the SLDDTR method achieves a lower LMSE than DTR at the same HE, although the difference is less clear at higher HEs. These observations suggest that using the log-domain parameterization directly has a detrimental effect on performance. Yet the same parameterization also allows easy incorporation of the symmetric constraint, which seems to be beneficial.

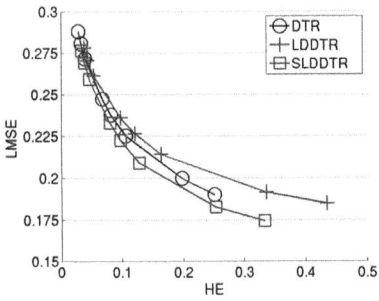

Fig. 1. The mean log-tensor image square error plotted against the mean transformation harmonic energy for registration of 42 subject pairs using the DTR, LDDTR and SLDDTR methods

Figure 2 shows an example of a single registration performed using all three methods with a single reasonable regularization parameter $\sigma_T = 1.4$. The visual correspondence of the warped DTIs these produce illustrate the similarity in performance.

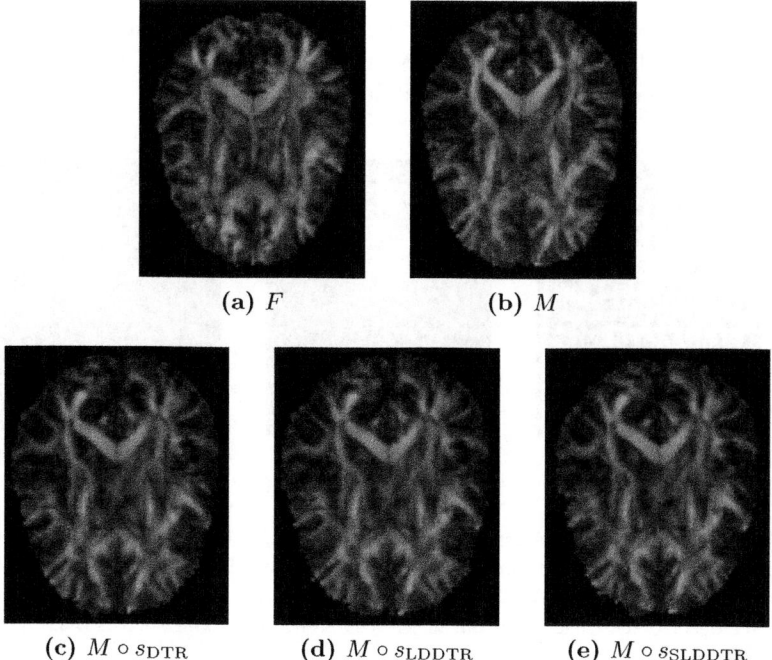

(a) F (b) M

(c) $M \circ s_{\text{DTR}}$ (d) $M \circ s_{\text{LDDTR}}$ (e) $M \circ s_{\text{SLDDTR}}$

Fig. 2. An example registration from the DTI of one subject (a) to another (b) using the DTR (c) (LMSE=0.280, HE=0.0623), LDDTR (d) (LMSE=0.199, HE=0.0881) and SLDDTR (e) (LMSE=0.200, HE=0.0742) methods using $\sigma_T = 1.4$. For (a-e) the image intensity represents fractional anisotropy and the color represents the principal axis of the tensor where red=left-right, green=posterior-anterior and blue=inferior-superior. In all cases, the same mid-axial slice is displayed using MedINRIA [19].

5.2 Performance on Synthetic Warps

In order to quantitatively compare the performance of the methods with a known ground truth, we create three random diffeomorphisms for each subject, apply them to the DTI of their respective subject and add noise to the warped DTIs. A single noisy warped DTI is generated according to the following scheme.

1. Create a random velocity field $\mathbf{v}_r$ by sampling a vector for each foreground voxel in the original DTI from $\mathcal{G}[\mathbf{0}, \sigma_r^2 \mathbf{I}]$.
2. Convolve $\mathbf{v}_r$ with $\mathcal{G}[\mathbf{0}, \sigma_s^2 \mathbf{I}]$ to give a smooth random velocity field $\mathbf{v}_s$.
3. Exponentiate $\mathbf{v}_s$ to give a random diffeomorphism $s_s = \exp(\mathbf{v}_s)$.
4. Warp the original DTI with s_s using FS reorientation.
5. Add noise drawn from $\mathcal{G}[\mathbf{0}, \sigma_n^2 \mathbf{I}]$ to the log-tensors in the warped DTI.

For our experiments, we find that using $\sigma_r^2 = 10^4$, $\sigma_s^2 = 7.25^2$ and $\sigma_n^2 = 0.005$ produces warps with similar properties to those found from pair-wise registration of the real data. Specifically, the mean displacement of the random warps is

3.403mm and their mean harmonic energy is 0.0915. Although the noisy warped DTIs are not necessarily anatomically believable, as demonstrated by a single example in Fig. 3, they do provide an opportunity to validate and explain previous observations from experiments on real data.

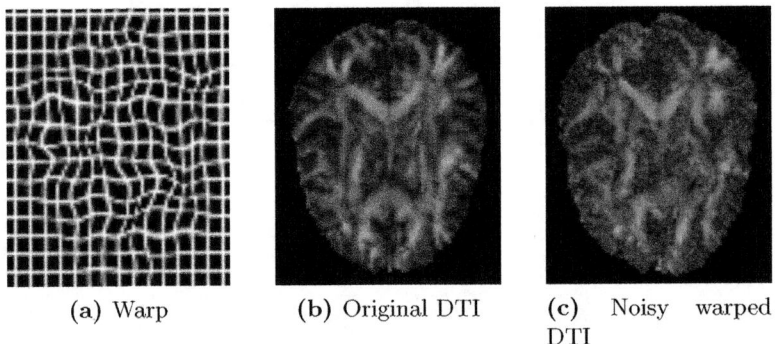

(a) Warp   (b) Original DTI   (c)   Noisy   warped DTI

Fig. 3. An example of a synthetic warp, represented here by its application to a regular grid image (a) (HE=0.0936), applied to the DTI of one subject (b) to produce a warped DTI to which noise is added (c) (LMSE=0.271). For the DTIs, the intensity and color maps are described in Fig. 2. In all cases, the same mid-axial slice is displayed using MedINRIA [19].

All registration methods are applied from the original image to the noisy warped images for each subject using the same range of regularization parameter values as before $\sigma_T = \{0.6, 0.8, \ldots, 2.0\}$. The DTR and LDDTR methods are also applied from the noisy images to the originals. As a ground truth is present in this experiment, we additionally consider the distance from the recovered deformation field to the true one $\text{dist}(s, s_{\text{true}}) = ||s - s_{\text{true}}||$, as well as the distance between their Jacobians $\text{dist}(J(s), J(s_{\text{true}})) = ||J(s) - J(s_{\text{true}})||$.

Figure 4 shows that at low HEs, all three methods exhibit very similar LMSEs. In accordance with this result, the distances between the transformations and their Jacobians are also relatively similar. At higher HEs, DTR produces a slightly lower LMSE than the LDDTR and SLDDTR methods, but this actually represents an increase in the distance from the true transformation.

The distance from the true transformations appears to be optimal for all methods at an HE of around 0.07. Here, the LDDTR method exhibits slightly better recovery of the true transformation than DTR, but this may occur simply because the synthetic warps really are parameterized by the velocity fields assumed by LDDTR. Yet the SLDDTR method, which makes the same assumption, recovers the true transformation even better than LDDTR at all HEs, which illustrates that the symmetric constraint is beneficial for DTI registration in the same way that has been previously demonstrated for scalar image registration [3]. Despite this, the Jacobian distances are relatively similar for all methods at all HEs. This suggests that the advantage of the symmetric constraint comes from capturing information in the transformation that is not locally linear.

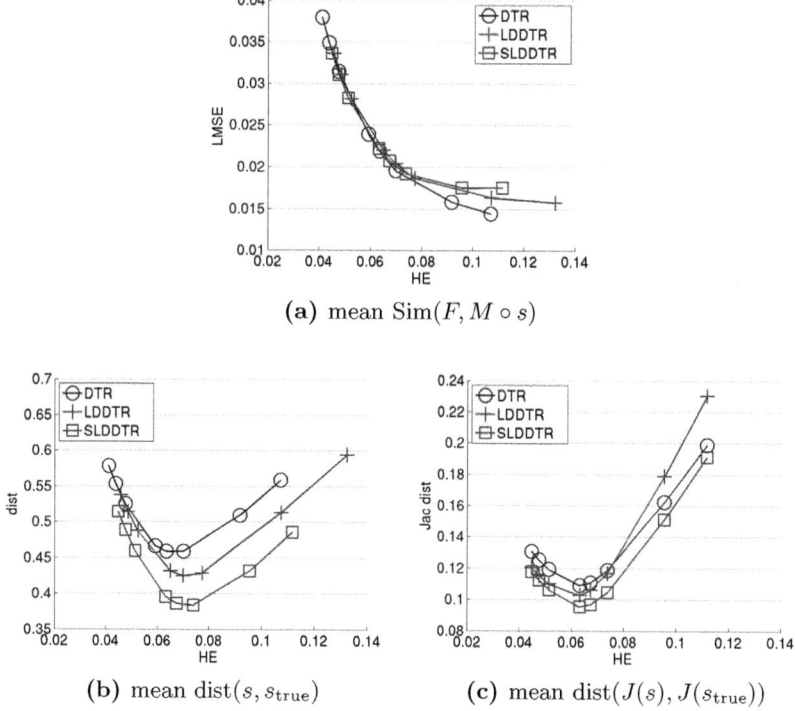

(a) mean $\mathrm{Sim}(F, M \circ s)$

(b) mean $\mathrm{dist}(s, s_{\mathrm{true}})$

(c) mean $\mathrm{dist}(J(s), J(s_{\mathrm{true}}))$

Fig. 4. The mean log-tensor image square error (a), mean distance between the re-covered and true transformations (b) and mean distance between their Jacobians (c) plotted against the mean transformation harmonic energy for registration of 42 subject pairs using the DTR, LDDTR and SLDDTR methods

6   Conclusions and Further Work

In this work, we have demonstrated that the log-domain parameterization of diffeomorphisms can be fully incorporated into the demons framework for non-linear registration of DTIs. While directly applying this parameterization with little regularization may reduce registration performance, this can be counter-acted by incorporating an inverse consistency constraint into the method. Fur-thermore, this extra constraint seems to improve performance a little beyond that of the original method.

Although the immediate contributions of this work are not revolutionary, they provide the essential foundations for proper statistical analysis of the structural deformations observable from DTI registration. In fact, the data used in this study are only a small subset from a larger collection of 180 subjects, pair-wise registration of which is currently being undertaken. The statistics from these registrations have the potential to demonstrate major modes of deformation and could also be reincorporated back into the method for statistical regularization through non-stationary convolution.

Other important variations on the DTR method are also possible. For example, [5] explains that as the DTR method must solve a large system anyway, we might as well directly solve the DTR equivalent of (1), thereby reducing the dependence on the regularization approximations made in the original demons framework. Additionally, we might also consider other ways of incorporating the symmetric constraint into the DTR method, such as [21] who find a single update from a symmetric energy for log-domain registration of scalar images. Although this means we could avoid solving two systems as in the projection approach, it means the single system to solve is larger and may be more easily subject to local minima. Time permitting, all these variations will be investigated prior to the future work described above, so that all the implications of DTI registration in the log-domain can be fully understood.

References

1. Pennec, X.: Statistical computing on manifolds: from riemannian geometry to computational anatomy. In: Nielsen, F. (ed.) Emerging Trends in Visual Computing. LNCS, vol. 5416, pp. 347–386. Springer, Heidelberg (2008)
2. Vercauteren, T., Pennec, X., Perchant, A., Ayache, N.: Diffeomorphic demons: Efficient non-parametric image registration. NeuroImage 45(1 Supp.1), S61–S72 (2009)
3. Vercauteren, T., Pennec, X., Perchant, A., Ayache, N.: Symmetric log-domain diffeomorphic registration: A demons-based approach. In: Metaxas, D., Axel, L., Fichtinger, G., Székely, G. (eds.) MICCAI 2008, Part I. LNCS, vol. 5241, pp. 754–761. Springer, Heidelberg (2008)
4. Basser, P.J., Mattiello, J., LeBihan, D.: MR diffusion tensor spectroscopy and imaging. Biophysical Journal 66(1), 259–267 (1994)
5. Yeo, B.T.T., Vercauteren, T., Fillard, P., Peyrat, J.M., Pennec, X., Golland, P., Ayache, N., Clatz, O.: DT-REFinD: Diffusion tensor registration with exact finite-strain differential. IEEE Transactions on Medical Imaging 28(12), 1914–1928 (2009)
6. Klein, A., Andersson, J., Ardekani, B.A., Ashburner, J., Avants, B., Chiang, M.C., Christensen, G.E., Collins, L.D., Gee, J., Hellier, P.: Evaluation of 14 nonlinear deformation algorithms applied to human brain MRI registration. NeuroImage 46(3), 786–802 (2009)
7. Thirion, J.P.: Image matching as a diffusion process: An analogy with Maxwell's demons. Medical Image Analysis 2(3), 243–260 (1998)
8. Cachier, P., Bardinet, E., Dormont, D., Pennec, X., Ayache, N.: Iconic feature based nonrigid registration: The PASHA algorithm. Computer Vision and Image Understanding 89(2-3), 272–298 (2003)
9. Arsigny, V., Commowick, O., Pennec, X., Ayache, N.: A log-Euclidean framework for statistics on diffeomorphisms. In: Larsen, R., Nielsen, M., Sporring, J. (eds.) MICCAI 2006. LNCS, vol. 4190, pp. 924–931. Springer, Heidelberg (2006)
10. Arsigny, V., Fillard, P., Pennec, X., Ayache, N.: Log-Euclidean metrics for fast and simple calculus on diffusion tensors. Magnetic Resonance in Medicine 56(2), 411–421 (2006)
11. Alexander, D.C., Pierpaoli, C., Basser, P.J., Gee, J.C.: Spatial transformations of diffusion tensor magnetic resonance images. IEEE Transactions on Medical Imaging 20(11), 1131–1139 (2001)

12. Renard, Y., Pommier, J., Fournie, M., Schleimer, B.: Gmm++,
    http://home.gna.org/getfem/gmm_intro.html
13. Hernandez, M., Olmos, S., Pennec, X.: Comparing algorithms for diffeomorphic registration: Stationary LDDMM and diffeomorphic demons. In: Pennec, X., Joshi, S. (eds.) Proc. MFCA 2008, pp. 24–35 (2008)
14. Bossa, M., Hernandez, M., Olmos, S.: Contributions to 3D diffeomorphic atlas estimation: Application to brain images. In: Ayache, N., Ourselin, S., Maeder, A. (eds.) MICCAI 2007, Part I. LNCS, vol. 4791, pp. 667–674. Springer, Heidelberg (2007)
15. Dru, F., Vercauteren, T.: An ITK implementation of the symmetric log-domain diffeomorphic demons algorithm. The Insight Journal (January-June 2009)
16. Fillard, P., Pennec, X., Arsigny, V., Ayache, N.: Clinical DT-MRI estimation, smoothing and fiber tracking with log-Euclidean metrics. IEEE Transactions on Medical Imaging 26(11), 1472–1482 (2007)
17. Mori, S., Oishi, K., Jiang, H., Jiang, L., Li, X., Akhter, K., Hua, K., Faria, A.V., Mahmood, A., Woods, R., Toga, A.W., Pike, G.B., Neto, P.R., Evans, A., Zhang, J., Huang, H., Miller, M.I., van Zijl, P., Mazziotta, J.: Stereotaxic white matter atlas based on diffusion tensor imaging in an ICBM template. NeuroImage 40(2), 570–582 (2008)
18. Ourselin, S., Roche, A., Prima, S., Ayache, N.: Block matching: A general framework to improve robustness of rigid registration of medical images. In: Delp, S.L., DiGoia, A.M., Jaramaz, B. (eds.) MICCAI 2000. LNCS, vol. 1935, pp. 557–566. Springer, Heidelberg (2000)
19. Toussaint, N., Souplet, J.C., Fillard, P.: MedINRIA: Medical image navigation and research tool by INRIA. In: Proc. MICCAI 2007 Workshop on Interaction in Medical Image Analysis and Visualization (2007)
20. Smith, S.M.: Fast robust automated brain extraction. Human Brain Mapping 17(3), 143–155 (2002)
21. Sabuncu, M.R., Yeo, B.T.T., van Leemput, K., Vercauteren, T., Golland, P.: Asymmetric image-template registration. In: Yang, G.-Z., Hawkes, D., Rueckert, D., Noble, A., Taylor, C. (eds.) MICCAI 2009. LNCS, vol. 5761, pp. 565–573. Springer, Heidelberg (2009)

Nonrigid Registration and Template Matching for Coronary Motion Modeling from 4D CTA

Dong Ping Zhang[1], Laurent Risser[1,2], Ola Friman[3], Coert Metz[4],
Lisan Neefjes[5], Nico Mollet[5], Wiro Niessen[4], and Daniel Rueckert[1]

[1] Department of Computing, Imperial College London, London, UK
[2] Institute for Mathematical Science, Imperial College London, London, UK
[3] Fraunhofer MEVIS, Universitaetsallee 29, 28359 Bremen, Germany
[4] Dept. of Medical Informatics and Radiology, Erasmus MC, Rotterdam, NL
[5] Dept. of Radiology and Cardiology, Erasmus MC, Rotterdam, NL

Abstract. In this paper, we present a method for coronary artery motion tracking in 4D cardiac CT angiogram data sets. The proposed method allows the construction of patient-specific 4D coronary motion model from pre-operative CTA which can be used for guiding totally endoscopic coronary artery bypass surgery (TECAB). The proposed approach consists of three steps: Firstly, the coronary arteries are extracted in the end-diastolic time frame using a minimal cost path approach. To achieve this, the start and end points of the coronaries are identified interactively and the minimal cost path between the start and end points is computed using A* graph search algorithm. Secondly, the cardiac motion is estimated throughout the cardiac cycle by using a non-rigid image registration technique based on a free-form B-spline transformation model and maximization of normalized mutual information. Finally, coronary arteries are tracked automatically through all other phases of the cardiac cycle. This is estimated by deforming the extracted coronaries at end-diastole to all other time frames according the motion field acquired in second step. The estimated coronary centerlines are then refined by template matching algorithm to improve the accuracy. We compare the proposed approach with two alternative approaches: The first approach is based on the minimal cost path extraction of the coronaries with start and end points manually identified in each time frame while the second approach is based on propagating the extracted coronaries from the end-diastolic time frame to other time frames using image-based non-rigid registration only. Our results show that the proposed approach performs more robustly than the non-rigid registration based method and that the resulting motion model is comparable to the motion model constructed from semi-automatic extractions of the coronaries in all time frames.

Keywords: Nonrigid Deformation, Computer Integrated Surgery, Intra-modality Registration, Motion Detection and Tracking.

1 Introduction

As one of the leading causes of death worldwide, coronary artery disease occurs due to the failure of the blood circulation to supply adequate oxygen and nu-

B. Fischer, B. Dawant, and C. Lorenz (Eds.): WBIR 2010, LNCS 6204, pp. 210–221, 2010.

trition to cardiac tissues. It is typically caused by the excessive accumulation of atheromatous plaques and fatty deposits within certain regions of the arteries which restricts the blood flow. To treat this disease, arteries or veins grafted from the patient's body are used to bypass the blockages and restore the supply to the heart muscle. Using image-guided robotic surgical system, totally endoscopic coronary artery bypass (TECAB) surgery techniques have been developed to allow clinicians to perform bypass surgery off-pump with three pin-hole incisions in the chest cavity through which two robotic arms and one stereo endoscopic camera are inserted. However, 20-30% conversion rates from TECAB surgery to the conventional invasive surgical approach [1,2] have been reported due to the vessel misidentification and mis-localization caused by the restricted field of view of the stereo endoscopic images.

The goal of our work is to construct a patient-specific 4D coronary artery motion model from preoperative cardiac Computed Tomography Angiography (CTA) sequences. By temporally and spatially aligning this model with intraoperative endoscopic views of the patient's beating heart, this can be used to assist the surgeon to identify and locate the correct coronaries during the TECAB procedures [3,4].

The recent advances in using CTA for the diagnosis of coronary artery disease diagnosis and surgical planning have attracted a wide range of studies. Extensive reviews on coronary artery segmentation are given in Schaap et al. [5] and Lesage et al. [6]. Although coronary artery segmentation has been well studied, constructing motion models of coronaries from pre-operative scans to assist the diagnosis and surgery is a topic which has received less attention.

In previous work, Shechter et al. [7,8] tracked coronary artery motion in a temporal sequence of biplane X-ray angiography images. In their approach, a 3D coronary model is reconstructed from extracted 2D centrelines in end-diastolic angiography images. The deformation throughout the cardiac cycle is then recovered by a registration-based motion tracking algorithm. The disadvantage is that 3D reconstruction of the coronary is required. An alternative approach for the extraction of the coronaries from cardiac CTA has been proposed by Metz et al. [9]: Here the coronaries are manually or semi-automatically identified at one time frame and then tracked throughout the cardiac cycle using non-rigid registration of the multi-phase cardiac CTA images. The restriction of this approach is that highly localized motion of the coronaries can not be fully recovered by the motion tracking of the entire heart.

In this paper, we present a novel approach for coronary motion tracking in cardiac CTA images which significantly improves the robustness of motion tracking and reduces the manual interactions. The proposed approach is based on a non-rigid registration of the CTA images which provides an initial estimation of the coronary motion. This estimation is then refined using template fitting algorithm that matches a tubular-like vessel model to the local image region. This simplifies the 4D motion modelling of coronaries significantly. Only one pair of the start and end points of each vessel in end-diastolic frame are manually identified. Once the start and end points have been identified, each coronary branch from the end-diastolic phase is extracted as the minimal cost path between both points. The proposed approach is compared to a nonrigid image registration based approach similar to the one presented by Metz *et al.* [9] and to manual tracking of the coronaries obtained from graph search at each time frame.

2 Method

We start from presenting the techniques used for pre-processing the images. The main methods are then organized in three parts. Firstly, using Euclidean distance as the heuristic term, A* graph search is performed at each phase in each dataset to extract the minimal cost path of coronaries, based on user-supplied start and end points for each vessel. The extracted results are used as ground truth for evaluating the coronary motion tracking methods. Secondly, we estimate the coronary motion using the hierarchy non-rigid registration of the CTA sequence. Thirdly, the minimal cost coronary paths at end-diastolic phase are transformed to other time points according to the deformation field. The deformed paths are resampled equidistantly and the points from each resampled path are used as initial guesses for vessel template fitting procedure. This enables the tracking of coronary motion without any further user interaction and also estimates the coronary radius at each fitting location. We then compare the template based approach with the non-rigid registration one.

2.1 Image Preprocessing

Before the coronary arteries are extracted their visibility in the cardiac CTA image sequences is enhanced by performing contrast limited adaptive histogram equalization [10]. This improves the contrast and enhances the coronary arteries. Note that this step is carried out for the entire image sequences so that intensities in all time frames are treated similarly and consistently.

Due to the ECG pulsing windows applied in the acquisition and reduced radiation dose [11], the signal-to-noise ration is varying in the multiple-phase 4D data sets. To improve the image quality, 4D anisotropic filtering [12] is used to reduce this noise and preserve the cardiac chamber boundaries and vessel structures. So after histogram equalization, we perform 4D anisotropic diffusion [12] to smooth the image sequence while preserving edges and other salient features. Again, the anisotropic diffusion filtering is performed for the entire 4D image sequence so that neighbouring time frames influence the diffusion at the current time frame.

For the template matching algorithm, minimum and maximum thresholds are used in order to reduce the effect of the presence of inhomogeneous background (e.g. air and tissue mixed region) or irrelevant neighboring structures (e.g. bone or metal implant). Multiple thresholds are selected automatically by 4D multi-level thresholding extended from Otsu's method [13] for each 4D data set. The intensities of the background voxels are increased so that they match the average myocardial intensity level. For the intensities above the upper threshold level, they are reduced to average myocardium intensity level too. One pair of thresholds is used for each 4D sequence.

2.2 Segmentation of Coronary Centerlines Using Graph Search

We first perform a coarse segmentation of the coronary arteries in the CTA image using a multiscale Hessian-based vessel enhancement filter [14]. The filter utilizes the 2nd-order derivatives of the image intensity after smoothing (using a Gaussian kernel) at multiple scales to identify bright tubular-like structures with various diameters. The six second-order derivatives of the Hessian matrix at each voxel are computed by convolving the image with second-order Gaussian derivatives at a pre-selected scale.

Assuming a 3D image function $I(\mathbf{x})$, the Hessian matrix at a given voxel $\mathbf{x}$ at scale σ is denoted as $H_\sigma(\mathbf{x})$. A vesselness term $V(\mathbf{x})$ is defined as in Frangi *et al.* [14] and is based on the eigenvalues and eigenvectors of $H_\sigma(\mathbf{x})$. The vesselness response is computed at a range of scales. The maximum response with the corresponding optimal scale is obtained for each voxel of the image. Once the vesselness at each voxel is computed, it can be used to define a minimal cost path between the start and end nodes.

The minimal cost path between the start node S and the end node E is obtained using the A* graph search algorithm [15] in the end-diastolic CTA image. The location of the pair of nodes S and E is specified semi-interactively. A uni-directional graph search algorithm evaluates the smallest cost from node S to current node $\mathbf{x}$ denoted as $g(\mathbf{x})$ and the heuristic cost from current node to node E denoted as $h(\mathbf{x})$ to determine which voxel to be selected as next path node. The algorithm finds the optimal path only if the heuristic underestimates the cost. In our approach, the Euclidean distance from $\mathbf{x}$ to E is used to calculate the heuristic cost term. We assess each candidate node by calculating the cost $f(\mathbf{x})$ as:

$$f(\mathbf{x}) = g(\mathbf{x}') + \frac{1}{V(\mathbf{x}) + \epsilon} + \delta h(\mathbf{x}). \tag{1}$$

where $g(\mathbf{x}')$ is the score of the previous node. To initialize the cost function, $g(\mathbf{x}')$ is set to be zero for the start node S. A small positive constant ϵ is added in order to avoid singularities. The parameter δ is estimated as the ratio of the minimum cost of the vessel to the Euclidean distance of the start and end nodes.

By using the heuristic term, the searching space is greatly reduced and the minimum cost path can be found in real-time. When node E is reached, the minimum cost path is reconstructed by tracing backwards to node S. The algorithm finds a minimal cost path consisting of an ordered set of discrete locations (voxels). After extraction of the path we estimate a B-spline representation of coronary centerlines that smoothly interpolates these voxel locations.

2.3 Non-rigid Image Registration for Estimating Coronary Motion

The motion of coronaries during the cardiac cycle is mainly caused by the expansion and contraction of the cardiac chambers. We use non-rigid image

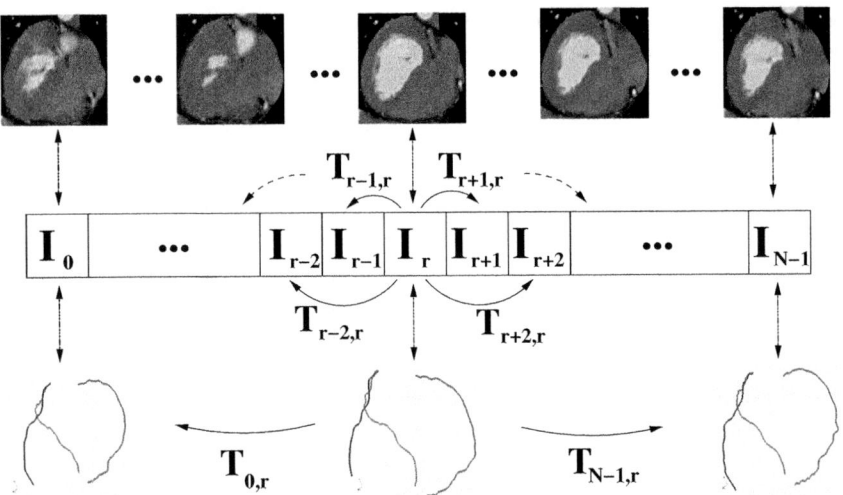

Fig. 1. Illustration of coronary motion tracking using a non-rigid registration approach. The bottom row shows the extracted coronary centerlines from I_r (in the middle) and the transformed centerlines for I_0 and I_{N-1} in the left and right. Right coronary artery is shown in red, left anterior descending artery in green, left circumflex artery in blue.

registration of the cardiac CTA sequence for a first approximation of the coronary motion throughout the cardiac cycle. In our application, we use a non-rigid image registration algorithm which employs a free-form deformation model based on cubic B-splines [16]. A series of registration steps is performed to register each time frame to the reference image at end-diastolic phase. Each registration proceeds in a multi-resolution fashion, starting with a control point spacing of 40mm and ending with a spacing of 5mm. The deformations derived from coarse level are used to initialize the finer level of registration. For each frame we use the registration result from the previous frame as initial estimation as shown in the middle row of Fig. 1. The non-rigid registration algorithm uses normalised mutual information as the similarity measure between time frames. A gradient descent optimization is used to find the optimal transformation. The extracted coronary arteries in the end-diastolic phase are propagated to the other cardiac phases by applying the deformations obtained from the finest registration step as illustrated in the bottom row of Fig. 1.

2.4   Coronary Motion Tracking Using Template Fitting

Combined with the deformation information obtained in Section 2.3, we propose a method for refining the tracking of the coronaries throughout the cardiac CTA sequence based on template localization and fitting. A tubular segment model [17,18] is adopted to map a spatial coordinate $\mathbf{x}$ to the intensity range $[0, 1]$ through a template function $M(\mathbf{x}; r, \mathbf{x}_0, \mathbf{v})$. The template function defines an ideal vessel segment centered at point $\mathbf{x}_0$ running in the direction of $\mathbf{v}$ with

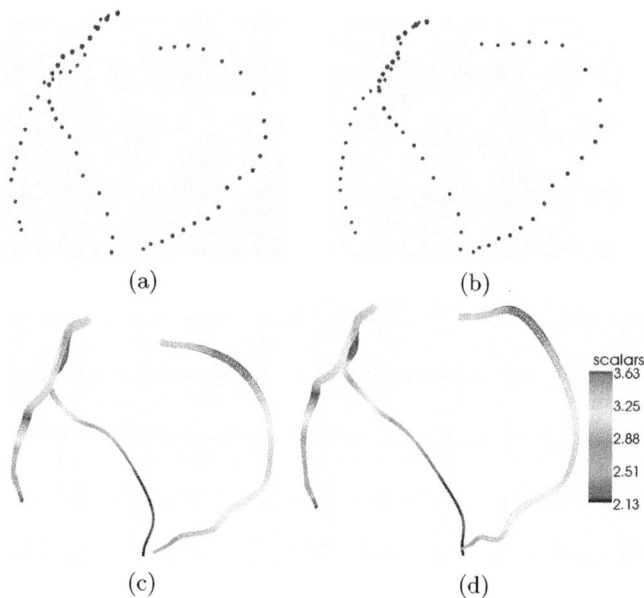

(a)   (b)

scalars
3.63

3.25

2.88

2.51

2.13

(c)   (d)

Fig. 2. Combination of non-rigid deformation and template matching. (b) shows the resampled coronary branches extracted at end-disatole as in Section 2.2. (d) shows the vessel lumen by chaining the fitted templates together at end-diastole. (a) shows estimation for the coronary at end-systole. (c) is coronary artery lumen obtained by fitting the templates with corresponding local region in end-systolic CTA image. The varying radii are represented by different colors as in the legend.

radius r. A vessel profile is defined to model the image intensity variation in the cross-sectional plane perpendicular to the vessel direction.

First, an equidistant sample of vessel points from each extracted coronary centerline (Section 2.2) at end-diastolic phase is chosen for refining the coronary segmentation as shown in Fig. 2 (b). Each point from these samples is used as the initial center for the template fitting procedure. For each point, the optimal vessel template together with the corresponding local contrast and local mean intensity parameters are obtained by solving the weighted least squared problem using Levenberg-Marquardt algorithm [18] in the end-diastolic time frame. This provide us a more detailed coronary segmentation with center location, radius, local contrast and mean intensity parameters for each template. By chaining these templates together, we obtain the coronary lumen at end-diastole as shown in Fig. 2 (d).

Given the coronary centrelines extracted in the end-diastolic time frame as shown in the middle bottom of Fig. 1, we can estimate the coronary center-line positions for other time frames by using the deformation information obtained in Section 2.3 to transform the end-diastolic extractions. An equidistant sample of vessel points are chosen from each vessel centerline at each non-end

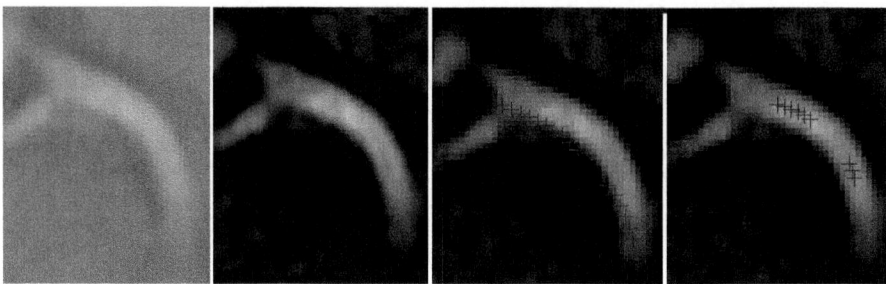

Fig. 3. Illustration of template position estimation and fitting. (a) A small region of CTA image containing right coronary artery. (b) after pre-processing. (c) the estimated right coronary artery position using non-rigid registration. Blue cross shows the estimated vessel centerlines. (d) The vessel centerlines after template fitting. The discontinuity of the centerline is due to that only one slice shown in 2D representation.

diastolic phase as the estimated locations of the centers of the vessel templates. The template fitting algorithm is performed on all these vessel points to provide an accurate match of the template with the local region. To achieve this, the template parameters are optimized again using Levenberg-Marquardt optimization. After this, the new discrete center points and their corresponding radii for each vessel is interpolated using B-spline. The coronary lumen is represented with a tubular mesh. This procedure is repeated in pair-wise order until the coronary lumen in all time frames is obtained. We then quantitatively measure the accuracy of these coronary lumen centerlines by assuming the minimal cost centerlines obtained in Section 2.2 as ground truth. We also compare their difference from the estimated centerlines using only non-rigid registration method as in Section 2.3.

To illustrate the procedure, segmented coronary lumen from two phases are shown in Fig. 2, together with the resampled minimal cost paths which are used as initialization for template matching. For illustration, in Fig. 3, a right coronary artery segment is randomly chosen from one image. It shows template matching improves the accuracy of the estimated centerlines.

3   Results and Evaluation

To assess the performance of the proposed motion tracking strategy we have performed experiments on eight cardiac CTA sequences. Each CTA sequence has twenty phases with various image dimensions ranging from $256 \times 256 \times 89$ to $512 \times 512 \times 335$ voxels. The voxel dimensions varies from $0.4 \times 0.4 \times 0.5$ mm^3 to $0.7 \times 0.7 \times 1.5$ mm^3. All datasets have various degrees of artifacts that affect the segmentation and registration procedure. In particular the fast motion of the heart in some time frames can lead to blurring or ghosting artifacts $e.g.$ around the coronary artery. As a result of this, in some cases, the non-rigid registration-based approach can only compensate for part of the deformation.

In order to have a gold standard to evaluate the two different motion modeling approaches, the left anterior descending artery (LAD), left circumflex artery (LCX) and right coronary artery (RCA) are extracted using the graph search algorithm (Section 2.2) from eight CTA sequences, P1, P2, P3, P4, P5, P6, P7 and P8. In all eight patients, the start and end points of the vessels have been identified manually and the results of the minimal cost path extraction have been judged as correctly falling inside the vessel lumen. The accuracy of these extractions are restricted by the shortcut effect as shown in [19]. The results are compared with motion estimates of the LAD, LCX and RCA as obtained using the non-rigid registration and template matching based approaches.

In order to assess the quality of motion tracking results, the distance between the semi-automatic extracted minimal cost centerline M and tracked coronary centerline U of each coronary branch in each time frame is measured. The distance is defined as,

$$D\left(M, U\right) = \frac{1}{N_M} \sum_{i=1}^{N_M} \|m_i - l(m_i, U)\|_2 + \frac{1}{N_U} \sum_{j=1}^{N_U} \|u_j - l(u_j, M))\|_2 \quad (2)$$

where N_M and N_U are the number of points representing vessel M and vessel U correspondingly. For each point $m_i \in M$, $l(m_i, U)$ calculates the closest point of m_i on the automatically extracted vessel U. Similarly, for each point $u_j \in U$, $l(u_j, M)$ defines the closest point of u_j on the vessel M.

The results are shown in Fig. 4. The total displacement of each coronary artery is computed as the distance between the minimal-cost centerline at end-diastole phase and the minimal-cost centerline at each other phase and is shown in the first column (a). The second column (b) shows the tracking error from purely non-rigid registration based approach. It is measured as the distance between centrelines estimated via non-rigid registration and the gold standard for each phase. The third column (c) shows the tracking error using the registration and template matching combined approach. It is measured as the distance between centrelines estimated via the proposed method and the gold standard for each phase.

We compare the accuracy of non-rigid registration based tracking method with the proposed approach in Table 1. The average motion is calculated as the average of the total displacements of each coronary artery for each patient. Mean error 1 shows the average residual motion for the non-rigid registration based tracking method. Mean error 2 shows the average residual motion for the non-rigid registration and template-matching based approach.

We also consider that the motion tracking is successful when the distance between modeled coronary and the minimal-cost path is under 1.4mm which is twice of the voxel size for most testing data sets. By considering this error threshold for right coronary artery motion modeling, 92% of vessel tracking are performed successfully by using our proposed method, comparing with 46% when using the purely non-rigid registration approach. By choosing 2.8 mm as threshold, all the right coronary tracking are successful in our method while the non-rigid registration approach produces 72% success rate. From Fig. 4 and Table 1, we can conclude that combining the non-rigid registration with the

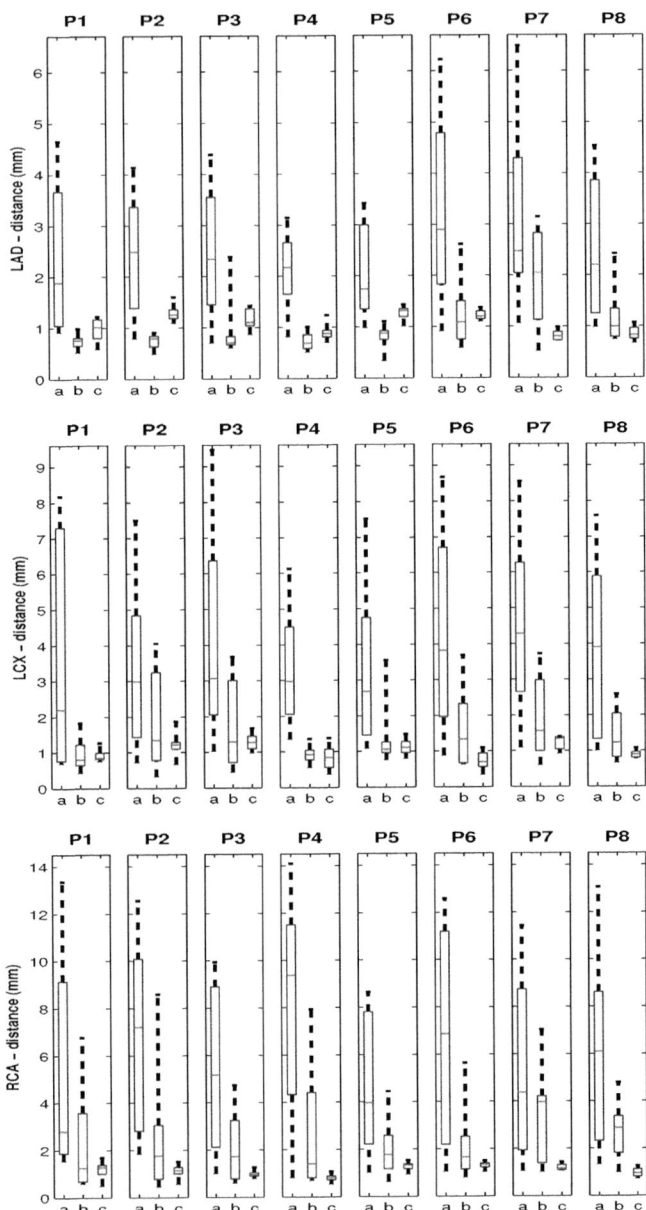

Fig. 4. Comparison of coronary motion tracking results. The total coronary displacement (LAD, LCX, RCA) is shown in column (a). The residual coronary displacement after non-rigid registration is shown in column (b) and after the combined registration and template-based tracking is shown in column (c). The results show that the proposed tracking method is able to model the coronary motion with acceptable errors (under 2 voxels) and in most cases it performed better.

Table 1. Average coronary motion and mean errors of motion tracking

LAD

	P1	P2	P3	P4	P5	P6	P7	P8
Average Motion (mm)	2.39	2.40	2.53	2.12	2.06	3.26	3.29	2.43
Mean error 1 (mm)	0.74	0.73	0.90	0.72	0.79	1.23	2.01	1.15
Mean error 2 (mm)	0.97	1.27	1.14	0.90	1.27	1.21	0.81	0.84

LCX

	P1	P2	P3	P4	P5	P6	P7	P8
Average Motion (mm)	3.41	3.23	4.42	3.28	3.10	4.31	4.47	3.92
Mean error 1 (mm)	0.92	1.81	1.77	0.90	1.31	1.61	1.89	1.45
Mean error 2 (mm)	0.90	1.19	1.28	0.84	1.12	0.72	1.21	0.89

RCA

	P1	P2	P3	P4	P5	P6	P7	P8
Average Motion (mm)	5.53	6.83	5.33	8.14	4.89	6.62	5.44	5.96
Mean error 1 (mm)	2.35	2.62	2.19	2.83	1.90	2.27	3.23	2.68
Mean error 2 (mm)	1.19	1.10	0.95	0.79	1.26	1.29	1.19	0.94

template matching together improve the motion tracking accuracy in most cases, particularly in the frames when the rapid cardiac motion occurs. The variance of tracking error is greatly reduced by using the proposed method.

4   Conclusions and Future Work

We have presented a novel approach for patient-specific coronary artery motion modeling from cardiac CTA sequences which combines the template matching and non-rigid registration algorithm. The proposed method has been tested on eight clinical CTA datasets and proved to be more robust than purely non-rigid registration approach. The limitation of this study is the lack of manual annotated coronary centerlines and lumen for the CTA images. By assuming the semi-automatically extracted minimal-cost paths as ground truth, the accuracy of the proposed tracking method is potentially under-estimated particularly for LAD and LCX. For more accurate evaluation, manual annotations are needed. However, it is very time-consuming and laborious to have all coronaries manually annotated in large CTA image. More importantly, in our application we focus more on the motion tracking of the coronaries from 4D pre-operative CTA scans. The vesselness based graph search algorithm provides us reliable and fast coronary artery extractions to be used as ground truth.

By constructing a 4D motion model of the coronaries from pre-operative cardiac images and aligning the 4D coronary model with the series of 2D endoscopic images acquired during the operation, we aim to assist the surgical planning and provide image guidance in robotic-assisted totally endoscopic coronary artery bypass (TECAB) surgery. Through this work, we expect to reduce the conversion rate from TECAB to conventional invasive procedures.

References

1. Mohr, F.W., Falk, V., Diegeler, A., Walther, T., Gummert, J.F., Bucerius, J., Jacobs, S., Autschbach, R.: Computer-enhanced "robotic" cardiac surgery: Experience in 148 patients. Journal of Thoracic and Cardiovascular Surgery 121(5), 842–853 (2001)
2. Dogan, S., Aybek, T., Andressen, E., Byhahn, C., Mierdl, S., Westphal, K., Matheis, G., Moritz, A., Wimmer-Greinecker, G.: Totally endoscopic coronary artery bypass grafting on cardiopulmonary bypass with robotically enhanced telemanipulation: Report of forty-five cases. Journals of Thoracic Cardiovascular Surgery 123, 1125–1131 (2002)
3. Figl, M., Rueckert, D., Hawkes, D., Casula, R., Hu, M., Pedro, O., Zhang, D.P., Penney, G., Bello, F., Edwards, P.: Augmented reality image guidance for minimally invasive coronary artery bypass. In: Proc. SPIE, vol. 6918 (2008)
4. Figl, M., Rueckert, D., Hawkes, D., Casula, R., Hu, M., Pedro, O., Zhang, D., Penney, G., Bello, F., Edwards, P.: Image guidance for robotic minimally invasive coronary artery bypass. Computerized Medical Imaging and Graphics 34, 61–68 (2009)
5. Schaap, M., Metz, C.T., van Walsum, T., van der Giessen, A.G., Weustink, A.C., Mollet, N.R., Bauer, C., Bogunovifa, H., Castro, C., Deng, X., Dikici, E., ODonnell, T., Frenay, M., Friman, O., Hernandez Hoyos, M., Kitslaar, P.H., Krissian, K., Kuhnel, C., Luengo-Oroz, M.A., Orkisz, M., Smedby, O., Styner, M., Szymczak, A., Tek, H., Wang, C., Warfield, S.K., Zambal, S., Zhang, Y., Krestin, G.P., Niessen, W.J.: Standardized evaluation methodology and reference database for evaluating coronary artery centerline extraction algorithms. Medical Image Analysis 13(5), 701–714 (2009)
6. Lesage, D., Angelini, E.D., Funka-Lea, G., Bloch, I.: A review of 3D vessel lumen segmentation techniques: Models, features and extraction schemes. Medical Image Analysis 13, 819–845 (2009)
7. Shechter, G., Devernay, F., Quyyumi, A., Coste-Maniere, E., McVeigh, E.: Three-dimensional motion tracking of coronary arteries in biplane cineangiograms. IEEE Transactions in Medical Imaging 22(4), 493–603 (2003)
8. Shechter, G., Resar, J.R., McVeigh, E.R.: Displacement and velocity of the coronary arteries: cardiac and respiratory motion. IEEE Transactions on Medical Imaging 25, 369–375 (2006)
9. Metz, C., Schaap, M., Klein, S., Neefjes, L., Capuano, E., Schultz, C., van Geuns, R.J., Serruys, P.W., van Walsum, T., Niessen, W.J.: Patient specific 4D coronary models from ECG-gated CTA data for intra-operative dynamic alignment of CTA with X-ray images. In: Yang, G.-Z., Hawkes, D., Rueckert, D., Noble, A., Taylor, C. (eds.) MICCAI 2009. LNCS, vol. 5761, pp. 369–376. Springer, Heidelberg (2009)
10. Zuiderveld, K.: Contrast limited adaptive histogram equalization. In: Graphics gems IV, pp. 474–485. Academic Press Professional, Inc., San Diego (1994)

11. Weustink, A.C., Mollet, N.R., Pugliese, F., Meijboom, W.B., Nieman, K., Heijenbrok-Kal, M.H., Flohr, T.G., Neefjes, L.A., Cademartiri, F., de Feyter, P.J., Krestin, G.P.: Optimal electrocardiographic pulsing windows and heart rate: Effect on image quality and radiation exposure at dual-source coronary CT angiography. Radiology 248(3), 792–798 (2008)

12. Weickert, J.: Anisotropic Diffusion In Image Processing. Teubner-Verlag, Stuttgart (1998)

13. Otsu, N.: A threshold selection method from gray-level histograms. IEEE Transactions on Systems, Man and Cybernetics 9(1), 62–66 (1979)

14. Frangi, A., Niessen, W., Hoogeveen, R., van Walsum, T., Viergever, M.: Model-based quantitation of 3D magnetic resonance angiographic images. IEEE Transactions on Medical Imaging 18(10), 946–956 (1999)

15. Hart, P.E., Nilsson, N.J., Raphael, B.: A formal basis for the heuristic determination of minimum cost paths. IEEE Transactions on Systems Science and Cybernetics 4(2), 100–107 (1968)

16. Rueckert, D., Sonoda, L.I., Hayes, C., Hill, D.L., Leach, M.O., Hawkes, D.J.: Nonrigid registration using free-form deformations: application to breast MR images. IEEE Transactions on Medical Imaging 18(8), 712–721 (1999)

17. Friman, O., Hindennach, M., Peitgen, H.O.: Template-based multiple hypotheses tracking of small vessels. In: 5th IEEE International Symposium on Biomedical Imaging: From Nano to Macro, pp. 1047–1050 (2008)

18. Friman, O., Hindennach, M., Khnel, C., Peitgen, H.O.: Multiple hypothesis template tracking of small 3d vessel structures. Medical Image Analysis (December 2009)

19. Li, H., Yezzi, A.: Vessels as 4d curves: Global minimal 4d paths to extract 3d tubular surfaces. In: Conference on Computer Vision and Pattern Recognition Workshop, CVPRW 2006, p. 82 (June 2006)

Cardiac Respiratory Motion Modelling by Simultaneous Registration and Modelling from Dynamic MRI Images

A.P. King, C. Buerger, and T. Schaeffter

Division of Imaging Sciences, King's College London, U.K.
andrew.king@kcl.ac.uk

Abstract. Motion models have been widely applied as a solution to the problem of organ motion in both image acquisition and image guided interventions. The traditional approach to constructing motion models from dynamic images involves first coregistering the images to produce estimates of motion parameters, and then modelling the variation of these parameters as functions of a surrogate value or values. Errors in this approach can result from inaccuracies in the image registrations and in the modelling process. In this paper we describe an approach in which the registrations of all images and the modelling process are performed simultaneously. Using numerical phantom data and 21 dynamic magnetic resonance imaging (MRI) datasets acquired from 7 volunteers and 7 patients, we demonstrate that our new technique results in an average reduction in motion model errors of 11.5% for the phantom experiments and 1.8% for the MRI experiments. This approach has the potential to improve the accuracy of motion estimates for a range of applications.

1   Introduction

Organ motion can cause problems in both image acquisition and image guided interventions. Motion during image acquisition can result in motion artefacts in reconstructed images. Motion during image guided interventions can cause a misalignment between the static preprocedure images used for guidance and the moving underlying anatomy. For 'repetitive' motion (i.e. motion due to the cardiac cycle or respiration) the motion is, at least partly, predictable. Therefore, motion models have been widely applied as a solution (e.g. [1,2,3]).

Such models are typically formed using 3-D motion estimates derived by coregistering images acquired at different points in the motion cycle (e.g. between end-expiration and end-inspiration in the breathing cycle). At the same time as the images are acquired, one or more motion 'surrogate' values are also measured. Examples of surrogate values for respiratory motion include navigator signals acquired during magnetic resonance imaging (MRI) scanning [1,3] and diaphragm translation estimated from fluoroscopic X-ray images [2,3]. A motion model is formed that models the variation of the 3-D motion parameters as

B. Fischer, B. Dawant, and C. Lorenz (Eds.): WBIR 2010, LNCS 6204, pp. 222–233, 2010.
© Springer-Verlag Berlin Heidelberg 2010

functions of these surrogate values. To apply the model, the surrogate values are subsequently measured and used as inputs to the model to predict 3-D motion fields.

Errors in predicting repetitive motion using motion models can result from inaccuracies in image registrations or from the modelling process itself. Traditionally, registration and modelling have been seen as separate processes and performed sequentially with no interaction between the two apart from the results of the image registrations being used as the input to the modelling process.

In this paper we propose an approach to motion model formation in which the image registration and the modelling phases are integrated. Our technique involves registering all images simultaneously and optimising the parameters of the motion model to maximise the similarity measure over all images. Previous related work includes [4], in which two 4D computed tomography (4DCT) datasets were spatiotemporally registered by adjusting the coefficients of a model formed from one of the datasets so that it matched the other dataset. A 4D-4D registration approach was also described in [5]. In [6] a motion consistency constraint was used in registering pairs of cardiac-cycle gated positron emission tomography (PET) images of the heart. Simultaneous registration of cardiac MRI images was demonstrated in [7] for the purposes of cardiac cycle motion estimation. In [8], thoracic respiratory motion was estimated from 4DCT using a 'trajectory constraint'. The optimal trajectory of each voxel was estimated over all images in the 4D dataset. We apply a similar concept to that employed in [7,8] to the problem of respiratory motion modelling of the heart from MRI data. Our aim is to construct the optimal motion model given a single set of dynamic images. We show that motion modelling errors can be reduced as a result of the integration of registration and modelling. We demonstrate our technique on respiratory motion models formed from numerical phantom data and dynamic cardiac MRI data.

2 Method and Materials

2.1 Method

In this section we first describe the traditional 'sequential' approach to registration and modelling, and then outline how this approach can be altered to perform 'simultaneous' registration and modelling. First, we define some terms:

- Our motion models are formed from a reference image, I_{ref} and N dynamic images $I_n, n \in [1 \dots N]$.
- We denote the similarity measure between 2 images as $Sim(I_A, I_B)$.
- We denote the surrogate values used in forming the model by s_n (we assume one value for each image).
  We define a D-dimensional vector of motion parameters estimated from image n as ϕ_n, e.g. $D = 6$ for rigid motion, $D = 9/12$ for affine motion, etc. The dth element of this vector is denoted by $\phi_{n,d}$.
- We denote by T_ϕ the transformation resulting from motion parameters ϕ.

- Our motion model is defined by a vector of P model parameters for each motion parameter d: $\gamma_d, d \in [1 \ldots D]$. For example, the model parameters γ_d could represent polynomial coefficients describing the variation of motion parameter d as a function of surrogate value.
- $F(\gamma_d, s)$ evaluates the model function defined by the P parameters, γ_d, and the surrogate value, s. For example, F could evaluate the polynomial function defined by coefficients γ_d at input value s.
- We denote by $T_{\gamma, s}$ the transformation produced using the motion model γ and surrogate value s. That is, the transformation resulting from the D predicted motion parameters, $F(\gamma_d, s), d \in [\ldots D]$.

Sequential registration and modelling. In the traditional sequential approach to registration and modelling the first step is to register all dynamic images to the reference image. For the nth dynamic image, an optimisation scheme is used to estimate the registration parameters,

$$\phi_n = \underset{\phi}{\operatorname{argmax}} \, Sim \left(T_\phi \left(I_{ref} \right), I_n \right) \tag{1}$$

Next, each motion parameter is modelled as a function of the surrogate values s_n. For example, using a least squares approach,

$$\tilde{\gamma}_d = \underset{\gamma_d}{\operatorname{argmin}} \sum_{n=1}^{N} \left(F \left(\gamma_d, s_n \right) - \phi_{n,d} \right)^2, d \in [1 \ldots D] \tag{2}$$

Finally, to apply the model, we predict the D motion parameters based on any given surrogate value s,

$$\tilde{\phi}_d = F \left(\gamma_d, s \right), d \in [1 \ldots D]. \tag{3}$$

where $\tilde{\phi}$ is the D-dimensional motion estimate vector. The predicted transformation for surrogate value s is $T_{\tilde{\phi}}$.

Simultaneous registration and modelling. Using our proposed simultaneous registration and modelling approach, we have a single step that performs registration of all images and motion modelling at the same time. For N dynamic images, our motion model is estimated as,

$$\tilde{\gamma} = \underset{\gamma}{\operatorname{argmax}} \frac{1}{N} \sum_{n=1}^{N} Sim \left(T_{\gamma, s_n} \left(I_{ref} \right), I_n \right) \tag{4}$$

That is, we perform an optimisation to directly estimate all $D \times P$ model parameters such that they would lead to predicted motion estimates that maximise the similarity measure over all N dynamic images. All that is required is a starting estimate for the model parameters and an optimisation scheme to maximise the term defined in (4). We will describe our approaches to these two issues in the following section.

The resulting motion model can be applied as before, using Equation (3).

2.2   Materials

We compare the performance of the traditional sequential and proposed simultaneous approaches to registration and modelling using a numerical phantom and dynamic cardiac MRI data. The phantom data allows us to control noise levels and the number of dynamic images whilst having knowledge of the gold standard motion model. The dynamic MRI images provide more realistic data with which to compare the performance of the two approaches.

Although, in principle, the general approach of simultaneous registration and modelling is applicable to any type of model or motion description, in this paper we demonstrate the technique using rigid/affine motion descriptions and polynomial functions for the model. We used rigid motion (6 degrees of freedom) for the phantom experiments and affine motion (9 degrees of freedom) for the dynamic MRI experiments. (Most previous work in the literature supports the view that an affine motion description is sufficient to describe cardiac respiratory motion, e.g. [1].) A pth order polynomial is defined by $p + 1$ coefficients. In this paper we used first order polynomials so the motion models comprised 12 coefficients in total for the phantom experiments and 18 coefficients for the dynamic MRI experiments. These represent the number of parameters to be optimised in equation (4) for the simultaneous approach. For optimisation, we used a steepest gradient ascent algorithm for both the sequential and simultaneous approaches. Currently, we use the model produced by the sequential approach as the starting estimate for the simultaneous optimisation. The mean squared difference was used as the similarity measure for both approaches.

Numerical phantom. The reference image for the numerical phantom consists of a large ellipse containing three smaller ellipses inside it (resolution $150 \times 150 \times 150$). The dynamic images were formed by transforming this reference image by rigid transformations produced by a known 'gold standard' motion model using regularly spaced integer surrogate values. Zero mean Gaussian noise of different standard deviations was added to the reference and dynamic images. Figure 1 shows sample clean and noisy reference and dynamic images.

Dynamic MRI data. The dynamic MRI data was acquired on a 1.5 Tesla cylindrical bore MRI scanner (Philips Achieva I/T) using a 3-D TFEPI sequence (cardiac triggered and gated at late diastole, typically, 100 dynamic images, 20 slices, TR = 10ms, TE = 4.9ms, flip angle = 20°, acquired voxel size $2.7 \times 3.6 \times 8.0$mm^3, acquired matrix size 128×77, reconstructed voxel size $2.22 \times 2.22 \times 4.0$mm^3, reconstructed matrix size 144×144, TFE factor 26, EPI factor 13, TFE acquisition time 267.9ms). This scan acquired a single volume every heartbeat, with each volume being acquired at an arbitrary respiratory position. A pencil-beam navigator was applied on the dome of the right hemi-diaphragm in the superio-inferior direction immediately before and after each dynamic acquisition. The averages of these lead and trail navigator values were used as the surrogate values for motion model formation. To form the motion models, one dynamic image (at end-expiration) was selected as a reference image and four others

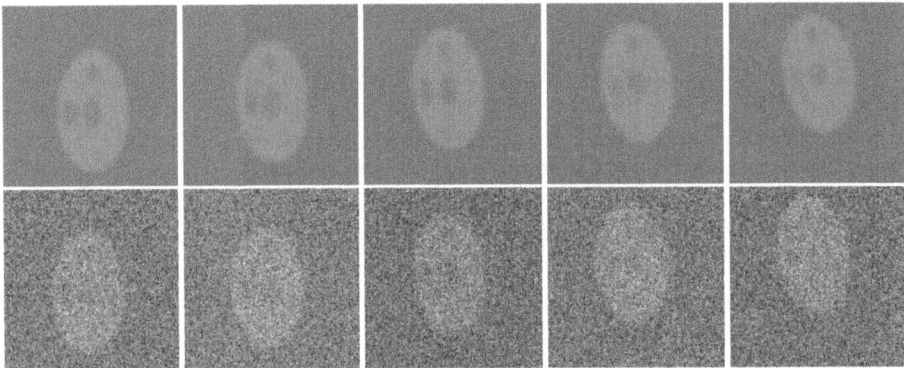

Fig. 1. The numerical phantom. Top row: no noise added. Bottom row: signal-to-noise ratio = 1.0. The left column shows the reference images and the next 4 columns show the dynamic images, each transformed from the reference image by rigid transformations generated by the gold standard motion model. All images show sample sagittal slices through a 3D volume.

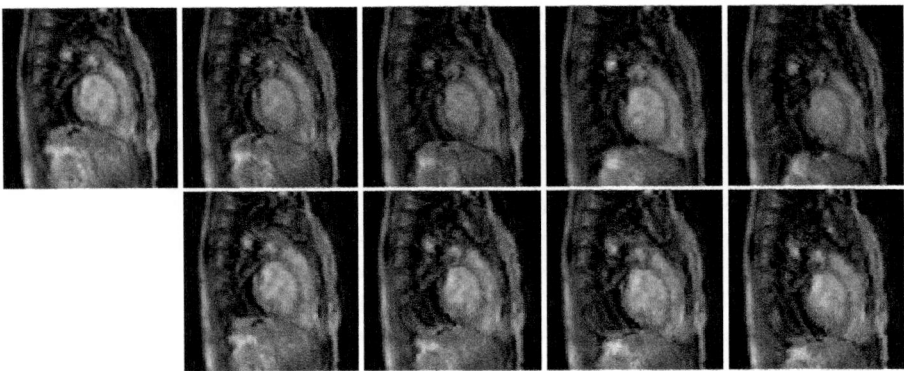

Fig. 2. The dynamic MRI data. Top row: original dynamic MRI images - the left image is the reference image and the next 4 images are the dynamic images. Bottom row: artificial MRI images for the 4 dynamics with known gold standard transformations. All images show sample sagittal slices through a 3D volume.

(evenly spaced between end-expiration and end-inspiration) as dynamic images. All selected dynamic images were acquired during the inspiration phase. For registration purposes, an elliptical mask was applied around the four chambers and major vessels of the heart in the reference image [3].

To order to accurately assess the performances of the sequential and simultaneous registration/modelling approaches, it is desirable to have gold standard motion fields for each dynamic image. To produce these, we first registered each dynamic MRI image to the reference image using a well-known freeform registration algorithm [9]. Next, the nonrigid motion field estimated by this algorithm was used to warp the reference image to produce new 'artificial' dynamic MRI images. These artificial MRI images are realistic but have known gold standard motion fields. The artificial MRI images were used to construct the motion models instead of the original MRI images. Figure 2 shows 4 original dynamic MRI image and the 4 corresponding artificial MRI images.

3   Results

For both the numerical phantom data and the dynamic MRI data we used the target registration error (TRE) as an error measure. To compute the TRE for a motion model we first defined a set of target points in the reference image. For the numerical phantom we defined target points at each alternate voxel inside the main ellipse (a total of 14802 points). For the dynamic MRI data we defined target points at each voxel inside the elliptical mask used for registration (typically a total of 10000-50000 points). Next, we formed motion models from the dynamic images using both the sequential and simultaneous registration/modelling techniques. For each dynamic image, we computed the root mean square (RMS) distance between the target points transformed using the gold standard transformation and the same points transformed using the transformation predicted by the motion model being tested. These RMS values were combined over all dynamics to produce a single RMS TRE value for the motion model.

3.1   Numerical Phantom

Numerical phantom datasets were produced consisting of 4, 8, 16 and 32 dynamic images. For each dataset, experiments were performed using 9 different noise standard deviations ranging from no noise up to a signal-to-noise ratio (SNR) of 1 (see Figure 1).

Figure 3 shows a summary of the TRE values for the sequential and simultaneous registration/modelling approaches for each dataset - the chart shows average TRE values over all 9 noise levels for each number of dynamic images. The improvements in average TRE for the 4, 8, 16 and 32 dynamic datasets were 22.3%, 5.7%, 2.9% and 14.0% respectively. Over all 36 experiments (9 noise levels for 4 different numbers of dynamic images) the TRE figures for the simultaneous approach showed a clear improvement over those for the sequential approach (0.88 +/- 0.6mm for the simultaneous approach against 0.99 +/- 0.68mm for the normal sequential approach, $p < 0.05$ in a two-tailed paired t-test). This represented an overall average improvement of 11.5%.

The motion models formed using the two approaches for a sample dataset are shown in Figure 4. Figure 4a shows the model formed using the sequential approach, and Figure 4b shows that formed using the simultaneous approach. The dotted black lines represent the constructed motion models, and the solid blue lines represent the gold standard motion model. We can see that the model formed using the simultaneous approach is closer to the gold standard than that formed using the sequential approach, particularly in the rotational parameters.

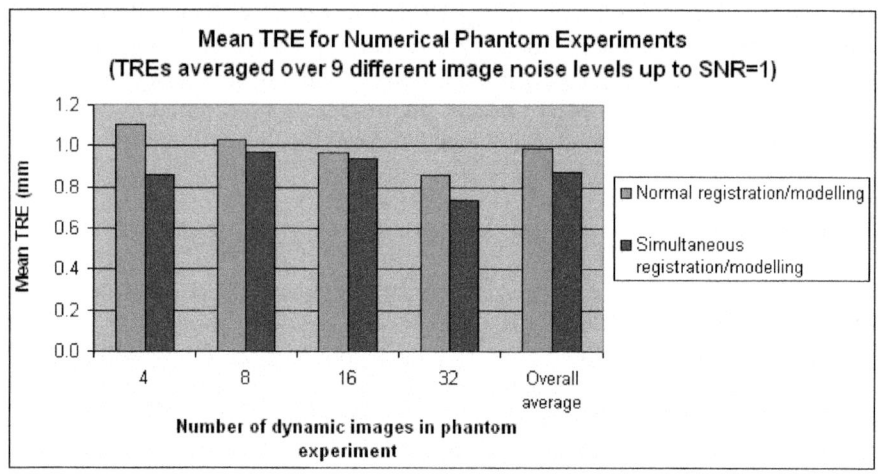

Fig. 3. Summary of target registration errors (TREs) for the numerical phantom experiments. The chart shows the mean TRE for datasets consisting of 4, 8, 16 and 32 dynamic images. The percentage improvements in mean TRE for the simultaneous registration/modelling approach were 22.3%, 5.7%, 2.9% and 14.0% respectively.

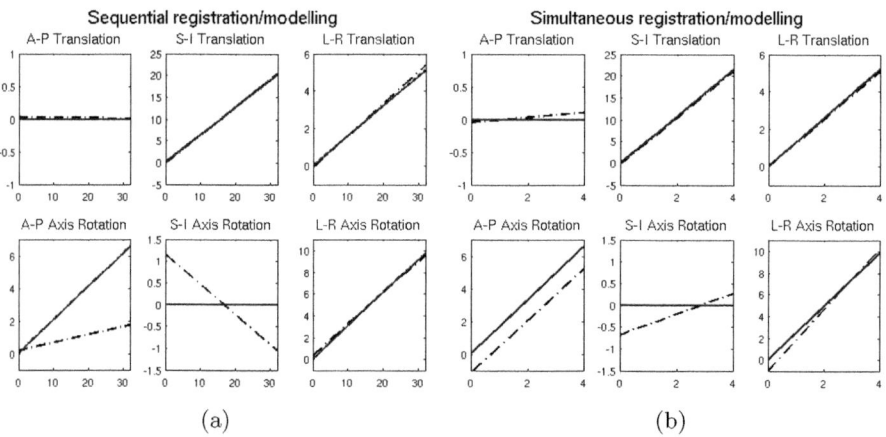

Fig. 4. Motion models for a sample numerical phantom dataset: (a) constructed using sequential registration/modelling; (b) constructed using simultaneous registration/modelling. There are 6 parameter plots in each figure, representing the 6 rigid body motion parameters: the anterior-posterior (A-P) translation; the superio-inferior (S-I) translation; the left-right (L-R) translation; and the three rotations about these axes. The gold standard motion model is shown using the solid blue lines in both figures. The black dotted lines represent the motion models constructed using the two approaches. The motion model constructed using the simultaneous approach is closer to the gold standard than the model constructed using the sequential approach.

The execution time (on a Dell Precision workstation featuring a 3.4GHz Quad-Core Intel Xeon processor) for constructing the motion models using the sequential approach varied between 13 minutes for 4 dynamics with no noise , up to 161 minutes for 32 dynamics with SNR = 1. Using the simultaneous approach, the execution times varied between 10 minutes and 96 minutes, although it should be noted that currently we use the sequential approach result as a starting estimate for the simultaneous approach.

3.2   Dynamic MRI Data

We ran experiments on the artificial dynamic MRI data acquired from 7 volunteers and 7 patients. The volunteers consisted of 1 female and 6 males and were aged between 20 and 32. Patients A and B were adult, aged 63 and 55, and were scanned as part of ongoing treatment for atrial fibrillation. Patients C-G were children, aged between 1 and 16, and were all undergoing treatment for congenital heart defects. Patients A, B and C were conscious and breathing freely during scanning. Patients D-G were all under general anaesthetic and had their breathing controlled by a ventillator. All volunteers underwent two dynamic MRI scans: one in which they breathed normally, and one in which they were instructed to breathe deeply. Separate motion models were constructed (using both sequential and simultaenous approaches) for the normal and deep breathing datasets. We acquired data for different breathing patterns because recent evidence in the literature has suggested that changes in breathing can lead to changes in the motion of internal organs [10]. For the patients only one dataset was acquired during normal breathing.

Table 1 summarises the results for the dynamic MRI datasets. Over all 21 datasets the average improvement for the simultaneous approach over the sequential approach was 1.8%. This improvement seems relatively small compared to the numerical phantom results. We believe that this is because of the larger voxel size of the dynamic MRI images, relative to the magnitude of the motion. The typical voxel size was $2.22 \times 2.22 \times 4.0$mm^3, compared to typical cardiac motions of 5-20mm during normal breathing. This introduces some uncertainty into the motion estimates and this effect may mask some of the improvement achievable from the simultaneous registration/modelling approach. This explanation is supported by the fact that the improvements were larger on the deep breathing datasets, in which the motion was larger relative to the voxel size. Nevertheless there was a clear reduction in errors over the 21 datasets (3.47 +/- 1.92mm for the simultaneous approach against 3.54 +/- 1.97mm for the normal sequential approach, $p < 0.01$ in a two-tailed paired t-test).

The execution times for constructing the motion models using the sequential approach varied between 45 and 103 seconds. For the simultaneous approach the execution times were between 70 and 230 seconds. These times are faster than those for the numerical phantom experiments because of the lower resolution of the dynamic MRI images.

Table 1. Motion model target registration errors (TREs) for dynamic MRI data acquired from 7 volunteers and 7 patients. The TRE figures were calculated over all 4 dynamic images for each dataset. Motion models were formed using the normal sequential approach to registration/modelling, and the proposed simultaneous approach. The right column shows the percentage improvement of the simultaneous approach over the sequential approach. A positive percentage indicates that the simultaneous approach had a lower TRE.

Subject	Breathing pattern	TRE of motion model(mm)		% improvement of simultaneous approach
		Sequential approach	Simultaneous approach	
Vol. A	Normal	4.73	4.71	+0.4%
	Deep	8.74	8.62	+2.2%
Vol. B	Normal	3.06	2.93	+4.3%
	Deep	3.26	3.33	-2.0%
Vol. C	Normal	2.44	2.34	+4.0%
	Deep	3.92	3.75	+4.4%
Vol. D	Normal	3.27	3.32	-1.4%
	Deep	3.8	3.67	+3.3%
Vol. E	Normal	2.08	2.07	+0.2%
	Deep	7.87	7.67	+2.5%
Vol. F	Normal	2.68	2.77	-3.1%
	Deep	4.52	4.3	+4.7%
Vol. G	Normal	2.59	2.66	-2.8%
	Deep	5.45	5.25	+3.7%
Pat. A (adult)	Normal	3.78	3.64	+3.8%
Pat. B (adult)	Normal	3.91	3.87	+1.0%
Pat. C (child)	Normal	1.88	1.84	+2.1%
Pat. D (child)	Normal	1.1	1.1	+0.6%
Pat. E (child)	Normal	1.01	0.99	+1.8%
Pat. F (child)	Normal	2.59	2.54	+2.0%
Pat. G (child)	Normal	1.61	1.56	+3.3%
Overall		3.54 +/- 1.97	3.47 +/- 1.92	+1.8%

4   Discussion

We have presented preliminary results for an approach to respiratory motion estimation and modelling in which the registrations of all dynamic images and the modelling process are performed simultaneously. Results on a numerical phantom and dynamic MRI data have suggested that modelling errors can be reduced using the proposed approach compared to the normal approach of registering each dynamic image separately and then subsequently modelling the variation of the estimated motion parameters. The numerical phantom experiments allowed us to test constructed motion models against a gold standard motion model. The dynamic MRI data was more realistic but had no gold standard motion model, only gold standard (nonrigid) motion fields for each dynamic image. This means that, in principle, it is possible to get a motion model error of zero for the numerical phantom experiments, whilst this will not be possible in most cases for the MRI experiments. Further validation and refinement of our technique is required, particularly with regard to the starting estimates for the model parameters and their optimisation, but we believe that this approach offers potential benefits to motion modelling, and has been relatively little explored in the literature.

The advantage of the simultaneous approach over the normal sequential approach is that it allows the registration to take advantage of prior knowledge of the 'smoothness' of the variation of the motion fields as a function of the surrogate value(s). The simultaneous registrations are constrained to find only solutions that are consistent with the constraints introduced by the motion model. This type of approach has previously been applied in image reconstruction. For example, in [11] free breathing CT data was reconstructed using a smooth motion constraint. The most similar techniques described in the literature are [7,8]. Our aim in this paper was to use a similar approach to estimate the optimal cardiac respiratory motion model given a sequence of dynamic images acquired at different points in the breathing cycle.

We used the mean squared difference as a similarity measure for both the numerical phantom and dynamic MRI experiments. Although more flexible similarity measures exist we believe that it was justified to use the mean squared difference because all of our registrations were intra-modality. We also used a relatively simple optimisation strategy (steepest gradient ascent) and motion model (first-order polynomials). We plan to investigate alternatives to these initial approaches in the future. For example, in recent years more sophisticated motion models have been proposed that can capture hysteresis effects [2,3] or the effects of different breathing patterns [10]. Also, currently we still use the result of the sequential approach as a starting estimate for the simultaneous approach. We plan to investigate alternative strategies for producing a starting estimate for the motion model, such as using a cross-population average breathing model.

The execution times for the sequential and simultaneous approaches are of the same order of magnitude. For the dynamic MRI experiments, each registration in the sequential approach involves optimising 9 parameters. This optimisation must be performed once for each dynamic image. For the simultaneous approach, using first-order polynomials, there is a single optimisation of 18 parameters (2 for each of the 9 affine motion parameters in the model). This leads to similar overall execution times. However, the rate at which execution time increases with respect to the number of model parameters is higher for the simultaneous approach. Therefore we believe that the technique as we describe it in this paper may only be feasible for relatively simple motion models, such as rigid or affine models. If this approach were to be applied to models based on freeform nonrigid registrations based on a large number of control points the execution time will become much larger. Clearly many organs exhibit motion that is more complex than rigid or affine motion descriptions are able to capture. We plan to tackle this issue by combining our simultaneous registration/modelling approach with a hierarchical local affine registration algorithm [12], enabling complex nonrigid motions to be captured by a combination of simpler affine motions.

The proposed simultaneous registration/modelling approach has potential application in a number of areas. For example, motion models have been applied in image-guided minimally invasive cardiac interventions [2,3] in which improved accuracy of respiratory motion prediction/correction could increase the utility of guidance information, therefore improving patient outcome. However, our intended application is thoracic motion-correction in a hybrid PET-MRI scanner. In this application improved motion predictions could lead to a reduction in motion artefacts in the resulting PET images, and consequently better resolution of tumours and other small structures. Overall, we believe that the technique we have described could offer potential benefits in a range of image acquisition applications and image guided interventions.

Acknowledgments

This work is part of the HYPERimage project which is supported by the European Union under the 7th framework program (201651).

References

1. Manke, D., Rosch, P., Nehrke, K., Bornert, P., Dossel, O.: Model evaluation and calibration for prospective respiratory motion correction in coronary MR angiography based on 3-D image registration. IEEE Transactions on Medical Imaging 21(9), 1132–1141 (2002)
2. Shechter, G., Shechter, B., Resar, J.R., Beyar, R.: Prospective motion correction of X-ray images for coronary interventions. IEEE Transactions on Medical Imaging 24(4), 441–450 (2005)
3. King, A.P., Boubertakh, R., Rhode, K.S., Ma, Y.L., Chinchapatnam, P., Gao, G., Tangcharoen, T., Ginks, M., Cooklin, M., Gill, J.S., Hawkes, D.J., Razavi, R.S., Schaeffter, T.: A subject-specific technique for respiratory motion correction in image-guided cardiac catheterisation procedures. Medical Image Analysis 13(3), 419–431 (2009)
4. Schreibmann, E., Thorndyke, B., Li, T., Wang, J., Xing, L.: Four-dimensional image registration for image-guided radiotherapy. Int. J. Radiation Oncology Biol. Phys. 71(2), 578–586 (2008)
5. Peyrat, J.M., Delingette, H., Sermesant, M., Pennec, X., Xu, C.Y., Ayache, N.: Registration of 4D time-series of cardiac images with multichannel diffeomorphic demons. In: Metaxas, D., Axel, L., Fichtinger, G., Székely, G. (eds.) MICCAI 2008, Part II. LNCS, vol. 5242, pp. 972–979. Springer, Heidelberg (2008)
6. Klein, G.J., Huesman, R.H.: Four-dimensional processing of deformable cardiac pet data. Medical Image Analysis 6(1), 29–46 (2002)
7. Shen, D., Sundar, H., Xue, Z., Fan, Y., Litt, H.: Consistent estimation of cardiac motions by 4D image registration. In: Duncan, J.S., Gerig, G. (eds.) MICCAI 2005. LNCS, vol. 3750, pp. 902–910. Springer, Heidelberg (2005)
8. Castillo, E., Castillo, R., Martinez, J., Shenoy, M., Guerrero, T.: Four-dimensional deformable image registration using trajectory modelling. Physics in Medicine and Biology 55, 305–327 (2010)

9. Rueckert, D., Sonoda, L.I., Hayes, C., Hill, D.L.G., Leach, M.O., Hawkes, D.J.: Non-rigid registration using free-form deformations: Application to breast MR images. IEEE Transactions on Medical Imaging 18(8), 712–721 (1999)

10. King, A.P., Rhode, K.S., Razavi, R.S., Schaeffter, T.R.: An adaptive and predictive respiratory motion model for image-guided interventions: Theory and first clinical application. IEEE Transactions on Medical Imaging 28(12), 2020–2032 (2009)

11. Hinkle, J., Fletcher, P.T., Wang, B., Salter, B., Joshi, S.H.: 4D MAP image reconstruction incorporating organ motion. In: Proceedings IPMI, pp. 676–687 (2009)

12. Buerger, C., Schaeffter, T., King, A.P.: Hierarchical adaptive local affine registration for respiratory motion estimation from 3-D MRI. In: Proceedings ISBI, pp. 1237–1241 (2010)

Model-Based Registration for Motion Compensation during EP Ablation Procedures

Alexander Brost[1], Rui Liao[2], Joachim Hornegger[1], and Norbert Strobel[3]

[1] Pattern Recognition Lab, Department of Computer Science,
Friedrich-Alexander-University Erlangen-Nuremberg, Erlangen, Germany
Alexander.Brost@informatik.uni-erlangen.de
[2] Siemens Corporate Research, Imaging and Visualization, Princeton, NJ, USA
[3] Siemens AG, Forchheim, Germany

Abstract. Radio-frequency catheter ablation (RFCA) has become an accepted treatment option for atrial fibrillation (Afib). RFCA of Afib involves isolation of the pulmonary veins under X-ray guidance. For easier navigation, two-dimensional X-ray imaging may take advantage of overlay images derived from static pre-operative 3-D data set to add anatomical details which, otherwise, would not be visible under X-ray. Unfortunately, respiratory and cardiac motion may impair the utility of static overlay images for catheter navigation. We developed a system for image-based 2-D motion estimation and compensation as a solution to this problem. It is based on 2-D catheter tracking facilitated by model-based registration of an ellipse-shaped model to fluorosocpic images. A mono-plane or a bi-plane X-ray C-arm system can be used. In the first step of the method, a 2-D model of the catheter device is computed. Respiratory and cardiac motion at the site of ablation is then estimated by tracking the catheter device in fluoroscopic images. The cost function of the registration step is based on the average distance of the model to the segmented circumferential mapping catheter using a distance map. In our experiments, the circumferential catheter was successfully tracked in 688 fluoroscopic images with an average 2-D tracking error of 0.59 mm $\pm$ 0.25 mm. Our presented method achieves a tracking rate of 10 frames-per-second.

1 Introduction

In the United States about two million people are affected by some form of atrial fibrillation (AF), making AF the most common sustained heart arrhythmia and a leading cause of stroke. Radio-frequency catheter ablation (RFCA) has become an accepted option for treating AF in today's electrophysiology (EP) labs, especially, if drug treatment has become ineffective [1,2]. RFCA of the pulmonary veins (PVs) usually requires fluoroscopic guidance. Unfortunately, X-ray images cannot distinguish soft tissue well. To address this issue, image integration combining pre-operative 3-D atrial CT data or MR volumes with the fluoroscopic images has been developed, commonly known as fluoroscopic overlay image guidance. The advantage of this strategy is the fused display of the actual, real-time fluoroscopic images

B. Fischer, B. Dawant, and C. Lorenz (Eds.): WBIR 2010, LNCS 6204, pp. 234–245, 2010.

together with the highly detailed soft-tissue images from CT or MRI [3,4,5,6]. In fact, state-of-the art C-arm systems [7,8], facilitate 3-D tomographic reconstruction. In other words, the fluoroscopic C-arm device itself can be used to obtain volumetric data sets, e.g., of the heart [9,10,11,12,13,14]. Since the 3-D data has been acquired on the same device that is used for 2-D X-ray imaging, initial registration of the 3-D data set to the 2-D fluoroscopic projection can be accomplished. The use of data sets from other modalities, e.g., CT, MR or even 3-D ultra-sound is possible. However, 2-D/3-D registration needs to be performed.

Current fluoroscopic overlay techniques are, however, static, i.e., they do not follow the heart while it beats and moves through the breathing cycle. To achieve a dynamic fused visualization, we need to take this motion into account. Unfortunately, there are few discernible features in typical EP fluoroscopic images. A first approach for 3-D respiratory motion compensation based on 3-D device tracking was proposed by the authors in [15,16], but this approach required continuous bi-plane fluoroscopy increasing the amount of X-ray dose. In this paper, we describe a method that requires only mono-plane fluoroscopy and therefore works in 2-D. To perform motion estimation, we still track the circumferential mapping catheter, a commonly available EP catheter. Since this device is often used for PV ablations, there is no need for additional instruments or fiducial markers. In addition, the mapping catheter is of unique shape, and it is one of the most prominent structures shown in EP fluoroscopy scenes, representing a good feature for robust tracking. During pulmonary vein isolation, the circumferential mapping catheter is typically fixed at the ostium of the PV that is to be ablated. Hence, by tracking the circumferential mapping catheter, we can obtain a motion estimate right at the ablation site. Once an estimate of the 2-D motion is available, we can, e.g., apply it to the static fluoroscopic overlay image to generate an animated representation of it moving in sync with the tracked device.

2 Two-Dimensional Model Generation

The circumferential mapping catheter on the imaging plane is extracted by manual clicking followed by fast marching in the first frame of the fluoroscopy sequence, as explained in [17]. This step provides the points $\mathbf{p}_i = (u_i, v_i)^T$ with $i = 1, \ldots, N$ of the catheter device. The 2-D ellipses are then calculated such that all ellipse points satisfy the linear equation [18]

$$au_i^2 + bu_iv_i + cv_i^2 + du_i + ev_i + f = 0 \tag{1}$$

with the 2-D coordinates u and v. The points $\mathbf{p}_i$ of the catheter are combined in a measurement matrix [19]

$$\mathbf{M} = \begin{pmatrix} u_1^2 & u_1v_1 & v_1^2 & u_1 & v_1 & 1 \\ \vdots & \vdots & \vdots & \vdots & \vdots & \vdots \\ u_i^2 & u_iv_i & v_i^2 & u_i & v_i & 1 \\ \vdots & \vdots & \vdots & \vdots & \vdots & \vdots \\ u_N^2 & u_Nv_N & v_N^2 & u_N & v_N & 1 \end{pmatrix}. \tag{2}$$

Then Eq. (1) can be rewritten as

$$\mathbf{M} \cdot \mathbf{f} = 0 \tag{3}$$

with the implicit ellipse parameters $\mathbf{f} = (a, b, c, d, e, f)^T$. As the points may not necessarily lie exactly on the ellipse to be fitted, we are looking for the ellipse parameters $\hat{\mathbf{f}}$ that minimize

$$\hat{\mathbf{f}} = \arg\min_{\mathbf{f}} ||\mathbf{M}\mathbf{f}||_2^2 \tag{4}$$

subject to

$$b^2 - 4ac < 0. \tag{5}$$

Errors in the points $\mathbf{p}_i$ used for the measurement matrix $\mathbf{M}$ lead to different estimated parameters $\hat{\mathbf{f}}$. Since a fast-marching algorithm is used to extract many points along the catheter in the fluoroscopic image, user errors due to inaccurate clicking, have rather little impact. Unfortunately, the constraint, $||\mathbf{f}||_2 = 1$, commonly used for ellipse fitting [19], does not necesarily guarantee an elliptic solution. Therefore, the method presented in [18] has been applied. It proposes to use the constraint $b^2 - 4ac < 0$ to assure an elliptical solution [20,21].

Given the implicit ellipse parameters $\hat{\mathbf{f}} = (\hat{a}, \hat{b}, \hat{c}, \hat{d}, \hat{e}, \hat{f})^T$, the explicit parameters can be calculated. To this end, we use the following substitution

$$(\hat{a}, \hat{b}, \hat{c}, \hat{d}, \hat{e}, \hat{f})^T = (\tilde{a}, 2\tilde{b}, \tilde{c}, 2\tilde{d}, 2\tilde{e}, \tilde{f})^T. \tag{6}$$

The center of the ellipse $\mathbf{q}_c = (u_c, v_c)^T$ is calculated by [22,23,24]

$$u_c = \frac{\tilde{b}\tilde{e} - \tilde{c}\tilde{d}}{\tilde{a}\tilde{c} - \tilde{b}^2} \tag{7}$$

$$v_c = \frac{\tilde{b}\tilde{d} - \tilde{a}\tilde{e}}{\tilde{a}\tilde{c} - \tilde{b}^2}. \tag{8}$$

The lengths of the semi-axes, l_1 and l_2, are then calculated by

$$l_1 = \sqrt{\frac{|2(\tilde{a}\tilde{c}\tilde{f} + 2\tilde{b}\tilde{d}\tilde{e} - \tilde{a}\tilde{e}^2 - \tilde{c}\tilde{d}^2 - \tilde{f}\tilde{b}^2)|}{|(\tilde{a}\tilde{c} - \tilde{b}^2) \cdot (\tilde{a} + \tilde{c} + \sqrt{(\tilde{c} - \tilde{a})^2 + 4\tilde{b}^2})|}} \tag{9}$$

$$l_2 = \sqrt{\frac{|2(\tilde{a}\tilde{c}\tilde{f} + 2\tilde{b}\tilde{d}\tilde{e} - \tilde{a}\tilde{e}^2 - \tilde{c}\tilde{d}^2 - \tilde{f}\tilde{b}^2)|}{|(\tilde{a}\tilde{c} - \tilde{b}^2) \cdot (-\tilde{a} - \tilde{c} + \sqrt{(\tilde{c} - \tilde{a})^2 + 4\tilde{b}^2})|}}. \tag{10}$$

The rotation within the 2-D image plane is given as

$$\gamma = \frac{1}{2} \arctan\left(\frac{2\tilde{b}}{\tilde{c} - \tilde{a}}\right). \tag{11}$$

The explicit ellipse parameters are summarized in Figure 1. Discrete sample points $\mathbf{q}_\theta$ of the ellipse can then be obtained by [25]

$$\mathbf{q}_\theta = \mathbf{q}_c + l_1 \cdot \cos\theta \cdot \mathbf{R}_\gamma \mathbf{e}_1 + l_2 \cdot \sin\theta \cdot \mathbf{R}_\gamma \mathbf{e}_2. \tag{12}$$

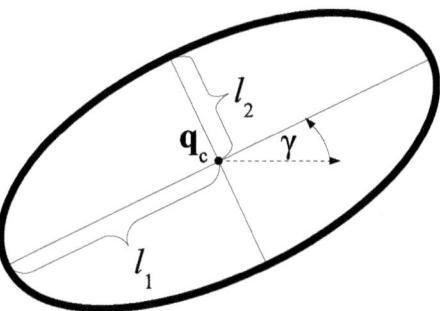

Fig. 1. An ellipse is described by its center, $\mathbf{q}_c$, its semi-axes, l_1 and l_2, and its rotation in the 2-D plane, γ

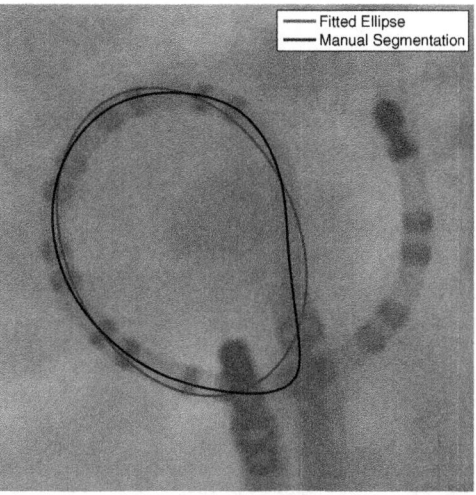

Fig. 2. Illustration of the model error for the first frame of clinical sequence 10. The manual segmentation is taken as a gold standard rerference. The resulting model error is 0.78 mm in this case. The model error is the difference between the manually outlined catheter and the fitted ellipse.

To this end, the parameter $\theta \in [0, 2\pi]$ is used for computing points along the ellipse, i.e., each θ produces a $\mathbf{q}_\theta$. The unit vectors of the coordinate system are called $\mathbf{e}_1 = (1, 0)^T$ and $\mathbf{e}_2 = (0, 1)^T$. The 2-D rotation matrix is denoted as

$$\mathbf{R}_\gamma = \begin{pmatrix} \cos\gamma & -\sin\gamma \\ \sin\gamma & \cos\gamma \end{pmatrix}. \tag{13}$$

The model may not always fit perfectly. The difference between model and the actual catheter is called model error. It is obtained by calculating the distance of the model to a gold standard segmentation in the first frame of a sequence.

The model error is the difference between the manually outlined catheter and the fitted ellipse. An illustration of this idea is presented in Figure 2.

3   Catheter Tracking by Registration

3.1   Feature Extraction and Distance Map Calculation

After the catheter model has been generated from the first frame of the fluoroscopic sequence, it is tracked throughout the remainder of the sequence. To speed up the computational efficiency and to minimize the influence of peripheral structures that could interfere with catheter tracking, the region of interest (ROI) for tracking is restricted to 400×400 pixels (on the 1024×1024 image) around the center of the tracked mapping catheter in the previous frame. Histogram equalization is further applied on the ROI to enhance the structure of the

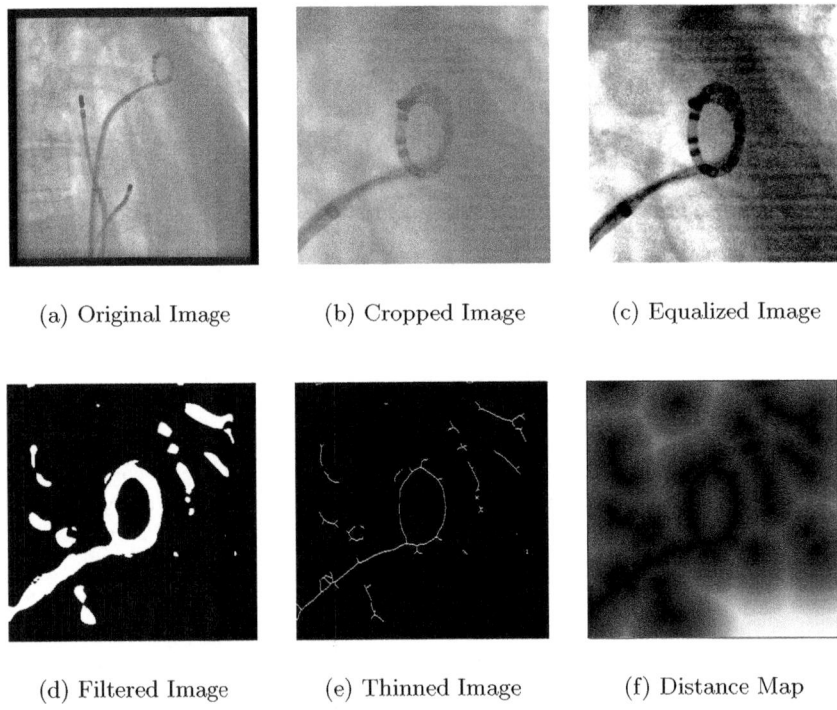

(a) Original Image   (b) Cropped Image   (c) Equalized Image

(d) Filtered Image   (e) Thinned Image   (f) Distance Map

Fig. 3. Image processing steps to enhance the elliptical structure of the catheter. This is needed to obtain a good registration. First, the acquired fluoroscopic image is cropped. The second step involves histogram equalization to enhance semi-transparent parts of the catheter. Afterwards, a vessel enhancement filter is applied to improve the structure of the catheter. It is then binarized using Otsu's method. As the catheter is usually wider than the model, a thinning algorithm is also applied. A distance map is computed next based on the thinned catheter representation. The final distance map provides a smooth image for model-based registration.

catheter. Next, a vessel enhancement filter as proposed in [26] is used to improve line-like structures such as the circumferential mapping catheter. The feature image is then binarized using Otsu's method [27] to facilitate segmentation of the mapping catheter. As the model has only a diameter of one pixel, we further apply a skeletonization algorithm as proposed in [28] to thin the segmentation. Finally, a distance map is calculated from the binarized image [29]. A distance map encodes the distance from a point to its closest feature point, that is the nonzero point representing the extracted mapping catheter in our binarized feature image. The distance transform offers an important advantage. It provides a denoised representation of the fluoroscopic image with a pronounced minimum around the shape of the mapping catheter. The distance map is denoted as $\mathbf{I}_{DT}$, with $\mathbf{I}_{DT}(\mathbf{p})$ returning the distance of pixel position $\mathbf{p}$ to the segmented catheter. The image processing steps are summarized in Figure 3.

3.2   Model-Based Registration

Circumferential catheter model tracking is achieved by performing model-based registration. The catheter model is translated by $\mathbf{t} = (\Delta_u, \Delta_v)$. The offset in u-direction is called $\Delta_u \in \mathbb{Z}$, and the offset in v-direction is referred to as $\Delta_v \in \mathbb{Z}$. The average distance between catheter model and segmentation in the fluoroscopic image is then considered as the cost value. It is calculated by using the distance map introduced above. The optimal translation $\hat{\mathbf{t}}$ is found by optimizing

$$\hat{\mathbf{t}} = \arg \min_{\mathbf{t}} \sum_{\theta} \mathbf{I}_{DT}(\mathbf{q}_\theta + \mathbf{t}) \tag{14}$$

with the distance map $\mathbf{I}_{DT}$ and θ as explained in the context of Eq. 12 above. The best parameters are found by nearest neighbor optimization, i.e., the position of the local optimum on a large scale is used as starting point for the next optimization on a smaller scale. We start with a 400×400 ROI and perform optimization with a step size of 16 pixels in each direction. Once we reach a local optimum, we reduce the step size to one pixel in u and v direction on a 16×16 sub-ROI. Since the shape of mapping catheters may not be exactly elliptical, a simple elliptical model may not always fit perfectly. Thanks to the properties of the distance map, we still end up with a good solution in most cases. A nearest neighbor optimizer is used to iteratively optimize the translational parameters. The estimated 2-D translation $\hat{\mathbf{t}}$ can be directly applied to the 2-D overlay to move it in sync with the tracked device.

4   Experimental Evaluation and Results

We evaluated our algorithm by calculating the tracking error for each X-ray image over seven different clinical fluoroscopy sequences that were acquired during EP procedures on an AXIOM Artis dBA C-arm system (Siemens AG, Forchheim, Germany). Although our data was acquired on a bi-plane system, our motion estimation approach is not restricted to such a system and will work

Table 1. Average tracking error for the clinical sequences used. The last row shows an average over all the 17 sequences. The total number of frames was 688.

No.	Mean ± Std.	Model Error
1	0.40 mm ± 0.04 mm	0.39 mm
2	0.80 mm ± 0.11 mm	0.67 mm
3	0.63 mm ± 0.13 mm	0.37 mm
4	0.47 mm ± 0.09 mm	0.37 mm
5	0.32 mm ± 0.04 mm	0.29 mm
6	0.63 mm ± 0.15 mm	0.30 mm
7	0.92 mm ± 0.26 mm	0.59 mm
8	0.63 mm ± 0.10 mm	0.56 mm
9	0.48 mm ± 0.05 mm	0.54 mm
10	1.05 mm ± 0.20 mm	0.87 mm
11	0.46 mm ± 0.07 mm	0.42 mm
12	0.77 mm ± 0.22 mm	0.53 mm
13	0.66 mm ± 0.11 mm	0.52 mm
14	0.55 mm ± 0.16 mm	0.35 mm
15	0.60 mm ± 0.12 mm	0.50 mm
16	0.69 mm ± 0.10 mm	0.58 mm
17	0.64 mm ± 0.15 mm	0.51 mm
μ	**0.59 mm ± 0.25 mm**	**0.49 mm**

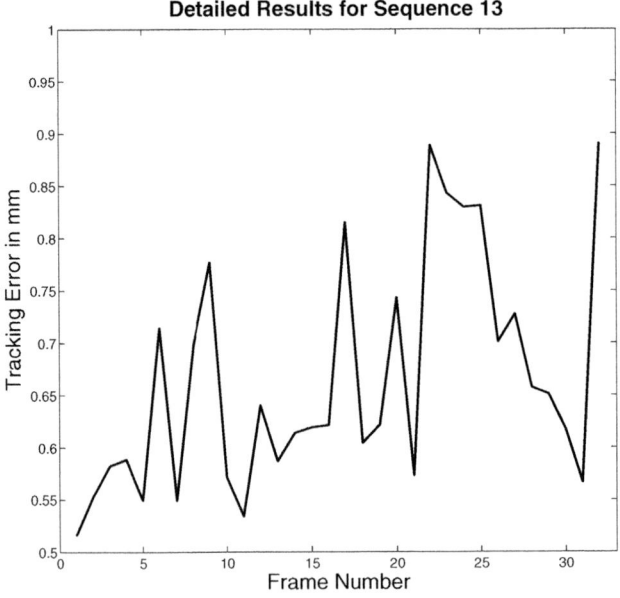

Fig. 4. Frame-by-frame tracking error in mm for sequence no. 13. The average tracking error is 0.66 mm ± 0.11 mm. The model error for this sequence is 0.52 mm.

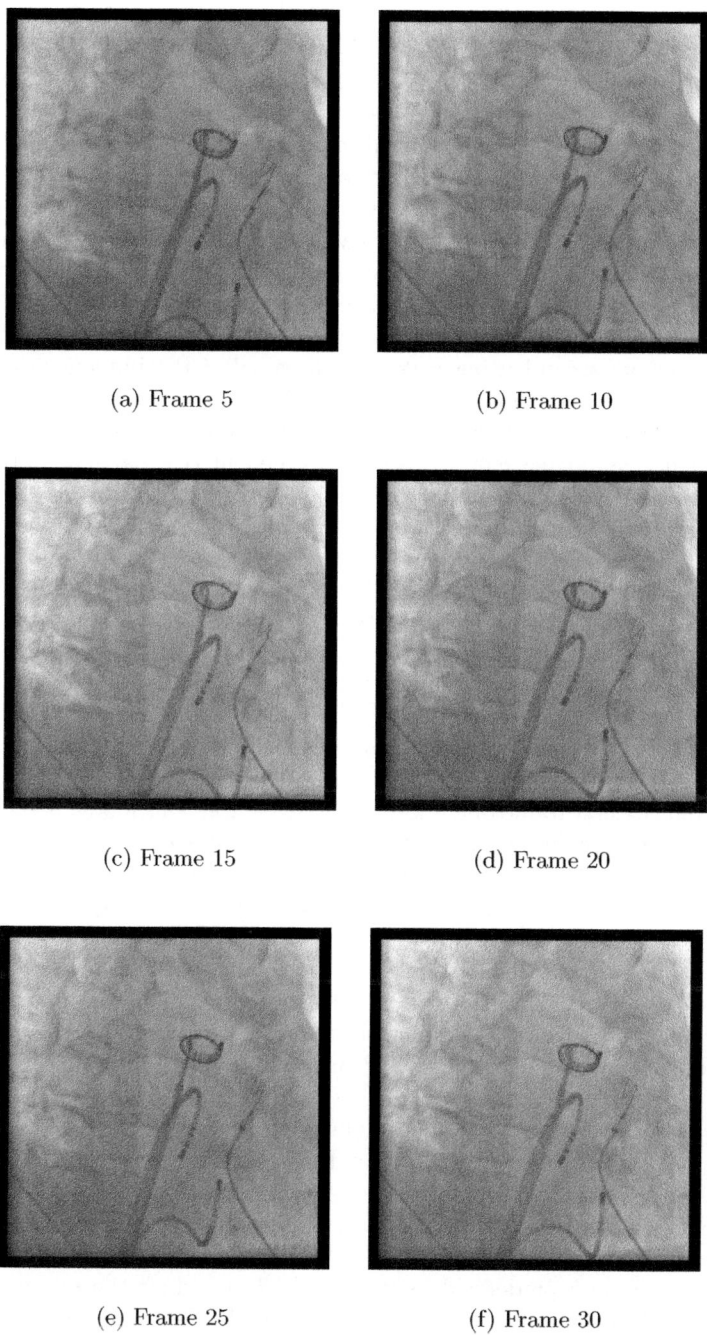

(a) Frame 5   (b) Frame 10

(c) Frame 15   (d) Frame 20

(e) Frame 25   (f) Frame 30

Fig. 5. Six frames of sequence no. 13. The red ellipse shows the tracked circumferential mapping catheter. It aligns well with the outer part of the (spiral) mapping catheter.

on a mono-plane device as well. We focus on a typical setup involving a circumferential mapping catheter and one ablation catheter only. The presence of other structures should not decrease the accuracy of our method, because we use an unique elliptical structure for registration. To evaluate the tracking error, we calculated the average distance of the forward tracked catheter model to a manually segmented circumferential mapping catheter. The manual catheter segmentation was supervised by a cardiologist, and we consider it our reference result. This distance was averaged over all frames of a particular sequence to arrive at an overall tracking error for each sequence. We tested our method on 17 clinical data sets. The results are summarized in Table 1. The average of the mean tracking error over all 17 sequences - 688 frames - was 0.59 mm. Figure 5 shows six frames of sequence 13. Our method currently achieves a frame rate of 10 frames-per-second using a (single threaded) CPU implementation. This is sufficiet for clinical applications. In addition to the tracking error, a model error can be calculated. The model error can be obtained from the first image of a sequence as no registration was performed in this particular frame. The model errors ranged between 0.31 mm and 0.78 mm. A detailed frame-by-frame tracking error for sequence no. 13 is presented in Fig. 4.

5   Discussion and Conclusions

We developed a method for respiratory and cardiac motion estimation for radio-frequency catheter ablation of atrial fibrillation. A C-Arm X-ray system is used to image a circumferential (or spiral) mapping catheter. Catheter tracking is based on a model-based registration framework. We start by estimating a catheter model from the first frame of a fluoroscopic sequence. This model is then tracked throughout the remainder of the sequence using model-based registration. The registration is based on a distance map derived from the fluoroscopic image of the catheter. Our experiments on clinical EP fluoroscopy sequences show that the mean 2-D tracking error is 0.59 mm including an average model error of 0.49 mm. Considering that breathing motion in typical EP fluoroscopy images is in the range of 15 mm and for for deep breathing in some patients up to 40 mm, our method has the potential to significantly improve the accuracy of fluoroscopy overlay techniques for EP navigation. The proposed method offers several advantages. First, it is workflow-friendly and does not require fiducial markers or additional contrast agent to be administered. Second, respiratory and cardiac motion is estimated directly at the ablation site. Due to the fact that registration is used, motion estimation and compensation is essentially done in one step. Third, we estimate the motion online and update it constantly from fluoroscopy with a frame rate up to 10 frames-per-second. Furthermore, we do not rely on a predefined motion model from which the real motion may deviate significantly during the procedure. Fourth, there are no restrictions on the 3-D data set that can be used as a fluoro overlay. A 3-D data set could come from MRI, CT or C-arm CT, e.g., *syngo* DynaCT Cardiac (Siemens AG, Forchheim, Germany). Unlike a previous approach that involved 3-D tracking based on bi-plane imaging [15,16], the proposed method tracks a device in a 2-D mono-plane fluoroscopic sequence. This method puts fewer restrictions on model generation and registration, since there is no second view to match against. As a consequence, it is possible to obtain a better fit of the model in the 2-D fluoroscopic images, i.e., a lower 2-D tracking error. However, this does not necessarily imply better 3-D tracking. Nevertheless, since the motion of the LA can be approximated by a 3-D rigid-body transform [30] and because the LA offers only limited space to move about, we expect that a 2-D motion estimate may offer an acceptable approximation. How well 2-D tracking of a device and a 3-D tracking, however, really relate to each other during EP procedures is subject of further studies.

Acknowledgements

The authors would like to thank Dr. med. Johannes Rieber for the gold-standard catheter segmentation, Andreas Wimmer for a tool to manually outline catheters easily, and Teri Moore for collecting the clinical data.

References

1. Cappato, R., Calkins, H., Chen, S.A., Davies, W., Iesaka, Y., Kalman, J., Kim, Y.H., Klein, G., Packer, D., Skanes, A.: Worldwide Survey on the Methods, Efficacy, and Safety of Catheter Ablation for Human Atrial Fibrillation. Circulation - Journal of the American Heart Association 111, 1100–1105 (2005)
2. Wazni, O.M., Marrouche, N.F., Martin, D.O., Verma, A., Bhargava, M., Saliba, W., Bash, D., Schweikert, R., Brachmann, J., Gunther, J., Gutleben, K., Potenza, E.P.D., Fanelli, R., Raviele, A., Themistoclakis, S., Rossillo, A., Bonso, A., Natale, A.: Radiofrequency ablation vs antiarrhythmic drugs as first-line treatment of symptomatic atrial fibrillation: a randomized trial. JAMA 293(21), 2634–2640 (2005)
3. Zagorchev, et al.: Rapid fusion of 2D x-ray fluoroscopy with 3D multislice CT for image-guided electrophysiology procedures. In: Proceedings of SPIE: Medical Imaging 2007, vol. 6509, p. 65092B (2007)
4. Sra, J., Narayan, G., Krum, D., Malloy, A., Colley, R., Bhatia, A., Dhala, A., Blanck, Z., Nangia, V., Akhtar, M.: Computed Tomography-Fluoroscopy Image Integration-Guided Catheter Ablation of Atrial Fibrillation. Journal of Cardiovascular Electrophysiology 18(4), 409–414 (2007)
5. Ector, J., Buck, S.D., Huybrechts, W., Nuyens, D., Dymarkowski, S., Bogaert, J., Maes, F., Heidüchel, H.: Biplane three-dimensional augmented fluoroscopy as single navigation tool for ablation of atrial fibrillation: Accuracy and clinical value. Heart Rhythm 5(7), 957–964 (2008)
6. Knecht, S., Skali, H., O'Neill, M.D., Wright, M., Matsuo, S., Chaudhry, G.M., Haffajee, C.I., Nault, I., Gijsbers, G.H.M., Sacher, F., Laurent, F., Montaudon, M., Corneloup, O., Hocini, M., Haissaguerre, M., Orlov, M.V., Jais, P.: Computed tomography-fluoroscopy overlay evaluation during catheter ablation of left atrial arrhythmia. Europace 10, 931–938 (2008)

7. Hertrich, P.H.: Practical Radiography - Principles and Applications, 1st edn. Publicis Corporate Publishing (May 2005)
8. Oppelt, A. (ed.): Imaging Systems for Medical Diagnostics, 2nd edn. Publicis Corporate Publishing (November 2005)
9. Orlov, M.V., Hoffmeister, P., Chaudhry, G.M., Almasry, I., Gijsbers, G.H.M., Swack, T., Haffajee, C.I.: Three-dimensional rotational angiography of the left atrium and esophagus: a virtual computed tomography scan in the electrophysiology lab? Heart Rhythm 4(1), 37–43 (2007)
10. Al-Ahmad, A., Wigstrm, L., Sandner-Porkristl, D., Wang, P.J., Zei, P.C., Boese, J., Lauritsch, G., Moore, T., Chan, F., Fahrig, R.: Time-resolved three-dimensional imaging of the left atrium and pulmonary veins in the interventional suite: A comparison between multisweep gated rotational three-dimensional reconstructed fluoroscopy and multislice computed tomography. Heart Rhythm 5(4), 513–519 (2008)
11. Nölker, G., Gutleben, K.J., Marschang, H., Ritscher, G., Asbach, S., Marrouche, N., Brachmann, J., Sinha, A.M.: Three-dimensional left atrial and esophagus reconstruction using cardiac C-arm computed tomography with image integration into fluoroscopic views for ablation of atrial fibrillation: Accuracy of a novel modality in comparison with multislice computed tomography. Heart Rhythm 5(12), 1651–1657 (2008)
12. Strobel, N., Meissner, O., Boese, J., Brunner, T., Heigl, B., Hoheisel, M., Lauritsch, G., Nagel, M., Pfister, M., Rührnschopf, E.P., Scholz, B., Schreiber, B., Spahn, M., Zellerhoff, M., Klingenbeck-Regn, K.: Imaging with Flat-Detector C-Arm Systems. In: Reiser, M.F., Becker, C.R., Nikolaou, K., Glazer, G. (eds.) Multislice CT (Medical Radiology / Diagnostic Imaging), 3rd edn., pp. 33–51. Springer, Heidelberg (2009)
13. Pruemmer, et al.: Cardiac C-arm CT: a unified framework for motion estimation and dynamic CT. IEEE Transactions on Medical Imaging 28(11), 1836–1849 (2009)
14. Lauritsch, et al.: Towards cardiac C-arm computed tomography. IEEE Transactions on Medical Imaging 28(7), 922–934 (2006)
15. Brost, A., Liao, R., Hornegger, J., Strobel, N.: 3-D Respiratory Motion Compensation during EP Procedures by Image-Based 3-D Lasso Catheter Model Generation and Tracking. In: Yang, G.-Z., Hawkes, D., Rueckert, D., Noble, A., Taylor, C. (eds.) MICCAI 2009. LNCS, vol. 5761, pp. 394–401. Springer, Heidelberg (2009)
16. Brost, A., Liao, R., Hornegger, J., Strobel, N.: 3D model-based catheter tracking for motion compensation in EP procedures, vol. 7625, 762507. SPIE, San Jose (2010)
17. Liao, et al.: Location Constraint Based 2D-3D Registration of Fluoroscopic Images of CT Volumes for Image-Guided EP Procedures. In: Proceedings of SPIE: Medical Imaging 2008, vol. 6918, p. 69182T (2008)
18. Halir, F.: Numerically Stable Direct Least Squares Fitting of Ellipses. In: Proceedings of the 6th Conference in Central Europe on Computer Graphics and Visualization, pp. 253–257 (1998)
19. Hartley, Z.: Multiple View Geometry in Computer Vision, 2nd edn. Cambridge University Press, Cambridge (2004)
20. Fitzgibbon, A., Pilu, M., Fisher, R.B.: Direct least square fitting of ellipses. IEEE Transactions on Pattern Analysis And Machine Intelligence 21(5), 476–480 (1999)
21. Fitzgibbon, A.W., Fisher, R.B.: A Buyer's Guide to Conic Fitting. In: BMVC 1995: Proceedings of the 6th British Conference on Machine Vision, Surrey, UK, vol. 2, pp. 513–522. BMVA Press (September 1995)

22. Bronstein, I.N., Semendjajew, K.A., Musiol, G., Mühlig, H.: Taschenbuch der Mathematik, 5th edn. Verlag Harri Deutsch, Thun und Frankfurt am Main (2001)
23. Poole, D.: Linear Algebra - A Modern Introduction, 1st edn. Brooks Cole (2002)
24. Zwillinger, D.: CRC Standard Mathematical Tables and Formulae, 31th edn. Chapman & Hall/CRC (2002)
25. Hearn, D., Baker, M.P.: Computer Graphics with OpenGL. Pearson Prentice Hall, London (2004)
26. Sato, et al.: 3D Multi-Scale Line Filter for Segmentation and Visualization of Curvilinear Structures in Medical Images. Medical Image Analysis 2(2), 143–168 (1998)
27. Otsu, N.: A Threshold Selection Method from Gray-Level Histograms. IEEE Transactions on Systems, Man, and Cybernetics 9(1), 62–66 (1979)
28. Cychosz, J.M.: Efficient Binary Image Thinning using Neighborhood Maps, pp. 465–473 (1994)
29. Breu, et al.: Linear time Euclidean distance transform algorithms. IEEE Transactions on Pattern Analysis and Machine Intelligence 17, 529–533 (1995)
30. Ector, et al.: Changes in Left Atrial Anatomy Due to Respiration: Impact on Three-Dimensional Image Integration During Atrial Fibrillation Ablation. Journal of Cardiovascular Electrophysiology 19(7), 828–834 (2008)

Spatial Information Encoded Mutual Information for Nonrigid Registration

Xiahai Zhuang, David J. Hawkes, and Sebastien Ourselin

Centre for Medical Image Computing, Department of Medical Physics and
Bioengineering, University College London
x.zhuang@ucl.ac.uk
http://www.cs.ucl.ac.uk/staff/x.zhuang/

Abstract. We propose a new nonrigid registration method based on
a unified framework of encoding spatial information in entropy measures. The encoding of spatial information improves nonrigid registration
against the problems caused by intensity distortion where the registration using traditional mutual information (MI) is challenged. Using this
encoding framework, we derive the new registration method, spatial information encoded mutual information (SIEMI). SIEMI registration has
a similar computation complexity as the registration using traditional MI
measures, but works significantly better in the nonrigid cases. We validated the registration method using brain MRI and dynamic contrast
enhanced MRI of the liver. The results showed that the proposed method
performed significantly better than the normalized mutual information
registration.

1 Introduction

Mutual information (MI) [1,2,3] is one of the most widely studied techniques
for biomedical image registration in the last fifteen years. The registration using
MI measures, including the normalized forms such as the normalized mutual
information (NMI) [4], has shown good robustness and wide applicability [5,6].
However, several recent works [7,8,9,10] showed that the traditional MI measures
may not be appropriate in many situations for nonrigid registration.

The first common situation happens in registering *in vivo* medical images,
which have *intensity non-uniformity* (INU), also referred to as intensity distortion or intensity bias. This INU results in the same tissue in different positions
having different intensity values, and thus some regions of the tissue having different *intensity classes*. Since patterns of INU fields vary in different images, the
inconsistency of intensity classes of one tissue in two images will lead to large
errors in nonrigid registration. Fig. 1 shows an example of registering two initially aligned brain MR images, where one contains INU while the other does
not. The nonrigid registration using NMI measure [4] generates a large erroneous
resultant deformation field. Fig. 1 (d) shows a more promising result using the
proposed method which will be described later. This method demonstrates a
much better robustness against the INU field.

B. Fischer, B. Dawant, and C. Lorenz (Eds.): WBIR 2010, LNCS 6204, pp. 246–257, 2010.
© Springer-Verlag Berlin Heidelberg 2010

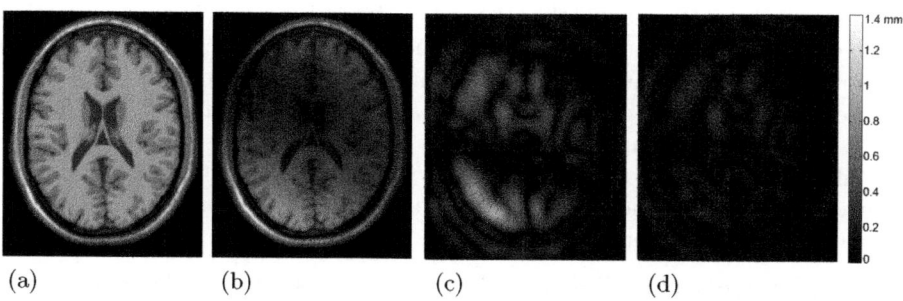

Fig. 1. (a) T1-weighted brain image without intensity non-uniformity (INU) and (b) the INU field computed from the subtraction of (a) and the image with INU. (c) is the resultant deformation field of registering (a) to the image with INU using NMI measure and (d) is the result using the proposed registration method. The color bar indicates the displacement magnitude in (c) and (d). Brain data downloaded from BrainWeb (www.bic.mni.mcgill.ca/brainweb/)

Other situations include the nonrigid registration of dynamic contrast enhanced MRI [11], perfusion MRI [12], and multi-modality images such as the CT-MR registration application [9]. It is still challenging to employ traditional MI measures for the nonrigid registration of these tasks.

To tackle the problems, Studholme *et al.* and Loeckx *et al.* proposed to consider the spatial coordinate as an extra channel of information and combine this information with the MI measure such as the regional mutual information (RMI) [7] and the conditional mutual information (cMI) [8,9]. The cMI measure was shown to be equivalent to the derived measure of RMI, referred to as RMI' in [7], by using a different Parzen window estimation function for the spatial variable [9,10]. Loeckx *et al.* further showed that the cMI registration performed better than the registration using the original RMI similarity form [9].

In this work, we extend the generalized weighting scheme for spatial information encoding in the previous work [10] to propose a new registration method. The weighting scheme is to vary the contribution of pixels to a set of joint histogram tables which are associated with a spatial variable. The registration measure, spatial information encoded mutual information (SIEMI), is a vector consisting of a set of entropy measures computed from these joint histogram tables.

The rest of the paper is organized as follows: Section 2 presents the SIEMI method; Section 3 provides the validation experiments, where discussion is also included; finally, our conclusions are given in Section 4.

2   Method

2.1   Definition of Terms and Notations

Intensity distribution: Intensity distribution describes the appearance and contrast of organs or tissues presented in a medical image.

Intensity class: We assume that the imaged intensity values in our registration images, such as MRI data, are related to the tissue types. Therefore, in an image scanned from n_{tis} types of tissues, n_{tis} intensity values should be presented. However, the intensity of one tissue normally has an intensity range in *in vivo* scans due to the non-uniformity of tissue property and noise. Also, a number of different tissues, referred to as a class of tissues, may have their intensity ranges overlapped. Hence, the intensity distribution is presented as n_C classes of intensity ranges, referred to as intensity classes.

Global intensity class linkage: The intensity class correspondence, reflecting the true joint intensity distribution of the two images, is normally unknown before registration due to the misalignment in local regions. By assuming the two images initially close to a true match and considering the local misalignment as noise, we can estimate this correspondence using the approximated joint intensity distribution from the global intensity information of the two images [13]. This global information, providing important guidance for correcting misaligned local regions, is referred to as *global intensity class linkage*.

Spatial variable s and local region Ω_s: Spatial variable s is an index of a set of spatial positions, $s = 1 \dots n_s$. The positions are defined according to the nonrigid transformation parameters. For example, in fluid registration each pixel (or voxel) can be defined as a value of spatial variable, while in free-form deformation (FFD) registration each control point can be defined as a value of s. It is commonly to define a local region Ω_s for s such as the user-defined cubic regions [7] or the local support volume of the FFD control point [8].

2.2   The Framework of Spatial Information Encoding

Spatial information encoding is achieved by varying the contribution of pixels to a set of joint histogram tables $\{\mathcal{H}_s\}$, from which a set of entropy measure $\{\mathcal{S}_s\}$ are computed, as illustrated in Fig. 2. The contribution is according to the spatial coordinate of the pixel and value of s.

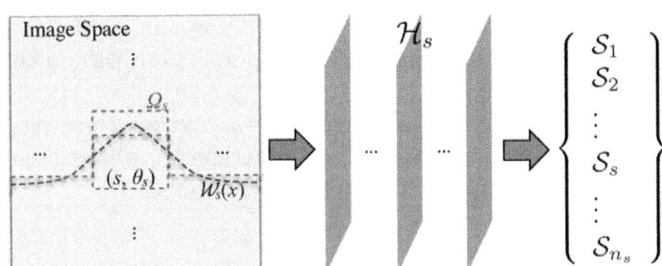

Fig. 2. The spatial variable s, associated local region Ω_s, transformation parameter θ_s, weighting function $\mathcal{W}_s(x)$, joint histogram table $\mathcal{H}_s$, and entropy measure $\mathcal{S}_s$. The spatial information encoded similarity measure is the vector representation of $\{\mathcal{S}_s\}$.

Let I_r be the reference image, I_f^T be the transformed floating image by transformation T, θ_s be a parameter of T, and Ω_s be the user-defined local region. Both θ_s and Ω_s are associated with the spatial variable s. To compute $\mathcal{S}_s$, we can estimate the local histogram using the information solely within the local region Ω_s, referred to as *local information*. However, the size of the local region Ω_s may be very small compared to the global volume Ω, which potentially leads to two problems. One is that the estimation of local probability distribution functions (PDFs) using a small number of sample points may lose the statistical power of the computed local entropy measure $\mathcal{S}_s$ [14,15]. The other is that this estimation of local PDFs may lose the global intensity class linkage [16,17]. Both of the two problems will result in reduced registration robustness using the local entropy measures.

To deal with the limitation of solely using local information, Likar and Pernus proposed to combine the local estimation with the global estimation [15]:

$$p_s(r,f) = wp_L + (1-w)p_G \; , \tag{1}$$

where $p_L = \frac{1}{N_L}\sum_{x\in\Omega_s}\omega_r(I_r(x))\omega_f(I_f^T(x))$ is estimated from Ω_s and $p_G = \frac{1}{N_G}\sum_{x\in\overline{\Omega}_s}\omega_r(I_r(x))\omega_f(I_f^T(x))$ is estimated from the complementary volume $\overline{\Omega}_s$, referred to as the *global information*; ω_r and ω_f are Parzen window estimation functions and N_L and N_G are the normalization factors. The weighting is set as $w = \frac{N_L}{N_L+N_G}$, proportional to the volume size of the local region Ω_s [15].

To assess the weights of each sample point $x\in\Omega$, Eq. (1) is rewritten:

$$p_s(r,f) = \frac{1}{N}\sum_{x\in\Omega_s}\omega(\circ)\frac{wN}{N_L} + \frac{1}{N}\sum_{x\in\overline{\Omega}_s}\omega(\circ)\frac{(1-w)N}{N_G} \; , \tag{2}$$

where $\omega(\circ) = \omega_r(I_r(x))\omega_f(I_f^T(x))$ and $N = N_L + N_G$. The weighting function is then given by:

$$\mathcal{W}_s(x) = \begin{cases} \frac{wN}{N_L}, & x\in\Omega_s \\ \frac{(1-w)N}{N_G}, & x\in\overline{\Omega}_s \end{cases} . \tag{3}$$

By using the setting in [15], the weights of all points $x\in\Omega$ are then the same, $\frac{wN}{N_L} = \frac{(1-w)N}{N_G} = 1$, resulting in the same value for all computed local measures, $\mathcal{S}_1 = \mathcal{S}_2 = \cdots = \mathcal{S}_{n_s}$, and no spatial information being encoded in $\{\mathcal{S}_s\}$.

Therefore, we can use $w \in [N_L/N, 1]$ to generalize the weighting scheme [10]. The weighting function is illustrated as the red dash-line in Fig. 2. This scheme has the mechanism of maintaining the global intensity class linkage as well as differentiating local regions in the computation of $\{\mathcal{S}_s\}$. However, the disadvantage is that all sample points within the local region Ω_s have the same weight, wN/N_L, regardless their different spatial coordinates.

Therefore, we propose to generalize the weighting scheme such that the value of $\mathcal{W}_s(x)$ should be monotonically decreasing with respect to the distance between x and the coordinate of s. This weighting function is illustrated as the blue dash-line in Fig. 2. The spatial variable associated joint histogram table is then given by:

$$\mathcal{H}_s(r, f) = \sum_{x \in \Omega} \omega_r(I_r(x))\omega_f(I_f^T(x))\mathcal{W}_s(x) \ . \tag{4}$$

Accordingly, the joint PDF is computed as $p_s(r, f) = \frac{1}{N_s}\mathcal{H}_s(r, f)$, where $N_s = \sum_{r,f} \mathcal{H}_s(r, f)$ is the normalization factor. Given $s = x$, the estimated PDF turns out to be similar to the local PDF in [13].

The derivative of $\mathcal{H}_s(r, f)$ with respect to a transformation parameter θ_t is given by:

$$\frac{\partial \mathcal{H}_s(r, f)}{\partial \theta_t} = \sum_{x \in \Omega_t} \frac{\partial \omega_f(I_f^T(x))}{\partial \theta_t}\omega_r(I_r(x))\mathcal{W}_s(x) \ , \tag{5}$$

where Ω_t is the local support volume of θ_t. The computation of $\partial \omega_f(I_f^T(x))/\partial \theta_t$ is the same as that in the traditional MI registration [1,2,3]. The computation complexity of Eq. (5) is $O(|\Omega_t|)$. Finally, the computation for marginal histogram tables and PDFs is similar, based on which MI or the normalized measures and their derivatives are computed.

2.3   Spatial Information Encoded Mutual Information

Similarity measure: The set of entropy measures $\{\mathcal{S}_s\}$ is computed from their associated PDFs. This computation results in a vector measure composed of $\{\mathcal{S}_s\}$ between the two registration images, as Fig. 2 shows. We refer to this measure as the *spatial information encoded mutual information* (SIEMI):

$$\mathrm{SIEMI} = \{\mathcal{S}_1, \mathcal{S}_2, \cdots, \mathcal{S}_s, \cdots, \mathcal{S}_{n_s}\}^{\mathrm{T}} \ , \tag{6}$$

To present a scalar value of SIEMI, one scheme is to compute the weighted sum of $\{\mathcal{S}_s\}$:

$$\mathrm{SIEMI}_{\mathrm{sum}} = \sum_s p(s)\mathcal{S}_s \ , \tag{7}$$

where $p(s) = N_s/\sum_t(N_t)$.

Alternatively, since SIEMI is a vector, the squared magnitude of the vector can be computed as a scalar similarity measure:

$$\mathrm{SIEMI}_{\mathrm{mag}} = \sum_s (\mathcal{S}_s)^2 \ . \tag{8}$$

The entropy measure $\mathcal{S}_s$ can be the joint entropy, MI, or the normalized forms such as NMI [4] and entropy correlation coefficient [2]. Studholme *et al.* [4] showed that NMI was robust to the changes in overlap volumes. Therefore, we use NMI for the implementation of $\mathcal{S}_s$ in this work. Noted that the results of using other MI forms may not be significantly different.

Driving forces and optimization of SIEMI: Given a nonrigid transformation parameter θ_s, the steepest ascent direction of registration using the scalar SIEMI is given by the derivative of SIEMI in Eq. (7) or Eq. (8) as follows:

$$
\begin{aligned}
\boldsymbol{F}_{SA}(\theta_s) &\equiv \frac{\partial \text{SIEMI}}{\partial \theta_s} \\
&= \sum_t \frac{\partial C(\mathcal{S}_t)}{\partial \theta_s}, \text{where } C(\mathcal{S}_t) \text{ is } (\mathcal{S}_t)^2 \text{ or } p(t)\mathcal{S}_t .
\end{aligned}
\tag{9}
$$

The computation complexity of Eq. (9) is $O(n_s \cdot |\Omega_s|)$, where n_s is the number of the spatial variable values. However, this computation may be practically too expensive when n_s is large, compared to only $O(|\Omega_s|)$ in standard MI.

Since SIEMI is a vector of $\{\mathcal{S}_s\}$, we propose to optimize each $\mathcal{S}_s$ with respect to θ_s using a direction of local ascent, resembling a greedy strategy:

$$
\boldsymbol{F}_{LA}(\theta_s) \equiv \partial \mathcal{S}_s / \partial \theta_s .
\tag{10}
$$

The computation complexity of Eq. (10) is now *significantly reduced* to $O(|\Omega_s|)$, which compares with $O(n_s|\Omega_s|)$ of Eq. (9). This *local ascent optimization* assumes that the optimization of each $\mathcal{S}_s$ would not deteriorate that of others, and thus would globally converge. The convergence of local ascent optimization, along with the comparisons with using global ascent optimization for SIEMI$_{\text{sum}}$, SIEMI$_{\text{mag}}$, and NMI, will be validated in Section 3.1.

2.4   Choices of $\mathcal{W}_s(x)$ and Unifying Existing Works

The spatial variable s is defined according to the nonrigid transformation model used in the registration. In this work, we employ the free-form deformations (FFDs) [5]. The value of s is defined to the index of the control points of FFD grids, and Ω_s is the local support volume of the control point.

Spatial information encoding is determined by the weighting scheme $\mathcal{W}_s(x)$. By using constant value such that $\mathcal{W}_s(x) = 1$, the computed measure $\mathcal{S}_s$ is identical to traditional entropy measure such as the MI or NMI.

By using the *boxcar* function, the 0-order B-spline function β^0:

$$
\mathcal{W}_s(x) = \begin{cases} 1, \text{ if } x \in \Omega_s \\ 0, \text{ otherwise} \end{cases}
\tag{11}
$$

the joint PDFs associated with s, $p_s(r, f)$, become the regional PDFs and the corresponding SIEMI$_{\text{sum}}$ is then given by:

$$
\text{SIEMI}_{\text{sum}}|_{\mathcal{W}_s=\beta^0, \mathcal{S}_s=\text{MI}} = \sum_s p(s) \sum_{r,f} p_s(r, f) \log \frac{p_s(r, f)}{p_s(r)p_s(f)} ,
\tag{12}
$$

which is identical to the derived RMI$'$ measure proposed in [7].

By using the cubic B-spline function β^3 such that:

$$
\mathcal{W}_s(x) = \beta^3_{\Delta_1}(x_1 - \phi_{s1})\beta^3_{\Delta_2}(x_2 - \phi_{s2})\beta^3_{\Delta_3}(x_3 - \phi_{s3}) ,
\tag{13}
$$

the joint PDFs associated with s become the conditional PDFs $p(r, f|s)$, where $x = [x_1, x_2, x_3]^T$ is the sample point's coordinate, $[\phi_{s1}, \phi_{s2}, \phi_{s3}]^T$ is the coordinate of the s corresponded FFD control point, and $[\Delta_1, \Delta_2, \Delta_3]$ are the FFD spacing in each dimension. SIEMI$_{\text{sum}}$ then becomes the cMI in [8,9].

In this study, we use the Gaussian kernel function for $\mathcal{W}_s(x)$, in 3D as follows:

$$\mathcal{W}_s(x) = Ae^{-\left(\frac{(x_1-\phi_{s1})^2}{2\sigma_1^2} + \frac{(x_2-\phi_{s2})^2}{2\sigma_2^2} + \frac{(x_3-\phi_{s3})^2}{2\sigma_3^2}\right)}, \tag{14}$$

where $A = 1$ and $[\sigma_1, \sigma_2, \sigma_3]$ are the standard deviations. In practice, the locality of the Gaussian function is set to the volume within three times the standard deviation. Therefore, $\mathcal{W}_s(x)$ using Eq. (14) is similar to the cubic B-spline function in Eq. (13), given $\sigma_i = \frac{2}{3}\Delta_i$, where Δ_i is the FFD spacing in each dimension.

The amount of information used in the computation of $\mathcal{H}_s$ in Eq. (4) is related to the non-zero-value domain of $\mathcal{W}_s(x)$. More information corresponds to better registration robustness, while more locality means higher achievable registration accuracy. A strategy to combine them is to start the registration using $\mathcal{W}_s(x)$ with a large non-zero-value domain such as the global space and hierarchically decrease the domain. This *hierarchy scheme* can be related to the multiresolution FFD registration [18] such as by setting the none-zero-value domain to the local support of the corresponding control point [8]. In this study, we set $\sigma_i = l\Delta_i$ to regularize the locality of $\mathcal{W}_s(x)$ in the multiresolution FFDs [18]. In this scheme, the information used in the computation of $\mathcal{H}_s$ can be extended to $(1.5l)^d$ times of the local support volume of the control points, where d is the dimension. We use $l \in [1, 2]$ in our experiments, where the smallest FFD spacing is 10 mm and the minimal number of sample points for the construction of histogram tables can be easily met [19].

We notice that there are applications which may need much finer spacing FFD registration. For this situation, we need to define $[\sigma_1, \sigma_2, \sigma_3]$ of Eq. (14) to be large enough to guarantee enough sample points for the construction of $\mathcal{H}_s$, such as σ_i=10mm when $l\Delta_i$<10mm.

It should be noted that the computation complexity of the optimization using Eq. (10) is not significantly increased along with the increased value of l. This is because it is determined by the size of local support volume as Eq. (5) shows.

3   Experiment

3.1   Global Steepest Ascent vs Local Ascent Optimization

Data: This experiment uses 2D brain MR T1 images, downloaded from Brain-Web to demonstrate the difference of SIEMI registration using the steepest ascent optimization, Eq. (9), and the local ascent optimization, Eq. (10). The steepest ascent optimization was applied to NMI, SIEMI using sum of $\{\mathcal{S}_s\}$, referred to as SIEMI$_{\text{sum}}^{\text{SA}}$, and SIEMI using magnitude of $\{\mathcal{S}_s\}$, referred to as SIEMI$_{\text{mag}}^{\text{SA}}$. The SIEMI registration using the local ascent optimization is referred to as SIEMI.

Table 1. The registration accuracy, given by warping index (WI), of the four schemes. The table also presents the p-values of the t-test between the registration accuracy of SIEMI and that of the other three methods, and the ratios of computation time (RCT) of the other three methods to that of the SIEMI.

	NMI	$SIEMI_{sum}^{SA}$	$SIEMI_{mag}^{SA}$	SIEMI
WI (0.01 mm)	23 ± 0.9	11 ± 0.6	11 ± 0.5	11 ± 0.7
P-value	<0.0001	0.462	0.662	—
RCT	0.60	160	144	1

One of the registration images did not have INU while the other had a 20% field. The initial transformations, regarded as the ground truth for the registration accuracy assessment, were combinations of scalings and FFD transformations [5] with 45×54 mm mesh spacing. Six different scaling values were chosen between [0.95, 1.05] and the FFD transformations moved the central control points either 15 mm or -15 mm at each direction, together generating 24 initial transformations. The *warping index*, root mean square (RMS) residual displacement error, of the initial transformation fields ranged between [3.47, 4.63] (3.90 ± 0.49) mm.

The registration used a series of concatenated isotropic FFDs with two levels (spacings 20mm and 10mm) [18,20]. The registration firstly employed 100 iteration steps for the 20 mm FFD level, and then 40 steps for the 10 mm FFD level. The warping index was calculated every 10 iteration steps.

Results: Fig. 3 (left) illustrates the mean warping indexes by the four registration methods. They are displayed in every 10 iteration steps. The mean accuracy is also displayed in Table 1 where the evidently small standard deviation values, all less than 0.01 mm, indicate the consistent performance of each registration scheme in the test cases. It is evident from Table 1 that NMI registration needed the least computation time, but it achieved a much worse warping index than the other three registration schemes.

For the SIEMI registration schemes, the computation of each iteration step in SIEMI was more than 100 times faster than those of $SIEMI_{sum}^{SA}$ and $SIEMI_{mag}^{SA}$, as Table 1 shows. The optimization of SIEMI is shown to converge twice to three times slower than $SIEMI_{sum}^{SA}$ and $SIEMI_{mag}^{SA}$ (Fig. 3 (left)), but it is still much faster in overall. Furthermore, there was no statistically significant difference in terms of registration accuracy between the use of the local ascent optimization and that of the two global steepest ascent schemes, as the p-value of the two tailed, paired t-test between SIEMI and $SIEMI_{sum}^{SA}$ was 0.462, and that between SIEMI and $SIEMI_{mag}^{SA}$ was 0.662.

3.2 Performance to Intensity Non-uniformity

Data: This experiment employs 3D brain MR images to study the performance of NMI and SIEMI registration in different magnitudes of INU fields. The MR

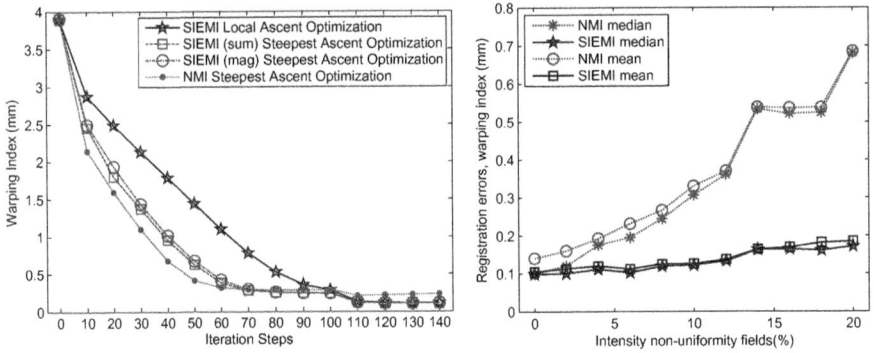

Fig. 3. The mean warping index of the 24 cases in every 10 iteration steps (left) and the mean and median values of the registration errors by SIEMI and NMI in the different intensity non-uniformity fields (right)

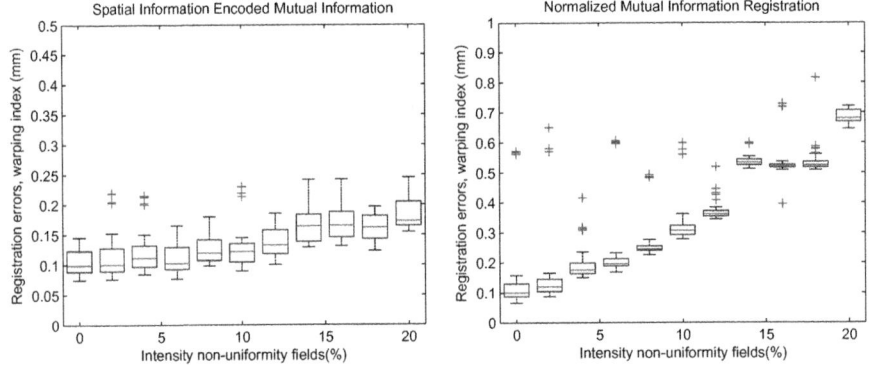

Fig. 4. The Box-and-Whisker diagrams of 48-case registration errors by SIEMI (left) and NMI registration (right) in different intensity non-uniformity fields

images were downloaded from the BrainWeb with 3% noise. Eleven levels of INU fields were generated, from 0% to 20%, using the equation $\mathcal{B} = a_1 x^2 + a_2 y^2 + a_3 z^3 + a_4 xy + a_5 xz + a_6 yz + a_7 x + a_8 y + a_9 z$, where $[x, y, z]$ is the pixel coordinate, and $\{a_i\}$ are random values in $[-1, 1]$. The magnitudes of the fields were normalized to the percentage of the intensity range of the original image. Forty-eight deformation fields were generated using the same method employed in Section 3.1, where the FFD mesh used in this experiment was 3D and with $45 \times 54 \times 45$ mm spacing. These initial deformations, warping index ranging from 0.31 mm to 6.27 mm (2.67 ± 1.49 mm), were used to generate 48 registration cases for each level of the INU fields.

SIEMI and NMI registration used the same transformation model, a series of concatenated isotropic FFDs with two levels (spacings 20mm and 10mm) [18,20].

Results: Fig. 4 plots the Box-and-Whisker diagrams of the warping index of the 48 registration cases by NMI and SIEMI in each level of INU fields, and Fig. 3

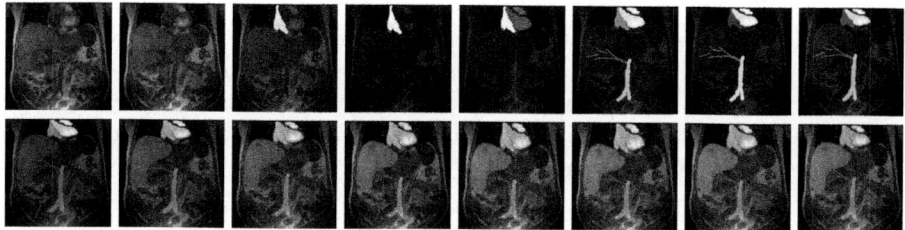

Fig. 5. One example of the simulated dynamic contrast enhanced MR data in 15 time points. The first one from the left of the upper row is the image without enhancement. The images from the second of the upper row to the second row are the dynamic enhanced data from time point one to fifteen.

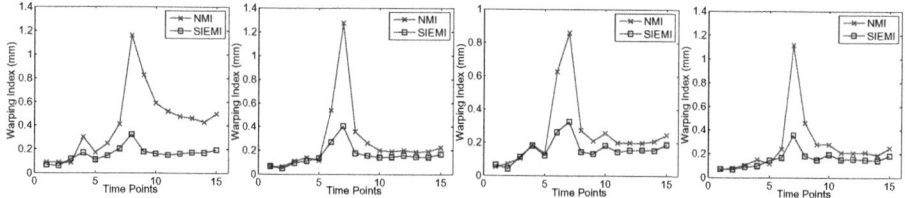

Fig. 6. The registration results, warping indexes, of the four simulated dynamic contrast enhancement MRI cases by SIEMI and NMI registration

(right) shows the mean and median numbers of them. The two registration methods achieved similar warping indexes in most of the cases in 0% INU level, but NMI had three outlier cases whose errors were larger than 0.5 mm. In the cases of images with INU, SIEMI registration performed with a fairly consistent mean warping index with respect to different levels of INU magnitudes, while NMI registration had radically increased registration errors when the INU became strong.

3.3   Application to Dynamic Contrast Enhanced MRI

Data: This experiment employs four sets of simulated DCE MRI data where the intensity values during flush-in of the contrast agent varied as a function of time and positions. Fig. 5 shows an example whose results are plotted in Fig. 6 (c). The DCE MRI data had simulated free-breathing motions which deformed the images. The four datasets had different magnitudes of motions. The images from different time points were all registered to a reference image, the MR image without enhancement, to correct the deformations in the liver. We calculated the warping index on the liver region.

Results: Fig. 6 plots the registration results. SIEMI performed evidently better than NMI, particularly between time points 5 to 10 when the contrast agent started to enter the liver region and changed the intensity values. The results also show that during the time points 1 to 5 when the contrast agent had not yet arrived the liver to change the intensity, NMI achieved similar warping indexes as SIEMI. From time point 10 to 15, the contrast agent in the liver was in late enhancement and the intensity distributions were more uniform. Therefore, NMI started to perform better than in the time points of enhancing. However, the accuracy was still not as good as that of SIEMI because there was still INU in the data due to the enhancement.

4   Conclusion

We have presented a new method, spatial information encoded mutual information measure (SIEMI), for nonrigid registration. This registration approach is based on the general spatial information encoding framework. We achieved the encoding using a weighting scheme to differentiate the contribution of pixels to the set of entropy measures which are associated with the spatial variable. The similarity measure of SIEMI is a vector which consists of the set of entropy measures. To efficiently search the optimum of this measure, we proposed to use the local ascent optimization scheme. The result showed that the local ascent was able to converge to similar accuracy and save up to two orders of magnitude computation time compared to the registration using the global ascent scheme.

SIEMI was particularly proposed to tackle the nonrigid registration problems caused by the intensity non-uniformity (INU) or enhancement in the images. We validated the method using brain MR data with different level of INU and dynamic contrast enhancement MRI of the liver. The results showed that SIEMI well overcame the problems and performed significantly better than the registration using normalized mutual information.

Acknowledgement

Xiahai Zhuang was funded by EPSRC grant GR/T11395/01. The authors thank Dr. Andrew Melbourne and Dr. David Atkinson for providing the DCE MRI.

References

1. Viola, P., Wells III, V.M.: Alignment by maximization of mutual information. International Journal of Computer Vision 24(2), 137–154 (1997)
2. Maes, F., Collignon, A., Vandermeulen, D., Marchal, G., Suetens, P.: Multimodality image registration by maximization of mutual information. IEEE Transactions of Medical Imaging 16(2), 187–198 (1997)
3. Wells III, W.M., Viola, P., Atsumi, H., Nakajima, S., Kikinis, R.: Multi-modal volume registration by maximisation of mutual information. Medical Image Analysis 1(1), 35–51 (1996)
4. Studholme, C., Hill, D.L.G., Hawkes, D.J.: An overlap invariant entropy measure of 3D medical image alignment. Pattern Recognition 32(1), 71–86 (1999)
5. Rueckert, D., Sonoda, L.I., Hayes, C., Hill, D.L.G., Leach, M.O., Hawkes, D.J.: Nonrigid registration using free-form deformations: Application to breast MR images. IEEE Transactions on Medical Imaging 18, 712–721 (1999)

6. Pluim, J.P.W., Maintz, J.B.A., Viergever, M.A.: Mutual information based registration of medical images: A survey. IEEE Transaction on Medical Imaging 22(8), 986–1004 (2003)
7. Studholme, C., Drapaca, C.S., Iordanova, B., Cardenas, V.: Deformation-based mapping of volume change from serial brain MRI in the presence of local tissue contrast change. IEEE Transactions on Medical Imaging 25(5), 626–639 (2006)
8. Loeckx, D., Slagmolen, P., Maes, F., Vandermeulen, D., Suetens, P.: Nonrigid image registration using conditional mutual information. In: Karssemeijer, N., Lelieveldt, B. (eds.) IPMI 2007. LNCS, vol. 4584, pp. 725–737. Springer, Heidelberg (2007)
9. Loeckx, D., Slagmolen, P., Maes, F., Vandermeulen, D., Suetens, P.: Nonrigid Image Registration Using Conditional Mutual Information. IEEE Transactions on Medical Imaging 29(1), 19–29 (2010)
10. Zhuang, X., Hawkes, D.J., Ourselin, S.: Unifying encoding of spatial information in mutual information for nonrigid registration. In: Information Processing in Medical Imaging. LNCS, vol. 5636, pp. 491–502. Springer, Heidelberg (2009)
11. Melbourne, A., Atkinson, D., White, M.J., Collins, D., Leach, M., Hawkes, D.: Registration of dynamic contrast-enhanced MRI using a progressive principal component registration (ppcr). Physics in Medicine and Biology 52, 5147–5156 (2007)
12. Li, C., Sun, Y.: Nonrigid registration of myocardial perfusion MRI using pseudo ground truth. In: Yang, G.-Z., Hawkes, D., Rueckert, D., Noble, A., Taylor, C. (eds.) MICCAI 2009. LNCS, vol. 5761, pp. 165–172. Springer, Heidelberg (2009)
13. Hermosillo, G., Chefd'Hotel, C.C., Faugeras, O.D.: Variational methods for multimodal image matching. International Journal of Computer Vision 50(3), 329–343 (2002)
14. Pluim, J.P.W., Maintz, J.B.A., Viergever, M.A.: Interpolation artefacts in mutual information-based image registration. Computer Vision and Image Understanding 77(2), 211–232 (2000)
15. Likar, B., Pernus, F.: A hierarchical approach to elastic registration based on mutual information. Image and Vision Computing 19, 33–44 (2001)
16. Zhuang, X., Rhode, K., Razavi, R., Hawkes, D.J., Ourselin, S.: A registration-based propagation framework for automatic whole heart segmentation of cardiac MRI. IEEE Transactions on Medical Imaging PP(99), 1 (in Press), doi:10.1109/TMI.2010.2047112
17. Zhuang, X., Rhode, K., Arridge, S., Razavi, R., Hill, D., Hawkes, D., Ourselin, S.: An atlas-based segmentation propagation framework using locally affine registration – application to automatic whole heart segmentation. In: Metaxas, D., Axel, L., Fichtinger, G., Székely, G. (eds.) MICCAI 2008, Part II. LNCS, vol. 5242, pp. 425–433. Springer, Heidelberg (2008)
18. Schnabel, J.A., Rueckert, D., Quist, M., Blackall, J.M., Castellano-Smith, A.D., Hartkens, T., Penney, G.P., Hall, W.A., Liu, H., Truwit, C.L., Gerritsen, F.A., Hill, D.L.G., Hawkes, D.J.: A generic framework for non-rigid registration based on non-uniform multi-level free-form deformations. In: Niessen, W.J., Viergever, M.A. (eds.) MICCAI 2001. LNCS, vol. 2208, pp. 573–581. Springer, Heidelberg (2001)
19. Klein, S., Staring, M., Pluim, J.P.W.: Evaluation of optimization methods for non-rigid medical image registration using mutual information and B-splines. IEEE Trans. Image Processing 16(12), 2879–2890 (2007)
20. Rueckert, D., Aljabar, P., Heckemann, R.A., Hajnal, J.V., Hammers, A.: Diffeomorphic registration using b-splines. In: Larsen, R., Nielsen, M., Sporring, J. (eds.) MICCAI 2006. LNCS, vol. 4191, pp. 702–709. Springer, Heidelberg (2006)

Normalized Measures of Mutual Information with General Definitions of Entropy for Multimodal Image Registration

Nathan D. Cahill

Center for Applied and Computational Mathematics,
School of Mathematical Sciences, Rochester Institute of Technology,
85 Lomb Memorial Drive, Rochester, NY 14618, USA
`nathan.cahill@rit.edu`

Abstract. Mutual information (MI) was introduced for use in multi-modal image registration over a decade ago [1,2,3,4]. The MI between two images is based on their marginal and joint/conditional entropies. The most common versions of entropy used to compute MI are the Shannon and differential entropies; however, many other definitions of entropy have been proposed as competitors. In this article, we show how to construct normalized versions of MI using any of these definitions of entropy. The resulting similarity measures are analogous to normalized mutual information (NMI), entropy correlation coefficient (ECC), and symmetric uncertainty (SU), which have all been shown to be superior to MI in a variety of situations. We use publicly available CT, PET, and MR brain images[1] with known ground truth transformations to evaluate the performance of the normalized measures for rigid multimodal registration. Results show that for a number of different definitions of entropy, the proposed normalized versions of mutual information provide a statistically significant improvement in target registration error (TRE) over the non-normalized versions.

Keywords: Image registration, mutual information, entropy.

1 Introduction

Collignon and Maes [1,2] and Viola and Wells [3,4] introduced the idea that multimodal images could be aligned by maximizing their mutual information (MI), which is an information measure that depends on the marginal and joint entropies of the underlying images. Since that introduction, much research has gone into understanding, applying, and generalizing this idea in a variety of ways. Pluim et al. [5] captured a snapshot of the state of the art in 2003, which showed that much progress had already been attained by that point.

---

[1] The images and data were provided as part of the project: "Retrospective Image Registration Evaluation," National Institutes of Health, Project Number 8R01EB002124-03, Principal Investigator, J. Michael Fitzpatrick, Vanderbilt University, Nashville, TN, USA.

B. Fischer, B. Dawant, and C. Lorenz (Eds.): WBIR 2010, LNCS 6204, pp. 258–268, 2010.

This paper focuses on two threads of investigation that emerged in the years after mutual information was introduced to the medical imaging community. One thread is the normalization of MI, in the form of Studholme's normalized MI (NMI) [6], Maes' entropy correlation coefficient (ECC) [1], or Melbourne's symmetric uncertainty (SU) [7], which have been empirically shown to improve registration accuracy and robustness to truncation of the images. The other thread is the use of different generalizations of entropy (Rényi and Tsallis entropies [8], cumulative residual entropy [9,10], and generalized survival exponential entropy [11]) to form the MI measure; such generalizations have also been shown to improve registration performance in various situations.

In this paper, we show that normalized versions of MI can be formed when MI is constructed from *any* of the definitions of entropy. Furthermore, we illustrate experimentally that such normalized versions in general outperform their unnormalized counterparts for the task of rigid registration of multimodal brain images. This idea generalizes some results in the literature that extend NMI for use with Rényi and Tsallis entropies [8] and extend NMI and ECC for use with cumulative residual entropy [12,13].

The remainder of this paper is organized as follows: section 2 describes various definitions of entropy, and section 3 provides a general framework for constructing MI from any of these definitions of entropy. Section 4 defines versions of NMI, ECC, and SU from any of the general definitions of entropy, and section 5 illustrates experimentally how these normalized versions of MI outperform their unnormalized counterparts. Finally, section 6 draws some conclusions and presents ideas for future work.

2   Measures of Entropy

In the context of probability theory, entropy describes the amount of uncertainty associated with a random variable. Shannon [14] considered an information source having components $L_1, L_2, \ldots, L_n$ with associated probabilities of occurrence $p_1, p_2, \ldots, p_n$, and he showed that the quantity:

$$H = -\sum_{i=1}^{n} p_i \log p_i \tag{1}$$

is a measure of the uncertainty in the outcome of a particular event. This measure is generalized to the case of a continuous random variable X with density $p(x)$ by the *differential* entropy:

$$H(X) = -\int_{-\infty}^{\infty} p(x) \ln p(x) \, dx \ . \tag{2}$$

A wide variety of competing measures of entropy have emerged in other contexts; a number of these measures that can be considered generalizations of Shannon or differential entropy are shown in Table 1. Rényi [15] presented a family of entropies that converge to the differential entropy as $\alpha \to 1$. Tsallis [16] proposed a family of entropies that is useful in describing non-additive systems. Exponential and generalized exponential entropies were introduced by Campbell [17] and Koski and Persson [18] and used for data compression. The Tsallis and exponential entropies converge to differential entropy as $\alpha \to 1$; the generalized exponential entropy can be thought of as being related to a generalized version of the Rényi entropy, both of which converge to differential entropy as $(\alpha, \beta) \to (1, 1)$.

Another type of entropy, the *cumulative residual* entropy (CRE), was presented by Rao *et al.* [19] and Wang *et al.* [9] in order to provide a way to accommodate random variables that do not have a defined density function. This is done by replacing the density function with the survival function $S(x) = P(|X| > x)$, and then defining the CRE as:

$$\varepsilon(X) = -\int_0^\infty S(x) \ln S(x)\, dx \ . \tag{3}$$

All of the generalizations of differential entropy listed in Table 1 can also be defined in terms of CRE, as shown in Table 2. Zografos and Nadarajah [20] presented and analyzed generalizations of CRE to Rényi, exponential, and generalized exponential entropy, and they named the latter two resulting quantities *survival exponential* and *generalized survival exponential* entropies.

Table 1. Differential entropy and generalizations

	Symbol	Definition
Differential	$H(X)$	$-\int_{-\infty}^{\infty} p(x) \ln p(x)\, dx$
Rényi	$H_\alpha^R(X)$	$\begin{cases} \dfrac{1}{1-\alpha} \ln \int_{-\infty}^{\infty} p^\alpha(x)\, dx, & \alpha \neq 1 \\ H(X), & \alpha = 1 \end{cases}$
Tsallis	$H_\alpha^T(X)$	$\begin{cases} \dfrac{1}{1-\alpha} \int_{-\infty}^{\infty} (p^\alpha(x) - p(x))\, dx, & \alpha \neq 1 \\ H(X), & \alpha = 1 \end{cases}$
Exponential	$H_\alpha^E(X)$	$\exp\left(H_\alpha^R(X)\right)$
Generalized Rényi	$H_{\alpha,\beta}^{GR}(X)$	$\begin{cases} \dfrac{1}{\beta - \alpha} \ln \dfrac{\int_{-\infty}^{\infty} p^\alpha(x)\, dx}{\int_{-\infty}^{\infty} p^\beta(x)\, dx}, & \alpha \neq \beta \\ \dfrac{-\int_{-\infty}^{\infty} p^\beta(x) \ln p(x)\, dx}{\int_{-\infty}^{\infty} p^\beta(x)\, dx}, & \alpha = \beta \end{cases}$
Generalized Exponential	$H_{\alpha,\beta}^{GE}(X)$	$\exp\left(H_{\alpha,\beta}^{GR}(X)\right)$

Table 2. Cumulative residual entropy (CRE) and generalizations

	Symbol	Definition
Cumulative Residual	$\varepsilon(X)$	$-\int_0^\infty S(x)\ln S(x)\,dx$
Rényi	$\varepsilon_\alpha^R(X)$	$\begin{cases} \dfrac{1}{1-\alpha}\ln\int_0^\infty S^\alpha(x)\,dx, \ \alpha \neq 1 \\[2mm] \varepsilon(X), \qquad\qquad \alpha = 1 \end{cases}$
Tsallis	$\varepsilon_\alpha^T(X)$	$\begin{cases} \dfrac{1}{1-\alpha}\int_0^\infty (S^\alpha(x) - S(x))\,dx, \ \alpha \neq 1 \\[2mm] \varepsilon(X), \qquad\qquad\qquad \alpha = 1 \end{cases}$
Exponential	$\varepsilon_\alpha^E(X)$	$\exp\!\left(\varepsilon_\alpha^R(X)\right)$
Generalized Rényi	$\varepsilon_{\alpha,\beta}^{GR}(X)$	$\begin{cases} \dfrac{1}{\beta-\alpha}\ln\dfrac{\int_0^\infty S^\alpha(x)\,dx}{\int_0^\infty S^\beta(x)\,dx}, \ \alpha \neq \beta \\[3mm] \dfrac{-\int_0^\infty S^\beta(x)\ln S(x)\,dx}{\int_0^\infty S^\beta(x)\,dx}, \ \alpha = \beta \end{cases}$
Generalized Exponential	$\varepsilon_{\alpha,\beta}^{GE}(X)$	$\exp\!\left(\varepsilon_{\alpha,\beta}^{GR}(X)\right)$

3   Measures of Mutual Information

Mutual information (MI) was introduced as a similarity measure for multimodal image registration by Collignon and Maes [1,2] and Viola and Wells [3,4]. MI can be defined in a number of ways (see Pluim et al. [5] for a comparison of the various definitions); we focus on two such definitions. The first defines the MI between two random variables X and Y in terms of their marginal (Shannon) entropies and their *joint* entropy $H(X,Y)$:

$$\mathrm{MI}(X,Y) = H(X) + H(Y) - H(X,Y) \ . \tag{4}$$

The second defines MI in terms of the *conditional* entropy:

$$\mathrm{MI}(X,Y) = H(X) - \mathrm{E}[H(X|Y)] \ . \tag{5}$$

Note that this notation for conditional entropy departs from other references; here, we consider $H(X|Y)$ to be a random variable that is a function of Y, namely,

$$H(X|Y) = -\int_{-\infty}^\infty p(x|Y)\ln p(x|Y)\,dx \ , \tag{6}$$

and $\mathrm{E}[H(X|Y)]$ to be the expected value of (6).

An analogous quantity to MI that uses CRE is the *cross cumulative residual entropy* (CCRE) of Wang et al. [10]:

$$\mathrm{CCRE}(X,Y) = \varepsilon(X) - \mathrm{E}[\varepsilon(X|Y)] \ . \tag{7}$$

CCRE was also investigated in [21] under the alternate name of *cumulative mutual information* (CMI). The conditional CRE $\varepsilon(X|Y)$ is a random variable that is a function of Y, namely,

$$\varepsilon(X|Y) = -\int_0^\infty S(x|Y)\ln S(x|Y)\,dx \quad , \tag{8}$$

where $S(x|Y) = P(|X| > x|Y)$.

One key difference between MI and CCRE is that MI is symmetric whereas CCRE is not (i.e., $\mathrm{MI}(X,Y) = \mathrm{MI}(Y,X)$ but $\mathrm{CCRE}(X,Y) \neq \mathrm{CCRE}(Y,X)$). However, CCRE can be easily symmetrized, yielding the *symmetric* CCRE:

$$\mathrm{SCCRE}(X,Y) = \frac{1}{2}\Big(\mathrm{CCRE}(X,Y) + \mathrm{CCRE}(Y,X)\Big)$$

$$= \frac{1}{2}\Big(\varepsilon(X) + \varepsilon(Y) - \mathrm{E}[\varepsilon(X|Y)] - \mathrm{E}[\varepsilon(Y|X)]\Big) \ . \tag{9}$$

The construction of SCCRE can be used to define a general form of mutual information for use with *any* definition of entropy. If we consider **H** to denote a placeholder for any of the definitions of entropy listed in Tables 1–2, we can define a general symmetric version of mutual information by:

$$\mathbf{H}\text{-MI}(X,Y) = \frac{1}{2}\Big(\mathbf{H}(X) + \mathbf{H}(Y) - \mathrm{E}[\mathbf{H}(X|Y)] - \mathrm{E}[\mathbf{H}(Y|X)]\Big) \ . \tag{10}$$

Using this general form (10), it is easily seen that H-MI and ε-MI are the specific forms of MI and SCCRE given in (5) and (9), respectively. Other specific forms of (10) have been explored in the medical image registration literature. H_α^R-MI and H_α^T-MI are similar to Rényi and Tsallis entropy based mutual information measures investigated by Wachowiak *et al.* [8], and ε_α^E-MI and $\varepsilon_{\alpha,\beta}^{GE}$-MI are symmetric versions of the SEE-MI and GSEE-MI measures introduced by Liao and Chung [11].

4   Normalized Measures of Mutual Information

Studholme *et al.* [6] argued that any image similarity measure should be invariant to changes in the overlap region through the course of registration. They showed that traditional MI does in fact vary with changing overlap, and they proposed the *normalized mutual information* (NMI) as an alternative:

$$\mathrm{NMI}(X,Y) := \frac{H(X) + H(Y)}{H(X,Y)} \quad . \tag{11}$$

Studholme *et al.* validated the invariance of NMI to changing overlap for some simple examples and illustrated how NMI exhibits better behavior than MI on the rigid registration of MR to CT and MR to PET volumes.

NMI is closely related to Astola's *entropy correlation coefficient* (ECC) [22], which is given by:

$$\mathrm{ECC}(X, Y) := \sqrt{2 - \frac{2H(X,Y)}{H(R) + H(Y)}} \quad . \tag{12}$$

Maes *et al.* [1] and Collignon [2] use the square of Astola's ECC for multimodal registration, which is equivalent to the *symmetric uncertainty* (SU) [7,23]:

$$\mathrm{SU}(X, Y) := \mathrm{ECC}(X, Y)^2 = 2 - \frac{2H(X,Y)}{H(R) + H(Y)} \quad . \tag{13}$$

In order to generalize these normalized versions of mutual information, we first recognize that $H(X,Y)$ and can be rewritten as:

$$H(X,Y) = \frac{1}{2}\Big(H(X) + H(Y) + \mathrm{E}[H(X|Y)] + \mathrm{E}[H(Y|X)]\Big) \quad . \tag{14}$$

Now, general forms of NMI, ECC, and SU can be defined analogously to the general mutual information (10). The resulting forms are shown in Table 3. It is straightforward to show that the use of differential entropy for **H** causes H-NMI, H-ECC, and H-SU to reduce to (11), (12), and (13), respectively.

A few specific examples of normalized MI measures that do *not* use differential entropy have been developed for use in medical image registration. Wachowiak *et al.* [8] investigated Rényi and Tsallis entropy based normalizations which are equivalent to H_α^R-NMI and H_α^T-NMI. Cahill *et al.* [12,13] showed that SCCRE exhibits the same overlap sensitivity problem as Studholme established with MI. Furthermore, they defined normalized versions of CRE-based MI called *normalized cross cumulative residual entropy* (NCCRE) and *cumulative residual entropy correlation coefficient* (CRECC), which are equivalent to ε-NMI and ε-ECC, respectively, and they established that NCCRE and CRECC exhibit the same type of improvement over SCCRE that NMI and ECC exhibit over MI.

Table 3. Normalized measures of MI with general definitions of entropy

Similarity Measure	Definition
H-NMI(X,Y)	$\dfrac{2\mathbf{H}(X) + 2\mathbf{H}(Y)}{\mathbf{H}(X) + \mathbf{H}(X) + \mathrm{E}\left[\mathbf{H}(X|Y)\right] + \mathrm{E}\left[\mathbf{H}(Y|X)\right]}$
H-ECC(X,Y)	$\sqrt{1 - \dfrac{\mathrm{E}\left[\mathbf{H}(X|Y)\right] + \mathrm{E}\left[\mathbf{H}(Y|X)\right]}{\mathbf{H}(X) + \mathbf{H}(Y)}}$
H-SU(X,Y)	$1 - \dfrac{\mathrm{E}\left[\mathbf{H}(X|Y)\right] + \mathrm{E}\left[\mathbf{H}(Y|X)\right]}{\mathbf{H}(X) + \mathbf{H}(Y)}$

5   Multimodal Rigid Registration Experiment

In order to illustrate the behavior of the various similarity measures on real-world data, we focus on the rigid registration case, and we use images from the Retrospective Image Registration Evaluation project. The RIRE project database contains CT, MR, and PET images for a variety of patients, and has a sequestered set of ground truth rigid body transformations that were computed from fiducial markers implanted in the skull. (The fiducial markers were removed from the images prior to retrospectively evaluating registration algorithms.) Results of the original RIRE study are provided by West *et al.*[24].

In this paper, we used the images from nine patient datasets. Each patient dataset contains MR images from some or all of the following protocols: T1-weighted, T2-weighted, PD-weighted, and rectified versions of the T1, T2, and PD-weighted images. Five of the nine datasets contain both CT and PET images in addition to the MR images. Two of the datasets contain CT but not PET images, and the remaining two datasets contain PET but not CT images. The CT images have resolution $0.65 \times 0.65 \times 4.0$ mm^3, the MR images have approximate resolution $1.25 \times 1.25 \times 4.0$ mm^3, and the PET images has resolution $2.59 \times 2.59 \times 8.0$ mm^3. For ease of computation, we resampled each image to $3.0 \times 3.0 \times 3.0$ mm^3 isotropic resolution.

Examples of some of the RIRE images are shown in Figures 1 and 2. Figure 1 shows axial views of the CT, MR-T1, and PET images from patient 5. Figure 2 illustrates overlayed isosurfaces of the CT (blue) and MR-T1 images from patient 4, both before (left) and after (right) rigid registration.

For each dataset, we rigidly registered the CT and/or PET image to all of the MR images. Rigid transformations were parameterized by three Euler angles and three translation parameters. Initial estimates of the solution were selected by translating the images to match their computed centroids. To constrain the parameters, we employed bounds of $\pm\pi/6$ radians on each Euler angle, and $\pm1/5$ of the width of the corresponding reference image dimension on each translation component. (We visually verified for each case that after the prealignment step is performed, the true rigid transformation parameters fall within these bounds.) For each dissimilarity measure, we carried out a bound-constrained optimization

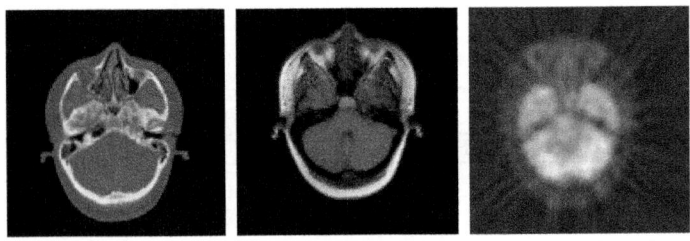

Fig. 1. Axial slices of CT, MR (T1-weighted) and PET images from the patient 5 dataset

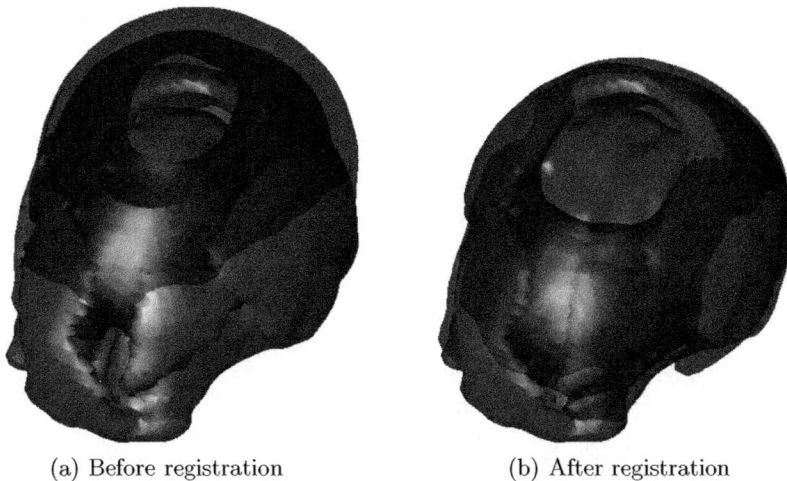

(a) Before registration   (b) After registration

Fig. 2. Isosurfaces of CT (blue) and MR-T1 (red) images of patient 4, before and after rigid registration

procedure using the active set algorithm employed by the `fmincon` function of MATLAB's Optimization Toolbox. All gradient vectors and Hessian matrices were estimated numerically via finite differences. The optimization was terminated when the maximum change in magnitude in any parameter was less than 10^{-4} or after 500 iterations, whichever occured first.

All probability densities (and joint densities) were estimated via histograms (and joint histograms) that were constructed with 32 (or 32×32) equally spaced bins. Linear (or bilinear) interpolation was used to accumulate partial weights in neighboring bins.

Registration is performed using the general versions of MI and ECC based on the original, Renyi, and Tsallis versions of differential entropy and CRE defined in Tables 1–2. Values of α are drawn from the set $\{0.5, 1, 2\}$.

5.1   Results

The performance of similarity measures on the various registration tasks is measured via Target Registration Error (TRE). For the RIRE project [24], a number of anatomically meaningful volumes of interest (VOI) were annotated. TRE is computed as the average Euclidean distance (in mm) between VOI centroids in the reference image and their predicted positions after registration.

Table 4 reports the mean, median, and standard deviation of the TRE values measured across the VOI's in every patient for various similarity measures.

We employed hypothesis testing to gauge the statistical significance of these results. Given similarity measures **H-MI** and **H-ECC**, the null hypothesis states that the TRE's from **H-MI** and **H-ECC** arise from the same distribution. The alternative hypothesis is that the TRE's from **H-MI** are "worse" than the TRE's

Table 4. Statistics of TRE (in mm) for CT/MR and PET/MR registration, aggregated across all patients

Measure	CT/MR Registration			PET/MR Registration		
	Mean TRE	Median TRE	Std. Dev. TRE	Mean TRE	Median TRE	Std. Dev. TRE
H-MI	2.0	1.8	1.0	6.6	3.1	8.3
H-ECC	2.3	2.0	1.3	3.1	2.8	1.6
$H_{1/2}^{R}$-MI	2.1	1.8	1.3	3.3	3.2	1.3
$H_{1/2}^{R}$-ECC	2.2	1.8	1.1	2.7	2.9	0.9
H_{2}^{R}-MI	24.0	27.5	14.9	6.4	3.6	7.6
H_{2}^{R}-ECC	13.6	2.9	15.0	4.0	2.8	4.7
$H_{1/2}^{T}$-MI	1.8	1.6	0.9	2.7	2.7	0.9
$H_{1/2}^{T}$-ECC	1.9	1.6	1.0	2.6	2.5	1.0
H_{2}^{T}-MI	5.4	3.4	6.0	6.2	2.9	8.1
H_{2}^{T}-ECC	6.2	4.6	6.2	4.4	2.6	5.9
ε-MI	3.2	3.0	1.7	3.6	3.4	2.2
ε-ECC	3.4	3.0	1.9	3.6	3.0	2.5
$\varepsilon_{1/2}^{R}$-MI	4.2	3.7	3.1	4.0	3.7	2.5
$\varepsilon_{1/2}^{R}$-ECC	4.4	4.4	2.1	3.8	3.3	2.3
ε_{2}^{R}-MI	13.2	11.3	14.9	5.2	3.3	5.0
ε_{2}^{R}-ECC	7.9	7.3	4.5	5.5	3.4	5.3
$\varepsilon_{1/2}^{T}$-MI	5.9	4.4	4.3	4.1	4.0	1.7
$\varepsilon_{1/2}^{T}$-ECC	3.1	3.0	1.8	3.2	3.3	1.3
ε_{2}^{T}-MI	14.6	14.4	10.2	14.3	11.6	13.9
ε_{2}^{T}-ECC	3.6	3.2	2.4	2.5	2.6	0.9

from **H-ECC**, in the sense that the c.d.f. values are smaller everywhere. Using the two-sample Kolmogorov-Smirnov test at a level $\alpha = 0.05$, we found that the null hypothesis can be rejected in favor of the alternative hypothesis for the following cases:

- CT/MR Registration: H_2^R, ε_2^R, $\varepsilon_{1/2}^T$, ε_2^T
- PET/MR Registration: H_2^R, $\varepsilon_{1/2}^T$, ε_2^T

When the same analysis was done with the roles of **H-MI** and **H-ECC** interchanged, there were no versions of **H** for which **H-MI** exhibited a statistically significant improvement over **H-ECC**.

This analysis indicates that in both the CT/MR and PET/MR registration cases, statistically significant improvements can be made by choosing the ECC versions of MI over MI itself when H_2^R, $\varepsilon_{1/2}^T$, or ε_2^T are selected for entropy. When ε_2^R is selected, a statistically significant improvement is made in CT/MR registration when ECC is used over MI.

6   Conclusion

In this article, we showed how to construct normalized versions of MI using a variety of definitions of entropy, including Rényi, Tsallis, exponential, generalized exponential, and cumulative residual entropy. The normalized similarity measures are analogous to NMI, ECC, and SU, which have previously been established to outperform MI in a variety of situations. To test the proposed normalized similarity measures, we used publicly available multimodal brain imaging data [24] that allowed us to perform CT/MR and PET/MR rigid registration and compare the results to known ground truth transformations. Results indicate statistically significant improvements in target registration error for a variety of the proposed similarity measures.

References

1. Maes, F., Collignon, A., Vandermeulen, D., Marchal, G., Suetens, P.: Multimodality Image Registration by Maximization of Mutual Information. IEEE Trans. Med. Imag. 16(2), 187–198 (1997)
2. Collignon, A.: Multi-modality Medical Image Registration by Maximization of Mutual Information. Ph.D. Thesis, Catholic University of Leuven, Leuven, Belgium (1998)
3. Viola, P.A.: Alignment by Maximization of Mutual Information. Ph.D. Thesis, Artificial Intelligence Laboratory, Massachusetts Institute of Technology (1995)
4. Viola, P.A., Wells III, W.M.: Alignment by Maximization of Mutual Information. Int. J. Comp. Vis. 24(2), 137–154 (1997)
5. Pluim, J.P.W., Maintz, J.B.A., Viergever, M.A.: Mutual-Information-Based Registration of Medical Images: A Survey. IEEE Trans. Med. Imag. 22(8), 986–1004 (2003)
6. Studholme, C., Hill, D.L.G., Hawkes, D.J.: An Overlap Invariant Entropy Measure of 3D Medical Image Alignment. Patt. Rec. 32, 71–86 (1999)
7. Melbourne, A., Hawkes, D., Atkinson, D.: Image Registration Using Uncertainty Coefficients. In: Proc. ISBI 2009, pp. 951–954 (2009)
8. Wachowiak, M.P., Smoliková, R., Tourassi, G.D., Elmaghraby, A.S.: Similarity Metrics Based on Nonadditive Entropies for 2D–3D Multimodal Biomedical Image Registration. In: Sonka, M., Fitzpatrick, J.M. (eds.) Proc. SPIE of Medical Imaging 2003: Image Processing, vol. 5032, pp. 1090–1100 (2003)
9. Wang, F., Vemuri, B.C., Rao, M., Chen, Y.: A New & Robust Information Theoretic Measure and Its Application to Image Alignment. In: Taylor, C.J., Noble, J.A. (eds.) IPMI 2003. LNCS, vol. 2732, pp. 388–400. Springer, Heidelberg (2003)
10. Wang, F., Vemuri, B.C.: Non-rigid Multi-modal Image Registration Using Cross-cumulative Residual Entropy. Int. J. Comp. Vis. 74(2), 201–205 (2007)
11. Liao, S., Chung, A.C.S.: Multi-modal Image Registration Using the Generalized Survival Exponential Entropy. In: Larsen, R., Nielsen, M., Sporring, J. (eds.) MICCAI 2006. LNCS, vol. 4191, pp. 964–971. Springer, Heidelberg (2006)
12. Cahill, N.D.: Constructing and Solving Variational Image Registration Problems. D.Phil. Thesis, Department of Engineering Science, University of Oxford (2009)
13. Cahill, N.D., Schnabel, J.A., Noble, J.A., Hawkes, D.J.: Overlap Invariance of Cumulative Residual Entropy Measures for Multimodal Image Alignment. In: Pluim, J.P.W., Dawant, B.M. (eds.) Proc. SPIE of Medical Imaging 2009: Image Processing, vol. 7259 (2009)

14. Shannon, C.E.: A Mathematical Theory of Communication. Bell Sys. Tech. J. 27, 379–423, 623–656 (1948)
15. Rényi, A.: On measures of entropy and information. In: Proc. 4th Berkeley Symp. Mathematical Statistics and Probability, Berkeley, CA, vol. I, pp. 547–561 (1961)
16. Tsallis, C.: Possible Generalizations of Boltzmann-Gibbs Statistics. J. Stat. Phys. 52, 479–487 (1988)
17. Campbell, L.L.: Exponential Entropy as a Measure of Extent of a Distribution. Zeitschr. für Wahrsch. und verw. Geb. 5, 217–255 (1966)
18. Koski, T., Persson, L.-E.: Some Properties of Generalized Exponential Entropies with Applications to Data Compression. Inf. Sci. 62(1-2), 103–132 (1992)
19. Rao, M., Chen, Y., Vemuri, B.C., Wang, F.: Cumulative Residual Entropy: A New Measure of Information. IEEE Trans. Inf. Th. 50(6), 1220–1228 (2004)
20. Zografos, K., Nadarajah, S.: Survival Exponential Entropies. IEEE Trans. Inf. Th. 51(3), 1239–1246 (2005)
21. Drissi, N., Chonavel, T., Boucher, J.M.: Generalized Cumulative Residual Entropy for Distributions with Unrestricted Supports. Res. Let. Sig. Proc. Article ID 790607, 2008 (2008)
22. Astola, J., Virtanen, I.: A Measure of Overall Statistical Dependence Based on the Entropy Concept. In: Proc. Univ. Vaasa. No. 91 (1983)
23. Witten, I.H., Frank, E.: Data Mining: Practical Machine Learning Tools and Techniques. Morgan Kaufmann, Amsterdam (2005)
24. West, J., et al.: Comparison and Evaluation of Retrospective Intermodality Brain Image Registration Techniques. J. Comp. Assist. Tom. 21(4), 554–566 (1997)

Nonlinear Elasticity Registration and Sobolev Gradients*

Tungyou Lin, Ivo Dinov, Arthur Toga, and Luminita Vese

University of California, Los Angeles, CA 90095-1555, USA

Abstract. We propose Mooney-Rivlin (MR) nonlinear elasticity of hyperelastic materials and numerical algorithms for image registration in the presence of landmarks and large deformation. An auxiliary variable is introduced to remove the nonlinearity in the derivatives of Euler-Lagrange equations. Comparing the MR elasticity model with the Saint Venant-Kirchhoff elasticity model (SVK), the results show that the MR model gives better matching in fewer iterations. To accelerate the slow convergence due to the lack of smoothness of the L^2 gradient, we construct a Sobolev H^1 gradient descent method [13] and take advantage of the smoothing quality of the Sobolev operator $(Id - \triangle)^{-1}$. The MR model with Sobolev H^1 gradient descent (SGMR) improves both matching criterion and computational time substantially. We further apply the L^2 and Sobolev gradient to landmark registration for multi-modal mouse brain data, and observe faster convergence and better landmark matching for the MR model with Sobolev H^1 gradient descent.

Keywords: image registration, landmarks, nonlinear elasticity, multi-modality, L^2 and Sobolev gradient, Mooney-Rivlin materials.

1 Introduction

In medical imaging, it is often useful to compare multi-modal images and combine the information for clinical studies of disease and for atlas-based identification and segmentation of anatomical structures. This is commonly done using image registration. To map a template image $T : \Omega \to \mathbb{R}$ to a reference image $R : \Omega \to \mathbb{R}$, $\Omega \subset \mathbb{R}^n$, we aim to find a smooth invertible transformation $\Phi(\mathbf{x}) = \mathbf{x} + \mathbf{u}(\mathbf{x})$ from Ω to itself, such that $T(\Phi(\mathbf{x})) \approx R(\mathbf{x})$ a.e. in Ω and $\Phi(x) = x$ on $\partial\Omega$, where $\mathbf{u}$ is the unknown displacement field. Since it is equivalent to find Φ or $\mathbf{u}$, we will seek the displacement $\mathbf{u}$ for two-dimensional planar images.

An extensive overview of registration models is given in [11], including parametric models such as landmark-based spline registration, and nonparametric models employing linear diffusion, linear elasticity, biharmonic and fluid regularization. Also, variational methods for regularization of the deformation, by linear

---

* Work funded by the National Institutes of Health through the NIH Roadmap for Medical Research, Grant U54 RR021813 entitled Center for Computational Biology.

B. Fischer, B. Dawant, and C. Lorenz (Eds.): WBIR 2010, LNCS 6204, pp. 269–280, 2010.
© Springer-Verlag Berlin Heidelberg 2010

elasticity or by diffusion tensor, using mutual information and other information-theoretic approaches, are presented in [4] in a theoretical framework. For models that deal with larger deformation, we refer to [2] for a well-known large deformation fluid registration method (not in variational form), and to a variational registration for large deformations (LDDMM) [1], [10]. The work [23], [24] presents a log-unbiased large deformation fluid registration. Besides fluid models, nonlinear elasticity regularization is implemented using the finite element method in [18] and [15]. Non-linear elasticity principles have also been used with the regularized gradient flow in [3]. As for landmark-based registration methods, we refer to [7], where a consistent landmark and intensity-based registration method is presented using thin-plate spline regularization (or biharmonic regularization). Another related reference is [21] where data fidelity, spline regularization and soft landmark constraints are combined, as in the present work.

In prior work [9], we have proposed the Saint Venant-Kirchhoff (SVK) nonlinear elasticity regularizer for image registration in the presence of landmarks. The operator splitting method was used for the numerical implementation. In the present work we improve the previous model in two ways: (i) we propose to use the Mooney-Rivlin regularization of hyperelastic materials, leading to a polyconvex functional, instead of the Saint Venant-Kirchhoff functional, which is not polyconvex [19] (theoretical condition important for existence of minimizers); (ii) we propose to use the Sobolev H^1 gradient descent [13] instead of the L^2 gradient descent, leading to improved results and computational speed.

2   Proposed Model for Planar Image Registration

The proposed energy functional consists of a dissimilarity measure DM, a regularizer REG, and a landmark penalty term LMP. The general form is given by: $J(\mathbf{u}) = DM_{T,R}(\mathbf{u}) + \alpha REG(\mathbf{u}) + \kappa LMP(\mathbf{u})$, where $\mathbf{u}$ is the unknown displacement vector field, $\alpha > 0$ and $\kappa \geq 0$ are penalty parameters.

2.1   Intensity Dissimilarity Measure

To minimize the pixel-by-pixel intensity dissimilarity between the reference R and the transformed template $T \circ \Phi$, we minimize the L^2 distance function $DM(\mathbf{u}) = \frac{1}{2} \int_{\Omega} |T(\mathbf{x} + \mathbf{u}(\mathbf{x})) - R(\mathbf{x})|^2 d\mathbf{x}$. Its Gâteaux-derivatives are $\frac{\partial DM(\mathbf{u})}{\partial u_p} = (T(\Phi(\mathbf{x})) - R(\mathbf{x}))T_{x_p}(\Phi(\mathbf{x}))$, where T_{x_p} denotes the intensity gradient component in the direction x_p, $p = 1, 2$.

2.2   Landmark Penalty Term

Let $\mathbf{x}^{R,k} = (x_1^{R,k}, x_2^{R,k})$ be the m landmark points extracted from R, and $\mathbf{x}^{T,k} = (x_1^{T,k}, x_2^{T,k})$ be those from T, $k = 1, 2, ..., m$. In Eulerian framework, where backward registration is done, the goal is to map $\mathbf{x}^{R,k}$ onto $\mathbf{x}^{T,k}$ by the transformation Φ. We enforce the spatial overlap of soft landmarks as optimality constraints in

the quadratic penalty method; precisely, we minimize the following landmark distance function: using $\Phi(\mathbf{x}) = \mathbf{x} + \mathbf{u}(\mathbf{x})$, $LMP(\mathbf{u}) = \frac{1}{2}\sum_{k=1}^{m}\|\mathbf{x}^{T,k} - \Phi(\mathbf{x}^{R,k})\|^2$.
Its Gâteaux-derivative is $\frac{\partial LMP(\mathbf{u})}{\partial u_p} = \begin{cases} x_p^{T,k} - x_p^{R,k} - u_p(\mathbf{x}^{R,k}), \ p = 1, 2, \\ 0 \ \text{if } \mathbf{x} \neq \mathbf{x}^{R,k}. \end{cases}$

2.3 Non-linear Elasticity Regularization

It is physically motivated to view the shape change of the image after transformation as the deformation of an elastic material under external force [11]. To allow large and smooth deformation, we minimize the energy functional consisting of a nonlinear elasticity regularizer based on the class of energy functions associated with hyper-elastic materials such as the Saint-Venant-Kirchhoff (SVK) materials and the Mooney-Rivlin (MR) materials [16].

Saint-Venant-Kirchhoff Elasticity. The SVK elasticity regularizer is $REG(\mathbf{u}) = \int_\Omega W(\epsilon(\mathbf{u}))d\mathbf{x}$, with $W(\epsilon) = \frac{\lambda}{2}(\text{trace}(\epsilon))^2 + \mu\text{trace}(\epsilon^2)$, where $\epsilon(\mathbf{u}) = \frac{1}{2}(\nabla\mathbf{u}^t + \nabla\mathbf{u} + \nabla\mathbf{u}^t\nabla\mathbf{u})$. It has been effective in conjunction with finite element methods in the field of Engineering for modeling membranes with large deformation and moderate strains [6], as well as in the medical field for the physical modeling of soft tissues [17]. However, the functional is not polyconvex [19,16] and thus the weak lower semicontinuity, necessary to establish existence of minimizers, cannot be induced; this theoretical drawback may be the cause of slower convergence when compared to the MR elasticity which has been proven to be polyconvex, guarantees existence of minimizers [5,19], and has an additional penalty term on the determinant of the Jacobian of the transformation, keeping it above 0.

Mooney-Rivlin Elasticity. The energy function associated with the MR elasticity is given by $\int_\Omega W(\mathbf{F})d\mathbf{x}$, with $W(\mathbf{F}) = c|\mathbf{F}|^2 + d|\text{adj}(\mathbf{F})|^2 + \Gamma(det(\mathbf{F}))$,
$\mathbf{F}(\nabla\mathbf{u}) = \begin{pmatrix} \partial_{x_1}(x_1 + u_1) \ \partial_{x_2}(x_1 + u_1) \\ \partial_{x_1}(x_2 + u_2) \ \partial_{x_2}(x_2 + u_2) \end{pmatrix}$, $det(\mathbf{F}) = (1+u_{1x_1})(1+u_{2x_2}) - u_{1x_2}u_{2x_1}$,
and Γ satisfies $\lim_{\varepsilon\to 0}\Gamma(\varepsilon) = \infty$ [16]. In two dimensions, $|F| = |\text{adj}(\mathbf{F})|$ and the MR model coincides with the Neo-Hookean model: $W(\mathbf{F}) = \eta|\mathbf{F}|^2 + \Gamma(det(\mathbf{F}))$. To encourage that $det(\mathbf{F}) \sim 1$ for smooth transformation, we further require $\lim_{\varepsilon\to 1}\Gamma(\varepsilon) = 0$. Since $-\log(\cdot)$ is convex and satisfies $\lim_{\varepsilon\to 0} -\log(\varepsilon) = \infty$, we construct the MR elasticity model with the log barrier method [14] for inequality constraints $det(\mathbf{F}) > 0 : \Gamma(det(\mathbf{F})) = -\gamma\log(det(\mathbf{F}))$, $\gamma > 0$, $\gamma \downarrow 0^+$. MR elasticity is theoretically more sound being polyconvex; it also enables us to build a unified minimization model with penalization $\Gamma(det(\nabla\Phi))$ during the minimization process to ensure $det(\nabla\Phi) > 0$ and $det(\nabla\Phi) \approx 1$ (see also [24]).

Gradient Approximation by Auxiliary Variable. To simplify the cumbersome Euler-Lagrange equations associated with the nonlinear elasticity regularizer, we apply, inspired from [12] and as in [9], the operator splitting method by introducing an auxiliary variable $\mathbf{V} = \begin{pmatrix} V_{11} & V_{12} \\ V_{21} & V_{22} \end{pmatrix}$ to approximate the gra-

dient $\nabla \mathbf{u} = \begin{pmatrix} \partial_{x_1} u_1 & \partial_{x_2} u_1 \\ \partial_{x_1} u_2 & \partial_{x_2} u_2 \end{pmatrix}$. In order to impose the soft constraint $V \approx \nabla \mathbf{u}$, we apply the quadratic penalty method and we reformulate the regularizer as:
$\int_\Omega REG_\beta(\mathbf{V}, \mathbf{u}) dx = \int_\Omega \left[W(F(\mathbf{V})) + \beta |\mathbf{V} - \nabla \mathbf{u}|^2 \right] dx = \int_\Omega \left[\eta((1 + V_{11})^2 + (1 + \right.$
$V_{22})^2 + V_{12}^2 + V_{21}^2) - \gamma \log((1 + V_{11})(1 + V_{22}) - V_{12} V_{21}) + \beta |\mathbf{V} - \nabla \mathbf{u}|^2 \left. \right] dx$, with $\gamma \downarrow 0^+$.
As $\beta \to \infty$, the quadratic penalty term $\to 0$, thus we expect $V \to \nabla \mathbf{u}$ in
the limit. The Gâteaux derivatives associated with $REG_\beta(\mathbf{V}, \mathbf{u})$ are given by:
$\frac{\partial REG_\beta(\mathbf{V}, \mathbf{u})}{\partial V_{pp}} = \eta[(1 + V_{pp}) - \frac{\gamma}{det(\mathbf{F})}(1 + V_{qq})] + \beta (V_{pp} - \frac{\partial u_p}{\partial x_p})$, $\frac{\partial REG_\beta(\mathbf{V}, \mathbf{u})}{\partial V_{pq}} =$
$\eta[V_{pq} + \frac{\gamma}{det(\mathbf{F})} V_{qp}] + \beta (V_{pq} - \frac{\partial u_p}{\partial x_q})$, $p, q = 1, 2$, $p \neq q$, $\frac{\partial REG_\beta(\mathbf{V}, \mathbf{u})}{\partial u_r} = \beta(\frac{\partial V_{r1}}{\partial x_1} +$
$\frac{\partial V_{r2}}{\partial x_2} - \triangle u_r)$, $r = 1, 2$. We notice that thanks to the auxiliary variable $\mathbf{V}$, the
nonlinearity in the derivatives of $\mathbf{u}$ has been removed.

2.4   The Combined Variational Formulation

Based on the above, we consider the combined unconstrained minimization

$$\min_{\mathbf{u}, \mathbf{V}} \left\{ J(\mathbf{u}, \mathbf{V}) = DM_{T,R}(\mathbf{u}) + \alpha REG_\beta(\mathbf{V}, \mathbf{u}) + \kappa LMP(\mathbf{u}) \right\}, \tag{1}$$

and the Gâteaux derivatives in $\mathbf{u}$ and $\mathbf{V}$ associated with (1), when $\kappa = 0$, are

$$\partial_{V_{pp}} J(\mathbf{u}, \mathbf{V}) = \int_\Omega \beta (V_{pp} - \partial_{x_p} u_p) + \alpha(1 + V_{pp}) - \frac{\gamma}{det(I + \mathbf{V})}(1 + V_{qq}) \, dx,$$

$$\partial_{V_{pq}} J(\mathbf{u}, \mathbf{V}) = \int_\Omega \beta (V_{pq} - \partial_{x_q} u_p) + \alpha V_{pq} - \frac{\gamma}{det(I + \mathbf{V})}(-V_{qp}) \, dx,$$

$$\partial_{u_r} J(\mathbf{u}, \mathbf{V}) = \int_\Omega (T(\mathbf{x} + \mathbf{u}(\mathbf{x})) - R(\mathbf{x})) \partial_{x_r} T + \beta(\partial_{x_1} V_{r1} + \partial_{x_2} V_{r2} - \triangle u_r) \, dx,$$

where $p, q, r = 1, 2$, $p \neq q$, I is the 2×2 matrix with all its entries 1, and
$det(I + \mathbf{V}) = (1 + V_{11})(1 + V_{22}) - V_{12} V_{21}$. When $\kappa > 0$, we add to the last
relation the Gâteaux-derivative from Section 2.2.

2.5   Sobolev H^1 Gradient Descent Method

We recall here the notion of Sobolev H^1 gradient for functionals, inspired from
Neuberger [13]. Let $\Omega \subset \mathbb{R}^2$ open, bounded, and connected, with Lipschitz
boundary, $\mathbf{u} \in \mathbf{H}^1(\Omega)^2 = \{ \mathbf{z} \in (\mathbf{L}^2(\Omega))^2 : \nabla \mathbf{z} \in \mathbf{L}^2(\Omega)^4 \}$ with $\mathbf{H}^1$ inner product
$\langle \cdot, \cdot \rangle$, and test function $\mathbf{v} \in \mathbf{H}_0^1(\Omega)^2$, and $L : \mathbb{R}^2 \times \mathbb{R}^4 \times \mathbb{R}^2 \to \mathbb{R}$ being C^1. To
solve the general minimization problem: $\min_{\mathbf{u} \in \mathbf{H}^1(\Omega)^2} J(\mathbf{u}) = \int_\Omega L(D\mathbf{u}(\mathbf{x}), \mathbf{x}) dx$,
$D\mathbf{z} = \begin{pmatrix} \mathbf{z} \\ \nabla \mathbf{z} \end{pmatrix}$, $\mathbf{z} \in \mathbf{H}^1(\Omega)^2$, we consider a gradient descent method defined by
the iteration $\mathbf{u}^{(s+1)} - \mathbf{u}^{(s)} = -\triangle t \nabla J(\mathbf{u}^{(s)})$, with $\mathbf{u}^{(0)} \in (\mathbf{H}^1(\Omega))^2$. The idea is

that J would decrease the fastest from $\mathbf{z}$ in the descent direction $-\nabla J(\mathbf{z})$, if $J(\mathbf{z})$ is well-defined and differentiable around $\mathbf{z}$. For each iterate $\mathbf{u}^{(s)}$ to remain in $(\mathbf{H}^1(\Omega))^2$, the directional derivative of J at $\mathbf{u}^{(s)}$ in the direction $\mathbf{v}$, $J'(\mathbf{u}^{(s)})\mathbf{v}$, must satisfy

$$J'(\mathbf{u}^{(s)})\mathbf{v} = \langle \nabla_S J(\mathbf{u}^{(s)}), \mathbf{v} \rangle_{\mathbf{H}^1(\Omega)^2}. \tag{2}$$

Neuberger [13] (see also Renka [20]) proved the existence of $\nabla_S J(\mathbf{z})$ and $\nabla_S J(\mathbf{z}) = \pi P(\nabla J)(D\mathbf{z})$, where $\pi \begin{pmatrix} f \\ g \end{pmatrix} = f$ for $f \in \mathbf{L}^2(\Omega)^2$, $g \in \mathbf{L}^2(\Omega)^4$, P is the orthogonal projection of $\mathbf{L}^2(\Omega)^2 \times \mathbf{L}^2(\Omega)^4$ onto $\left\{ D\mathbf{z} = \begin{pmatrix} \mathbf{z} \\ \nabla \mathbf{z} \end{pmatrix} : \mathbf{z} \in \mathbf{H}^1(\Omega)^2 \right\}$. To see how the Sobolev $\mathbf{H}^1$ gradient descent is more suitable for our purpose, we examine the construction of the $\mathbf{L}^2$ gradient. With $L = L(\mathbf{z}, \mathbf{p}, \mathbf{x})$, $\mathbf{p} = (p_1, p_2)$, $p_k = \partial_{x_k} \mathbf{z}$, $\mathbf{z} = (z_1, z_2)$, and $\mathbf{x} = (x_1, x_2)$, we derive the $\mathbf{L}^2$ gradient associated with the $\mathbf{L}^2$ inner product as follows:

$$J'(\mathbf{u})\mathbf{v} = \int_\Omega \sum_{k=1,2} \partial_{z_k}(L(\mathbf{u}, \nabla\mathbf{u}, \mathbf{x}))\mathbf{v} + \sum_{k=1,2} \partial_{p_k}(L(\mathbf{u}, \nabla\mathbf{u}, \mathbf{x}))\partial_{x_k}\mathbf{v} \, d\mathbf{x}$$

$$= \int_\Omega \left[\nabla_{\mathbf{z}}(L(\mathbf{u}, \nabla\mathbf{u}, \mathbf{x})) - \sum_{k=1,2} \partial_{x_k}\left(\partial_{p_k}(L(\mathbf{u}, \nabla\mathbf{u}, \mathbf{x})) \right) \right] \mathbf{v} \, d\mathbf{x}$$

$$= \int_\Omega \left[\nabla_{\mathbf{z}}(L(\mathbf{u}, \nabla\mathbf{u}, \mathbf{x})) - \nabla_{\mathbf{x}}\left(\nabla_{\mathbf{p}}(L(\mathbf{u}, \nabla\mathbf{u}, \mathbf{x})) \right) \right] \mathbf{v} \, d\mathbf{x}$$

$$= \int_\Omega \begin{pmatrix} Id & (-\nabla_{\mathbf{x}}) \end{pmatrix} \begin{pmatrix} \nabla_{\mathbf{z}}(L(\mathbf{u}, \nabla\mathbf{u}, \mathbf{x})) \\ \nabla_{\mathbf{p}}(L(\mathbf{u}, \nabla\mathbf{u}, \mathbf{x})) \end{pmatrix} \mathbf{v} \, d\mathbf{x}$$

$$= \langle \tilde{D}^t \nabla L(D\mathbf{u}, \mathbf{x}), \mathbf{v} \rangle_{\mathbf{L}^2(\Omega)^2}, \text{ where } \tilde{D} = \begin{pmatrix} Id \\ -\nabla_{\mathbf{x}} \end{pmatrix}. \tag{3}$$

Thus the $\mathbf{L}^2$ gradient, $\nabla_{\mathbf{L}^2} J(\mathbf{u}) = \tilde{D}^t \nabla L(D\mathbf{u}, \mathbf{x})$ at $\mathbf{u}^{(s)}$ must be in $\mathbf{H}^1(\Omega)^2$, requiring second-order derivatives of $u^{(s)}$ being in $\mathbf{L}^2(\Omega)$. When these strong smoothness conditions on $\mathbf{u}$ and $\tilde{D}^t \nabla L(D\mathbf{u}, \mathbf{x})$ do not hold, the L^2 gradient descent is theoretically ill-posed and may result in numerical instability. Due to this drawback of L^2 gradient, we want to consider the Sobolev $\mathbf{H}^1$ gradient, $\nabla_S J(\mathbf{u}) = \pi P(\nabla J)(D\mathbf{u})$, for a more sound and efficient model. To construct the Sobolev $\mathbf{H}^1$ gradient descent method, we start with the relation between the $\mathbf{L}^2$ and the Sobolev $\mathbf{H}^1$ inner product, which is given by $\langle a, b \rangle_{\mathbf{H}^1} = \langle a, b \rangle_{\mathbf{L}^2} + \langle \nabla a, \nabla b \rangle_{\mathbf{L}^2} = \langle a, b \rangle_{\mathbf{L}^2} - \langle \triangle a, b \rangle_{\mathbf{L}^2} = \langle (Id - \triangle)a, b \rangle_{\mathbf{L}^2}$, where Id is the identity operator, $\triangle$ is the Laplacian operator and the second equality comes from Green's formula. Now, let $a = (\nabla_S J)(\mathbf{u})$ and $b = \mathbf{v}$, a smooth test function with compact support, we then obtain the following relation:

$$\langle (\nabla_S J)(\mathbf{u}), \mathbf{v} \rangle_{\mathbf{H}^1(\Omega)^2} = \langle ((Id - \triangle)\nabla_S J)(\mathbf{u}), \mathbf{v} \rangle_{\mathbf{L}^2(\Omega)^2}. \tag{4}$$

Combining (2), (3), and (4), we obtain

$$\langle \nabla_{\mathbf{L}^2} J(\mathbf{u}), \mathbf{v} \rangle_{\mathbf{L}^2(\Omega)^2} = \langle \nabla_S J(\mathbf{u}), \mathbf{v} \rangle_{\mathbf{H}^1(\Omega)^2} = \langle ((Id - \triangle)\nabla_S J)(\mathbf{u}), \mathbf{v} \rangle_{\mathbf{L}^2(\Omega)^2},$$

or, equivalently,

$$(Id - \triangle)^{-1}\langle \nabla_{\mathbf{L}^2} J(\mathbf{u}), \mathbf{v}\rangle_{\mathbf{L}^2(\Omega)^2} = \langle \nabla_S J(\mathbf{u}), \mathbf{v}\rangle_{\mathbf{H}^1(\Omega)^2}.$$

2.6   Solving the Euler-Lagrange Equations

First, we solve the Euler-Lagrange equations in $\mathbf{V}$ associated with (1) by the L^2 gradient descent method:

$$V_{pq}^{(s+1)}(\mathbf{x}) = V_{pq}^{(s)}(\mathbf{x}) + \triangle t[-\partial_{V_{pq}} J(\mathbf{u}, \mathbf{V})(\mathbf{x})], \tag{5}$$

where $p, q = 1, 2$, $p \neq q$, s is the iteration index. With the updated $\mathbf{V}$ and its derivatives, we then solve the Euler-Lagrange equations in $\mathbf{u} = (u_1, u_2)$ by the Sobolev gradient descent method:

$$u_r^{(s+1)}(\mathbf{x}) = u_r^{(s)}(\mathbf{x}) + \triangle t(Id - \triangle)^{-1}[-\partial_{u_r} J(\mathbf{V}, \mathbf{u})(\mathbf{x})], \quad r = 1, 2. \tag{6}$$

To solve equation (6), we let $\mathbf{B} = (B_1, B_2) = (-\partial_{u_1} J, -\partial_{u_2} J) \in \mathbf{L}^2(\Omega)^2$ and let $\mathbf{W} = (W_1, W_2) \in \mathbf{H}^1(\Omega)^2$ be the unique function which satisfies

$$\int_\Omega \mathbf{W} \cdot \mathbf{h} + \nabla \mathbf{W} \cdot \nabla \mathbf{h} \; dx = \int_\Omega \mathbf{B} \cdot \mathbf{h} \; dx, \; \forall \mathbf{h} \in \mathbf{H}^1(\Omega)^2. \tag{7}$$

To numerically solve (7), we discretize the system

$$\mathbf{W} - \triangle \mathbf{W} = \mathbf{B} \text{ in } \Omega, \; \nabla \mathbf{W} \cdot \nu = 0 \text{ on } \partial\Omega, \tag{8}$$

where ν is the exterior unit normal on $\partial\Omega$. We solve for $\mathbf{W}$ by a finite difference semi-implicit scheme

$$\mathbf{W}^{(s+1)}(i, j) = \mathbf{B}^{(s)}(i, j) + \left(\frac{\mathbf{W}^{(s)}(i+1, j) - 2\mathbf{W}^{(s+1)}(i, j) + \mathbf{W}^{(s)}(i-1, j)}{(\triangle x)^2} \right.$$
$$\left. + \frac{\mathbf{W}^{(s)}(i, j+1) - 2\mathbf{W}^{(s+1)}(i, j) + \mathbf{W}^{(s)}(i, j-1)}{(\triangle x)^2} \right). \tag{9}$$

and then use the updated $\mathbf{W}$ to advance the displacement field $\mathbf{u}$ by

$$u_r^{(s+1)}(\mathbf{x}) = u_r^{(s)}(\mathbf{x}) + \triangle t W_r^{(s+1)}, \; r = 1, 2. \tag{10}$$

The main steps of the algorithm for the Sobolev $\mathbf{H}^1$ gradient MR elasticity registration model, abbreviated as SGMR, are given in Algorithm 1.

3   Numerical Results and Comparisons

In this section, we compare the SVK L^2 gradient descent model [9] with the proposed MR model (L^2 and Sobolev gradient descent variants), on (i) real human brain MRI data where the template has been artificially deformed from the reference (the ground truth deformation is known); and on (ii) real mouse data with landmarks for matching gene expression data to MRI mouse brain atlas. All images are in two dimensions.

3.1   Ground Truth Test

We consider the "ground truth test" without the landmark penalty term (purely intensity based registration). Tagare et al. in [22] selected a 2D coronal brain MRI slice as the undistorted image R; R is then artificially distorted by a known diffeomorphism $f : (x_1, x_2) \mapsto (y_1, y_2)$ to produce $T = R \circ f$. The two images are shown in Fig.1. We perform the registration and calculate the error between $\Psi(x_1, x_2) = (x_1 - u_1, x_2 - u_2)$ and $f(x_1, x_2)$ in Frobenius norm scaled by the image size to see which model gives the smallest error from the true map f. We calculate the distance between Ψ and the diffeomorphism f because our registration model is in the Eulerian framework based on the backward registration $T \circ \Phi = R$; that is, our deformation vector field moves from $(\Phi^{-1}(\tilde{y}_1), \Phi^{-1}(\tilde{y}_2)) \in \Omega_R$ to $(\tilde{y}_1, \tilde{y}_2) \in \Omega_T$ while T is in fact the image under transformation. We also calculate the inverse of the determinant of the deformation gradient because it corresponds to the transformation from T to $T \circ \Phi \sim R$. Table 1 lists the registration results of the ground truth test by SVK ($\lambda = 6$, $\mu = 1$), MR ($\alpha = 500$, $\gamma = 0.01$), and SGMR ($\alpha = 4$, $\gamma = 10$), all using Matlab linear interpolation. We observe that the Sobolev $\mathbf{H}^1$ gradient model, SGMR, requires smaller penalty parameter β, achieves higher fidelity while taking about 95% fewer iterations and about 96% shorter total running time. For SVK and MR models, we observe that larger penalty parameter β does produce smoother transformation though with even larger iteration number; however, the smoothing qualities of the operator

---

Algorithm 1

Input: Reference Image R of size $M \times N$; Template Image T of size $M \times N$;
Output: Transformed Template Image T1 of size $M \times N$;
Initialization: $G_{x_1}^{(0)} \leftarrow (1:M)' * ones(1, N)$, $G_{x_2}^{(0)} \leftarrow ones(M, 1) * (1:N)$;
$u_p \leftarrow zeros(M, N)$, $p = 1, 2$; $V_{pq} \leftarrow zeros(M, N)$, $p, q = 1, 2$;
$\partial_{x_r} u_p \leftarrow zeros(M, N)$, $r, p = 1, 2$; $\partial_{x_r} V_{pq} \leftarrow zeros(M, N)$, $r, p, q = 1, 2$;
while $max(|\mathbf{u}^{(s+1)} - \mathbf{u}^{(s)}|) < tol$ **do**
    $\mathbf{V}^{(s+1)} \leftarrow (5)$;
    for $i = 2$ to $(M - 1)$, $j = 2$ to $(N - 1)$ **do**
        $\partial_{x_r} V_{pq}^{(s+1)}(i, j) \leftarrow \frac{V_{pq}^{(s+1)}(i+1, j) - V_{pq}^{(s+1)}(i-1, j)}{2\triangle x}, p, q = 1, 2$;
    end for
    for $i = 2$ to $(M - 1)$, $j = 2$ to $(N - 1)$ **do**
        $\mathbf{W}^{(s+1)} \leftarrow (9)$; $u_r^{(s+1)} \leftarrow (10)$; $r = 1, 2$;
    end for
    for $i = 2$ to $(M - 1)$, $j = 2$ to $(N - 1)$ **do**
        $\partial_{x_1} u_p(i, j) \leftarrow \frac{u_p(i+1, j) - u_p(i-1, j)}{2\triangle x}, \partial_{x_2} u_p(i, j) \leftarrow \frac{u_p(i, j+1) - u_p(i, j-1)}{2\triangle x}, p = 1, 2$;
    end for
    for $i = 2$ to $(M - 1)$, $j = 2$ to $(N - 1)$ **do**
        $det(\nabla \Phi)^{(s+1)}(i, j) \leftarrow (1 + \partial_{x_1} u_1^{(s+1)}(i, j))(1 + \partial_{x_2} u_2^{(s+1)}(i, j)) - \partial_{x_2} u_1^{(s+1)}(i, j) \partial_{x_1} u_2^{(s+1)}(i, j)$;
    end for
    $G_{x_p}^{(s+1)} = x_p + u_p^{(s+1)}$, $p = 1, 2$; $T1^{(s+1)} \leftarrow interpolate(T, G_{x_1}^{(s+1)}, G_{x_2}^{(s+1)})$;
end while

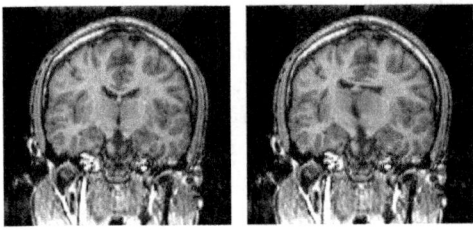

Fig. 1. Reference R (left), template T (right).

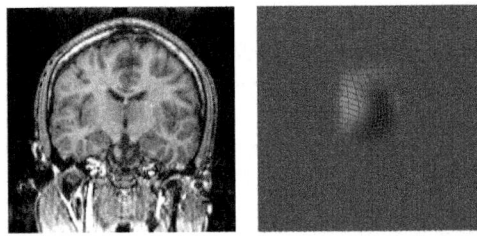

Fig. 2. Transformed template (left) and $det(\nabla\Phi)^{-1}$ (right) with the deformed grid in red lines by SGMR

$(Id - \triangle)^{-1}$ makes it possible to have smooth transformations with substantially fewer iterations and shorter total running time, and the choice of β affects fidelity more than the computation time. Fig.2 contains the transformed template $T \circ \Phi \sim R$ and the inverse of the determinant of the deformation gradient $\nabla\Phi$ together with the level lines of Φ by the Sobolev $\mathbf{H}^{-1}$ gradient model. We see that the transformed template resembles the reference image and this corresponds to the small error from the ground truth. The level lines of Φ are quite smooth and the areas divided by the deformed grid are regular enough; this is also consistent with the fact that the inverse of the determinant of the deformation gradient $\nabla\Phi$ is well away from zero, thus computing a smooth transformation.

Table 1. Ground truth test results by SVK, MR, and SGMR. Image size is 186×197 and the intensity range is $(0, 90)$ for both R and T. Iteration stops when $max(|\mathbf{u}^{(s+1)} - \mathbf{u}^{(s)}|) < tol$. itn is the iteration number and ttltime is the total running time.

	dt	β	$\frac{\|\Psi - f\|_{fro}}{M*N}$	range($det(\nabla\Phi^{-1})$)	itn	ttltime
SVK	0.1	1,500	0.0032300	(0.38715, 2.0274)	8,035	355 sec.
MR	0.1	1,300	0.0032044	(0.37464, 2.0392)	7,469	309 sec.
SGMR	**0.001**	**500**	**0.0030889**	**(0.36242, 2.1392)**	**289**	**14 sec.**

3.2   Mouse Gene Expression to MRI Mouse Atlas Registration

Neuroscientists have been categorizing brain cells using molecular biology for the past 20 years. With the complete genome sequencing of many organisms and advanced technology in DNA experiments, the full range of gene expression across the brain has become a useful tool for neuroscientists to understand the classification and function of neuron types in the brain.

Gene Expression Data. To facilitate gene expression analysis, Stanford University has developed some complementary DNA (cDNA)-deposited glass slides, called the microarrays, where messenger ribonucleic acid (mRNA) from two sources, one controlled and one treated, labeled with different fluorescent dyes, is passed onto for synthesization. The fluorescence signal from each mRNA population is then evaluated and used to calculate the expression ratio. The microarrays are suitable for analysis of up to 10,000 cDNA clones per array and each data point produced by such a microarray hybridization represents the expression ratio of the treated expression level over the controlled expression level.

Standard Atlases. Lee *et al.* [8] constructed a standard atlas space with stereotaxic coordinates for the postnatal day 0 mouse brains from atlases generated by the average of eight co-registered MR image volumes; they have shown that the generated atlases statistically represent diversity across a population and, as a result, provide a stable framework for image registration. Image registration is commonly used in correlating multi-modal data, such as mapping the information from the gene expression data to the anatomical structure represented by the standard atlas.

Mouse Data Landmark Registration. As in [9], we use the standard mouse brain atlas as a common and unbiased framework and map gene expression data to the atlas in order to facilitate the integration of anatomic, genetic, and physiologic observations from multiple subjects in a common space. In the case of mapping gene expression data to atlas, we want to match anatomically or geometrically significant features in the template image with those corresponding ones in the reference image. The images that we test here are of size 200×200 pixels with the landmark points marked in red for the reference and in green

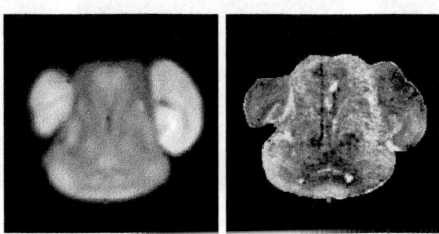

Fig. 3. Reference R (left) and template $\tilde{T}$ (right) after histogram equalization, with landmark points marked in red and green respectively

for the template. Since the original template image has an interior with very low contrast, we perform histogram equalization on the template image so that the intensity histogram of the output image matches a specified histogram such as the histogram of the reference image. Therefore, the pair of images that we actually work with are the original reference R and a template $\tilde{T}$ with its intensity histogram matched with the reference, shown in Fig.3. Although R and T for the mouse data are of different modalities (MRI atlas and gene expression), it was shown in [9] with SVK model that the L^2 similarity measure can still be used, and that the mutual information between T and R increases versus iterations.

We apply the intensity and landmark based SVK [9], MR, and SGMR registration models to the above pair of images and obtain the following convergence results. The transformed templates by the three models are given in Fig.4.

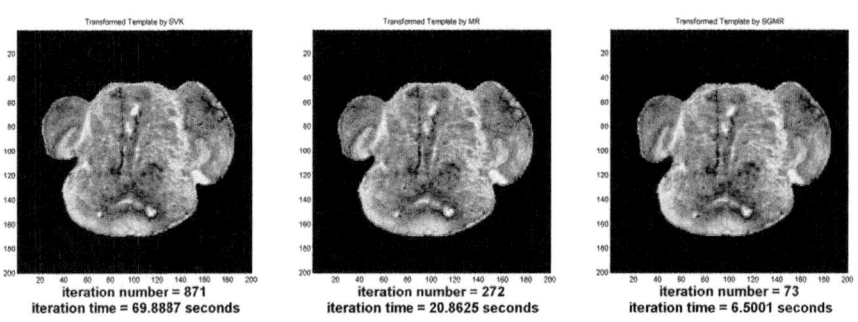

Fig. 4. Transformed template images by SVK, MR and SGMR from left to right, with iteration number and total running time denoted underneath

Besides that the MR model is more computationally efficient than the SVK model, we also observe that the SGMR model renders largest deformation with respect to shape while requiring smallest iteration number and shortest total running time among the three models. This is the expected effect of the smoothing quality of the Sobolev H^1 gradient on the convergence to minimizers. We do

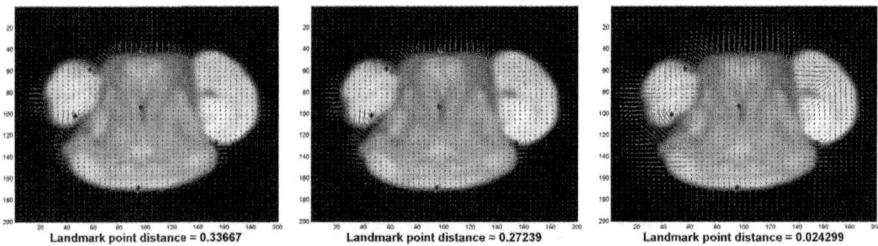

Fig. 5. Distortion maps in Euler framework by SVK, MR and SGMR from left to right, with landmark distance denoted underneath

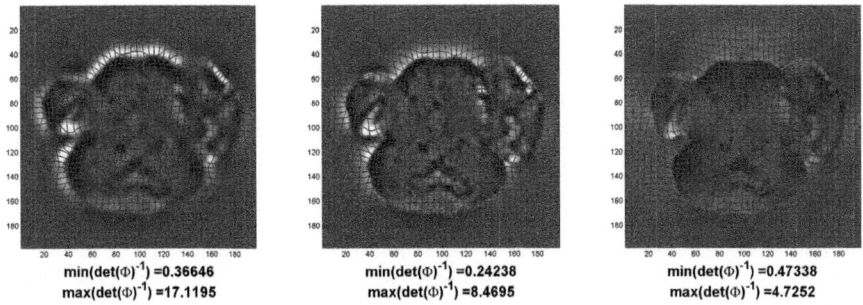

min(det(Φ)⁻¹) =0.36646
max(det(Φ)⁻¹) =17.1195

min(det(Φ)⁻¹) =0.24238
max(det(Φ)⁻¹) =8.4695

min(det(Φ)⁻¹) =0.47338
max(det(Φ)⁻¹) =4.7252

Fig. 6. Determinant of inverse Jacobian by SVK, MR and SGMR from left to right, with range of values of determinant denoted underneath

not compute the dissimilarity between the reference and the transformed template here, but we calculate the distance between the landmark points in ℓ^2 norm divided by p, the number of landmark points. Fig.5 shows the distortion maps by the three models plotted in red vectors originating from $\Phi^{-1}(x_1, x_2) \in R$ to $(y_1, y_2) \in \tilde{T}$ with the transformed landmark points $\mathbf{x}^{R,k} + \mathbf{u}(\mathbf{x}^{R,k})$ marked in blue moving from $\mathbf{x}^{R,k}$ (marked in red) to $\mathbf{x}^{\tilde{T},k}$ (marked in green). The SGMR model gives the smallest landmark distance in accordance with the largest deformation. Despite the large deformation, the deformation gradient remains smooth. Fig.6 shows plots of the determinant of the inverse Jacobian, where the expansion and shrinkage of areas are indicated by lighter and darker gray levels and all results use the same gray scale. The grid consists of level lines of Φ.

We see that the SGMR model renders the least contrastive gray-scale color map and the smallest range of determinant; this indicates it gives the smoothest deformation.

4   Conclusion

As predicted, possibly due to the theoretical disadvantage for not being poly-convex, the SVK model requires more iterations to converge while rendering still larger landmark distance than the MR and SGMR models. With the Sobolev $\mathbf{H}^1$ gradient operator applied to the Euler-Lagrange equations in the displacement vector field $\mathbf{u}$ modeled by MR elasticity, we have seen substantial improvement in fidelity, deformation smoothness, and convergence rate due to the smoothing quality of $(Id - \triangle)^{-1}$.

References

1. Beg, F., Miller, M., Trouvé, A., Younes, L.: Computing Large Deformation Metric Mappings via Geodesic Flows of Diffeomorphisms. IJCV 61(2), 139–157 (2005)
2. Christensen, G., Rabbitt, R., Miller, M.: Deformable Templates Using Large Deformation Kinematics. IEEE TIP 5(10), 1435–1447 (1996)

3. Droske, M., Rumpf, M.: A Variational Approach to Non-Rigid Morphological Registration. SIAM Applied Mathematics 64(2), 668–687 (2004)
4. Faugeras, O., Hermosillo, G.: Well-Posedness of Two Nonrigid Multimodal Image Registration Methods. SIAM Applied Mathematics 64(5), 1550–1587 (2004)
5. Fusco, N., Leone, C., Verde, A., March, R.: A Lower Semi-Continuity Result for Polyconvex Functionals in SBV. Proceedings of the Royal Society of Edinburgh 136A, 321–336 (2006)
6. Gil, A.: FEM for Prestressed Saint Venant-Kirchhoff Hyperelastic Membranes. In: Textile Composite and Inflatable Structures, pp. 123–142. Springer, Heidelberg (2005)
7. Johnson, H.J., Christensen, G.E.: Consistent Landmark and Intensity-Based Image Registration. IEEE TMI 21(5), 450–461 (2002)
8. Lee, E., Jacobs, R., Dinov, I., Leow, A., Toga, A.: Standard Atlas Space for C57BL/6J Neonatal Mouse Brain. Anat. Embryol (Berl) 210(4), 245–263 (2005)
9. Lin, T., Le Guyader, C., Lee, E.-F., Dinov, I., Thompson, P.M., Toga, A.W., Vese, L.A.: Gene to mouse atlas registration using a landmark-based nonlinear elasticity smoother. In: SPIE MI, Image Processing, vol. 7259 (2009)
10. Miller, M.I., Trouvé, A., Younes, L.: On the Metrics and Euler-Lagrange Equations of Computational Anatomy. Annu. Rev. B. Eng. 4, 375–405 (2002)
11. Modersitzki, J.: Numerical Methods for Image Registration. Oxford University Press, Oxford (2004)
12. Negrón Marrer, P.V.: A Numerical Method for Detecting Singular Minimizers of Multidimensional Problems in Nonlinear Elasticity. Numerische Mathematik 58(1), 135–144 (1990)
13. Neuberger, J.: Sobolev Gradients and Differential Equations. LNM, vol. 1670. Springer, Heidelberg (1997)
14. Nocedal, J., Wright, S.J.: Numerical Optimization. Springer, Heidelberg (1999)
15. Peckar, W., Schnörr, C., Rohr, K., Stiehl, H.S.: Parameter-Free Elastic Deformation Approach for 2D and 3D Registration Using Prescribed Displacements. Journal of Mathematical Imaging and Vision 10(2), 143–162 (1999)
16. Pedregal, P.: Variational Methods in Nonlinear Elasticity. SIAM, Philadelphia (2000)
17. Picinbono, G., Delingette, H., Ayache, N.: Non-Linear Anisotropic Elasticity for Real-Time Surgery Simulation. Graphical Models 65, 305–321 (2003)
18. Rabbitt, R.D., Weiss, J.A., Christensen, G.E., Miller, M.I.: Mapping of Hyperelastic Deformable Templates Using the Finite Element Method. In: Proceedings SPIE, vol. 2573, pp. 252–265 (1995)
19. Raoult, A.: Non-Polyconvexity of the Stored Energy Function of A Saint Venant-Kirchhoff Material. Application of Mathematics 31(6), 417–419 (1986)
20. Renka, R.: Constructing Fair Curves and Surfaces with a Sobolev Gradient Method. Computer Aided Geometric Design 21, 137–149 (2004)
21. Sorzano, C.O.S., Thévenaz, P., Unser, M.: Elastic Registration of Biological Images Using Vector-Spline Regularization. IEEE T. Biom. Eng. 52(4), 652–663 (2005)
22. Tagare, H., Groisser, D., Skrinjar, O.: A geometric theory of symmetric registration. In: IEEE CVPRW 2006 (2006)
23. Yanovsky, I., Osher, S., Thompson, P., Leow, A.: Log-Unbiased Large-Deformation Image Registration. VISAPP 1, 272–279 (2007)
24. Yanovsky, I., Osher, S., Thompson, P., Leow, A.: Topology Preserving Log-Unbiased Nonlinear Image Registration: Theory and Implementation. CVPR, 1–8 (2007)

Author Index